CHILDHOOD ADVERSITY AND DEVELOPMENTAL EFFECTS

International and Cross-Disciplinary Perspectives

CHILDHOOD ADVERSITY AND DEVELOPMENTAL EFFECTS

International and Cross-Disciplinary Perspectives

Edited by
Lisa Albers Prock, MD, MPH

AAP APPLE
ACADEMIC
PRESS

Apple Academic Press Inc.	Apple Academic Press Inc.
3333 Mistwell Crescent	9 Spinnaker Way
Oakville, ON L6L 0A2	Waretown, NJ 08758
Canada	USA

©2015 by Apple Academic Press, Inc.

First issued in paperback 2021

Exclusive worldwide distribution by CRC Press, a member of Taylor & Francis Group

No claim to original U.S. Government works

ISBN 13: 978-1-77463-384-7 (pbk)
ISBN 13: 978-1-77188-110-4 (hbk)

Library of Congress Control Number: 2014953554

Library and Archives Canada Cataloguing in Publication

Childhood adversity and developmental effects: international and cross-disciplinary perspectives/edited by Lisa Albers Prock, MD, MPH.

Includes bibliographical references and index.
ISBN 978-1-77188-110-4 (bound)
1. Children and violence. 2. Violence--Health aspects. 3. Child abuse. 4. Psychic trauma in children. 5. Child mental health. 6. Child development--Social aspects. I. Prock, Lisa Albers, editor

| HQ784.V55C45 2015 | 303.6083 | C2014-907045-4 |

Apple Academic Press also publishes its books in a variety of electronic formats. Some content that appears in print may not be available in electronic format. For information about Apple Academic Press products, visit our website at **www.appleacademicpress.com** and the CRC Press website at **www.crcpress.com**

ABOUT THE EDITOR

LISA ALBERS PROCK, MD, MPH

Dr. Prock is a Developmental Behavioral Pediatrician at Children's Hospital (Boston) where she co-founded and directs the Adoption Program and works in the Developmental Medicine Center. She is a co-director of the Translational Neuroscience Center at Boston Children's Hospital, and she is the director of Developmental Behavioral Pediatric Services at Children's Hospital and Harvard Medical School, where her responsibilities include Clinical Director of the Developmental Behavioral Pediatrics Fellowship Program. She also is active in international health and resident/fellow education. She attended college at the University of Chicago, medical school at Columbia University and received a master's degree in public health from the Harvard School of Public Health. At the end of her training, she worked as a primary care pediatrician at a community health center and as an inpatient hospital physician. After obtaining a public health degree in International Health, she lived and worked in Cambodia where she taught pediatrics and studied the epidemiology of tuberculosis in children. She returned to Boston for further training in general pediatrics and development as a Dyson Fellow at Children's Hospital.

Dr. Prock is currently involved in translational research efforts as the Principal Investigator for four clinical trials working with adolescents and young adults with Fragile X Syndrome. She is also co-director of the clinical arm of the Translational Neuroscience Center at Boston Children's Hospital, a multidisciplinary collaboration to accelerate the translation of basic science findings into clinical meaning for children with developmental disabilities and their families. Dr. Prock has also combined her clinical interests in child development and international health with advocacy for children, particularly in the areas of foster care and adoption. She has been working with adoptees (both domestic and international) involved in medical, residential and educational settings since 1991.

Her research interests include the long-term developmental, behavioral and emotional concerns of adoptees. She has co-authored several original publications, edited several reference volumes, and written numerous articles. She has been a board member for several nonprofit organizations, including the Center for Family Connections, a family therapy organization specializing in issues for foster-care and adoptive families; Adoptive Families Together, a parent support group specific to adoptive families; and the Treehouse Foundation, a foster family empowerment program. She has received numerous local and national awards for her work with children and families, most recently the 2004 United States Congressional Angel in Adoption Award. She is a past chairperson of the American Academy of Pediatrics Section on Adoption and Foster Care and current executive committee member of the American Academy of Pediatrics Council on Foster Care, Kinship and Adoption.

CONTENTS

ACKNOWLEDGMENT AND HOW TO CITE

The editor and publisher thank each of the authors who contributed to this book. The chapters in this book were previously published in various places in various formats. To cite the work contained in this book and to view the individual permissions, please refer to the citation at the beginning of each chapter. Each chapter was read individually and carefully selected by the editor; the result is a book that provides a nuanced look at the outcomes of childhood adversity around the world. The chapters included examine the following topics:

- Written from a completely American perspective, Chapter 1 provides a comprehensive overview of the compendium topic, as represented within the United States, offering prevalence numbers, definitions, a summary of research, and discussion of the related factors social workers need to consider in relation to this issue.
- The authors of Chapter 2 provide parallel information to that offered in the previous chapter, though in less depth, for German society instead of American.
- In Chapter 3, we shift our attention to Canada, where the authors consider the connections between childhood adversity and adult homelessness, offering social workers a better understanding of how two population groups intersect and in fact may need to be perceived holistically rather than as two separate social issues.
- In Chapter 4, the authors provide a fascinating discussion of how school teachers' "disciplinary style" within Yemen society may actually be a form of emotional abuse that is facilitated by socio-cultural factors.
- China's one-child families create a particular environment within which to consider the problem of child abuse. The authors of Chapter 5 underline China's unique societal demands that make it difficult to compare the prevalence of this issue to other regions of the world, while offering a foundation and direction for further research.
- The first of two chapters examining the effect of war on children, the authors of Chapter 6 focus on trans-generational mental health issues. Their findings did not support the hypothesis that parental PTSD is associated with children's mental health. Instead, mental health issues in children are closely associated with trans-generational maternal violence (violence tak-

ing place within the household rather than in the larger surrounding society). These findings indicate that children may be surprisingly resilient to war (societal, large-scale violence), at least on an emotional level, while extremely vulnerable to small-scale intra-family violence.

- In Chapter 7, the authors suggest findings that may appear to be contradictory to those offered in the previous chapter. However, these authors include a wider perspective than only mental-health consequences, finding that disease, malnutrition, and impaired development may all be trans-generational effects of war. The scope of this article is wider, including many historical conflicts, with the consequence that associations may be harder to interpret.

- Chapter 8 provides another look at China's specific societal milieu, this one connecting negative pressures found within Chinese society with suicidal behaviors. The authors point out that because this is a cross-sectional study, only correlations can be reached, rather than causal relationships.

- Unsurprisingly, the authors of Chapter 9 find that Chinese children exposed to sexual abuse are as likely as Western children (specifically American and Australian) to experience mental health consequences.

- In Chapter 10, the authors take advantage of South Africa's unique population demographics to reach implications regarding the intersection between childhood trauma, ethnicity, and obesity.

- The unique study in Chapter 11 looks at the association between childhood adversity and geriatric cognitive dysfunction. This possible connection between two seemingly widely separated groups, both serviced by social workers, provides fertile ground for future research and understanding. This study, however, is limited by the small size and specificity of its sample (child laborers).

- Chapter 12 provides a cross-country study of the connections between childhood abandonment and educational outcomes, the research is interesting, but doesn't separate out the socioeconomic effects of abandonment as a causal factor in learning outcome. It does underline the need for intervention within low-income communities where there are numerous orphans and abandoned children.

- The authors of Chapter 13 reach the conclusion that school-based interventions may not be most effective, at least as treatment (rather than prevention). They recommend further research into the potential of parental interventions to help treat and prevent the adverse mental health consequences of childhood trauma in war-torn regions. As with chapter 6, the research indicates children's vulnerability to domestic, intra-family factors over those in the larger society.

- The American-based research presented in Chapter 14 indicates the effectiveness of cognitive behavioral therapy as a treatment for children who have experienced childhood adversity. The treatment requires trained professionals, but research like this supports the value of such training, as well as encourages social workers to refer clients to professionals who do have this training. The article includes a helpful list of contacts for training and consultation, as well as an implementation guide.

LIST OF CONTRIBUTORS

Amal S. S. Ba-Saddik
Department of Behavioral Sciences, Faculty of Medicine & Health Sciences, Aden University, P.O. Box 6165 (Khormaksar), Aden, Yemen

Marion Birch
Medact, London, UK

Elmar Brähler
Department of Medical Psychology and Medical Sociology, University of Leipzig, Leipzig, Germany

Andrea Burri
Department of Psychology, University of Zurich, Zurich, Switzerland

Min Cai
Huzhou No.3 Hospital, Huzhou, Zhejiang, People's Republic of China

Yiyun Cai
Huashan Hospital of Fudan University, Shanghai, People's Republic of China

Guibing Chen
Huaian No.3 Hospital, Huaian, Jiangsu, People's Republic of China

Jing Chen
Huashan Hospital of Fudan University, Shanghai, People's Republic of China

Mingxi Chen
Key Laboratory of Adolescent Cyberpsychology and Behavior (CCNU), Ministry of Education, Wuhan, China; School of Psychology, Central China Normal University, Wuhan, China

Yiping Chen
Clinical Trial Service Unit, Oxford, United Kingdom

Yunchun Chen
Xijing Hospital of No.4 Military Medical University, Xian, Shaanxi, People's Republic of China

Enzhao Cong
Shanghai Mental Health Center, Shanghai Jiaotong University School of Medicine, Shanghai, People's Republic of China

Hong Deng
Mental Health Center of West China Hospital of Sichuan University, Chengdu, Sichuan, People's Republic of China

Delan Devakumar
Institute for Global Health, University College London, London, UK

Jicheng Dong
Qingdao Mental Health Center, Qingdao, Shandong, People's Republic of China

Bo Du
Hebei Mental Health Center, Baoding, Hebei, People's Republic of China

Thomas Elbert
Department of Psychology, University of Konstanz, 78457 Konstanz, Germany

Maya Escueta
Terry Sanford Institute of Public Policy, Duke University, Durham, NC, USA

Xiang Fang
Fuzhou Psychiatric Hospital, Fuzhou, Fujian, People's Republic of China

Jonathan Flint
Wellcome Trust Centre for Human Genetics, Oxford, United Kingdom

J. Forbes
UCT/MRC Research Unit for Exercise Science and Sports Medicine, Department of Human Biology, University of Cape Town, Cape Town, South Africa

Chengge Gao
No. 1 Hospital of Medical College of Xian Jiaotong University, Xian, Shaanxi, People's Republic of China

Jingfang Gao
Chinese Traditional Hospital of Zhejiang, Hangzhou, Zhejiang, People's Republic of China

Shugui Gao
Ningbo Kang Ning Hospital, Ningbo, Zhejiang, People's Republic of China

Heide Glaesmer
Department of Medical Psychology and Medical Sociology, University of Leipzig, Leipzig, Germany

J. H. Goedecke
UCT/MRC Research Unit for Exercise Science and Sports Medicine, Department of Human Biology, University of Cape Town, Cape Town, South Africa; South African Medical Research Council, Parow, South Africa

Danhua Gu
Weihai Mental Health Center, Weihai, Shandong, People's Republic of China

Guixiong Gu
Pediatrics Research Institution of Suzhou University, Suzhou, China

Baowei Ha
Liaocheng No.4 Hospital, Liaocheng, Shandong, People's Republic of China

Abdullah S. Hattab
Department of Social Medicine &Public Health, Faculty of Medicine &Health Sciences, Aden University, P.O. Box 6165 (Khormaksar), Aden, Yemen

Winfried Häuser
Department of Internal Medicine, Klinikum Saarbrücken, Saarbrücken, Germany; Department of Psychosomatic Medicine, Technische Universität München, Munich, Germany

Xiaohong Hong
Mental Health Center of Shantou University, Shantou, Guangdong, People's Republic of China

Chunmei Hu
No.3 Hospital of Heilongjiang Province, Beian, Heilongjiang, People's Republic of China

Jian Hu
Harbin Medical University, Haerbin, Heilongjiang, People's Republic of China

Jing Hua
Shanghai First Maternity and Infant Hospital, Tongji University School of Medicine Shanghai, Shanghai, China

Guoping Huang
Sichuan Mental Health Center, Mianyang, Sichuan, People's Republic of China

Benjamin Iffland
Department of Psychology, Bielefeld University, Postbox 100131, 33501 Bielefeld, Germany

xiv   List of Contributors

Guoqing Jiang
Chongqing Mental Health Center, Chongqing, People's Republic of China

Joop T. V. M. de Jong
Amsterdam Institute of Social Science Research, University of Amsterdam, Amsterdam, the Nether-
lands; Boston University School of Medicine, Boston, USA; Rhodes University, Grahamstown, South
Africa

Mark J. D. Jordans
Department of Research & Development, HealthNet TPO, Amsterdam, the Netherlands; Centre for
Global Mental Health, Institute of Psychiatry, Kings College London, London, UK

Kenneth S. Kendler
Virginia Institute for Psychiatric and Behavioral Genetics, Department of Psychiatry, Virginia Com-
monwealth University, Richmond, Virginia, United States of America

Ivan H. Komproe
Department of Research & Development, HealthNet TPO, Amsterdam, the Netherlands; Faculty for
Behavioral & Social Sciences, Utrecht University, Utrecht, the Netherlands

Sandy Krammer
Department of Psychology, University of Zurich, Zurich, Switzerland

Gongying Li
Mental Health Institute of Jining Medical College, Jining, Shandong, People's Republic of China

Kan Li
Mental Hospital of Jiangxi Province, Nanchang, Jiangxi, People's Republic of China

Yi Li
Dalian No.7 Hospital, Dalian, Liaoning, People's Republic of China

Yi Li
Wuhan Mental Health Center, Wuhan, Hubei, People's Republic of China

Yihan Li
Wellcome Trust Centre for Human Genetics, Oxford, United Kingdom

Youhui Li
No.1 Hospital of Zhengzhou University, Zhengzhou, Henan, People's Republic of China

Wei Liang
Psychiatric Hospital of Henan Province, Xinxiang, Henan, People's Republic of China

Lanfen Liu
Shandong Mental Health Center, Jinan, Shandong, People's Republic of China

Tiebang Liu
Shenzhen Kang Ning Hospital, Shenzhen, Guangdong, People's Republic of China

Tieqiao Liu
No.2 Xiangya Hospital of Zhongnan University, Changsha, Hunan, People's Republic of China

Xiaojuan Liu
Tianjin First Center Hospital, Tianjin, People's Republic of China

Ying Liu
The First Hospital of China Medical University, Shenyang, Liaoning, People's Republic of China

Zhengrong Liu
Anshan Psychiatric Rehabilitation Hospital, Anshan, Liaoning, People's Republic of China

Robert D. Macy
International Trauma Center & Harvard School of Medicine, Boston, MA, USA

Andreas Maercker
Department of Psychology, University of Zurich, Zurich, Switzerland

Qiyi Mei
Suzhou Guangji Hospital, Suzhou, Jiangsu, People's Republic of China

Huaqing Meng
No.1 Hospital of Chongqing Medical University, Chongqing, People's Republic of China

Wei Meng
Department of Epidemiology, Public Health School, Fudan University, Shanghai, China; Key Laboratory of Public Health Safety, Ministry of education, Shanghai, China

Guodong Miao
Guangzhou Brain Hospital (Guangzhou Psychiatric Hospital), Guangzhou, Guangdong, People's Republic of China

Akm Moniruzzaman
Faculty of Health Sciences, Simon Fraser University, 8888 University Drive, Burnaby, British Columbia, Canada

Zhe Mu
Shanghai Urban Environmental Meteorology Center, Shanghai, China; The Medical School of Tongji University, Shanghai, China

Aline Ndayisaba
HealthNet TPO Burundi, Bujumbura, Burundi

Frank Neuner
Department of Psychology, Bielefeld University, Postbox 100131, 33501 Bielefeld, Germany

Prudence Ntamutumba
HealthNet TPO Burundi, Bujumbura, Burundi

Bright I. Nwaru
School of Health Sciences, University of Tampere, Tampere, Finland

Karen O'Donnell
Terry Sanford Institute of Public Policy, Duke University, Durham, NC, USA; Center for Health Policy, Duke Global Health Institute, Duke University, 2812 Erwin Rd., Suite 403, Durham, North Carolina 27705, USA; Center for Child and Family Health, Duke University, Durham, NC, USA

Jan Ostermann
Center for Health Policy, Duke Global Health Institute, Duke University, 2812 Erwin Rd., Suite 403, Durham, North Carolina 27705, USA

David Osrin
Institute for Global Health, University College London, London, UK

Jiyang Pan
No.1 Hospital of Jinan University, Guangzhou, Guangdong, People's Republic of China

Runde Pan
Guangxi Longquanshan Hospital, Liuzhou, Guangxi, People's Republic of China

Michelle L. Patterson
Faculty of Health Sciences, Simon Fraser University, 8888 University Drive, Burnaby, British Columbia, Canada

Ping Qin
National Center for Register-based Research, University of Aarhus, Aarhus, Denmark; National Center for Suicide Research and Prevention, Institute of Clinical Medicine, University of Oslo, Oslo, Norway

Maria Roth
Department of Psychology, University of Konstanz, 78457 Konstanz, Germany

Hong Sang
Changchun Mental Hospital, Changchun, Jilin, People's Republic of China

Jianhua Shen
Tianjin Anding Hospital, Tianjin, People's Republic of China

Zhenming Shen
Tangshan No.5 Hospital, Tangshan, Hebei, People's Republic of China

Jianguo Shi
Xian Mental Health Center, Xian, Shaanxi, People's Republic of China

Shenxun Shi
Shanghai Mental Health Center, Shanghai Jiaotong University School of Medicine, Shanghai, People's Republic of China; Huashan Hospital of Fudan University, Shanghai, People's Republic of China

Keti Simmen-Janevska
Department of Psychology, University of Zurich, Zurich, Switzerland

Heather Sipsma
Department of Women, Children, and Family Health Science, University of Illinois at Chicago College of Nursing, Chicago, IL, USA

Eva S. Smallegange
Department of Childhood and Educational Sciences, University of Amsterdam, Amsterdam, the Netherlands

Julian M. Somers
Faculty of Health Sciences, Simon Fraser University, 8888 University Drive, Burnaby, British Columbia, Canada

Egbert Sondorp
Royal Tropical Institute, Amsterdam, Netherlands

Yan Song
Mudanjiang Psychiatric Hospital of Heilongjiang Province, Mudanjiang, Heilongjiang, People's Republic of China

D. J. Stein
South African Medical Research Council, Parow, South Africa

Jing Sun
Nanjing Brain Hospital, Nanjing, Jiangsu, People's Republic of China

Ming Tao
Xinhua Hospital of Zhejiang Province, Hangzhou, Zhejiang, People's Republic of China

Wietse A. Tol
Department of Mental Health, Johns Hopkins Bloomberg School of Public Health, 624 N Broadway, Hampton House R863, Baltimore, MD 21205-1996, USA; Department of Research & Development, HealthNet TPO, Amsterdam, the Netherlands

Gang Wang
Beijing Anding Hospital of Capital University of Medical Sciences, Beijing, People's Republic of China

Xiaoping Wang
Renmin Hospital of Wuhan University, Wuhan, Hubei, People's Republic of China

Xumei Wang
ShengJing Hospital of China Medical University, Shenyang, Liaoning, People's Republic of China

Xueyi Wang
First Hospital of Hebei Medical University, Shijiazhuang, Hebei, People's Republic of China

Jonathan C.K. Wells
Childhood Nutrition Research Centre, Institute of Child Health, University College London, London, UK

Kathryn Whetten
Terry Sanford Institute of Public Policy, Duke University, Durham, NC, USA; Center for Health Policy, Duke Global Health Institute, Duke University, 2812 Erwin Rd., Suite 403, Durham, North Carolina 27705, USA; Department of Community and Family Medicine, Duke University, Durham, NC, USA

Wenyuan Wu
Tongji University Hospital, Shanghai, People's Republic of China

Zhuochun Wu
Department of Epidemiology, Public Health School, Fudan University, Shanghai, China; Key Laboratory of Public Health Safety, Ministry of education, Shanghai, China

Donglin Yang
Jining Psychiatric Hospital, Jining, Shandong, People's Republic of China

Lijun Yang
Jilin Brain Hospital, Siping, Jilin, People's Republic of China

Sen Yang
Key Laboratory of Adolescent Cyberpsychology and Behavior (CCNU), Ministry of Education, Wuhan, China; School of Psychology, Central China Normal University, Wuhan, China

Zhiqi You
Key Laboratory of Adolescent Cyberpsychology and Behavior (CCNU), Ministry of Education, Wuhan, China; School of Psychology, Central China Normal University, Wuhan, China

Fengyu Yu
Harbin No.1 Special Hospital, Haerbin, Heilongjiang, People's Republic of China

Jinbei Zhang
No. 3 Hospital of Sun Yat-sen University, Guangzhou, Guangdong, People's Republic of China

Kerang Zhang
No.1 Hospital of Shanxi Medical University, Taiyuan, Shanxi, People's Republic of China

Qiwen Zhang
Hainan Anning Hospital, Haikou, Hainan, People's Republic of China

Wei Zhang
Daqing No.3 Hospital of Heilongjiang Province, Daqing, Heilongjiang, People's Republic of China

Yutang Zhang
No.2 Hospital of Lanzhou University, Lanzhou, Gansu, People's Republic of China

Zhen Zhang
No.4 Hospital of Jiangsu University, Zhenjiang, Jiangsu, People's Republic of China

Hui Zhong
Anhui Mental Health Center, Hefei, Anhui, People's Republic of China

Zongkui Zhou
Key Laboratory of Adolescent Cyberpsychology and Behavior (CCNU), Ministry of Education, Wuhan, China; School of Psychology, Central China Normal University, Wuhan, China

INTRODUCTION

Child protection is a cross-cultural, global concern. It affects children re-siding in countries and societies regardless of wealth and culture. Child wellbeing is a matter of concern to professionals from an equally wide spectrum, from mental health workers to justice system employees, social workers to policy makers, and physicians to childcare workers.

The statistics are staggering. According to World Health Organization figures, approximately 20 percent of women and 5–10 percent of men re-port being sexually abused as children, while 25–50 percent of all children report being physically abused. Between one-quarter and one-half of all children in the world report severe and frequent physical abuse. Not all trauma is direct; witnessing violence, whether domestic or political, can be just as damaging to children. Between 133 and 275 million children worldwide are estimated to witness domestic violence annually, while even more are traumatized by war: 12 million are left homeless because of war, more than 1 million are orphaned or separated from their parents, and as many as 10 million are psychologically traumatized (UNICEF fig-ures, 2006). Developmentally significant adversity may occur in a child's home, school or community setting.

Children are particularly vulnerable to the ravages of war. According to a United Nations study on children in war by Graca Machel, "The physi-cal, sexual and emotional violence to which [children] are exposed shat-ters their world. War undermines the very foundations of children's lives, destroying their homes, splintering their communities and breaking down their trust in adults." This is truly a developmental trauma, one which will require coordinated and informed efforts from the international commu-nity to heal.

Developmental trauma has a long reach, one that extends across many aspects of physical and mental health, beginning with an impact on cel-lular DNA. In the brain, trauma has a profound impact on the intricate neuronal networks that impact an individual by shaping behavior, evoking emotions, determining reactions to danger, and building relationships with others. Cross-cultural research into brain-body science offers new insights into the impact of early trauma on physical and mental health because of neurobiological and epigenetic changes.

The neurobiology of childhood trauma is now integral to the daily clinical practice of professionals from many fields, including educators, social workers, mental health professionals, family and substance abuse counselors, police, caregivers, and criminal justice service providers. Developments in the neurosciences provide insight into the ways in which trauma impacts the emotional, cognitive, social, and biological forces that shape human development. As more and more researchers delve into this issue, professionals from many fields can gain new understanding of the ways in which trauma has specific consequences for the central nervous system and determination of "self," which has implications for society as a whole. Research offers suggestions and possibilities for helping children recover from the effects of violence, disruption, and neglect. We can use findings from this research to work together, across disciplines and cultures, to build a safer world for our children.

All providers working with children should routinely consider:

- Gathering a focused history of potential exposure to neglect, emotional, physical and sexual abuse
- The potential risk factor of childhood abuse/neglect for later behavioral emotional/behavioral/mental health concerns

Lisa Albers Prock, MD, MPH

Neglect accounts for over three-quarters of confirmed cases of child maltreatment in the United States—far more than physical or sexual abuse—but it continues to receive less attention from practitioners, researchers, and the media. Some reasons may be that neglect is not well understood and is difficult to identify, prevent, and treat effectively. Chapter 1, originally published by the Child Welfare Information gateway, is a bulletin for professionals that addresses the scope of the problem of child neglect as well as its consequences, reviews definitions and strategies for assessing neglect, presents lessons learned about prevention and intervention, and suggests sources of training and informational support.

Representative data about the frequency of child maltreatment is needed in order to estimate the extent of the problem in the wider population as well as to provide the basis for interpretation of frequency rates in clinical samples. However, previous representative studies on the frequency of child maltreatment in Germany and other countries were limited as they focused on the assessment of physical and sexual abuse whilst emotional forms of maltreatment were ignored. In addition, previous studies applied scales that had not been validated against external criteria. Chapter 2, by Iffland and colleagues, provides a cross-sectional study, where standardized questionnaires were administered to a representative sample of the German population. Maltreatment in childhood and adolescence was assessed using the German version of the Childhood Trauma Questionnaire. Empirically derived threshold values for the five different types of child maltreatment including emotional maltreatment were applied to determine presence of abuse and neglect. Complete data was available from N = 2,500 subjects. Prevalence rates were 13.9% for emotional neglect, 10.2% for emotional abuse, 12.0% for physical abuse, 48.4% for physical neglect, and 6.2% for sexual abuse. Differences between sexes were found for the frequency of sexual abuse. Although the analysis in this chapter has found lower rates of child maltreatment than previous reports that used less well validated criteria, the results of this study confirm that child abuse, with its many different facets, is a significant problem in Germany.

It is well documented that childhood abuse, neglect and household dysfunction are disproportionately present in the backgrounds of homeless adults, and that these experiences adversely impact child development and a wide range of adult outcomes. However, few studies have examined the cumulative impact of adverse childhood experiences on homeless adults with mental illness. Chapter 3, by Patterson and colleagues examines adverse events in childhood as predictors of duration of homelessness, psychiatric and substance use disorders, and physical health in a sample of homeless adults with mental illness. This study was conducted using baseline data from a randomized controlled trial in Vancouver, British Columbia for participants who completed the Adverse Childhood Experiences (ACE) scale at 18 months follow-up (n = 364). Primary outcomes included current mental disorders; substance use including type, frequency and severity; physical health; duration of homelessness; and vocational functioning. In multivariable regression models, ACE total score independently predicted a range of mental health, physical health, and substance use problems, and marginally predicted duration of homelessness. Adverse childhood experiences are overrepresented among homeless adults with complex comorbidities and chronic homelessness. The findings are consistent with a growing body of literature indicating that childhood traumas are potent risk factors for a number of adult health and psychiatric problems, particularly substance use problems. Results are discussed in the context of cumulative adversity and self-trauma theory.

Emotional abuse is central to other forms of abuse. The primary objective of Chapter 4, by Ba-Saddik and colleagues, was to estimate the prevalence of emotional abuse among pupils in basic education schools and the risk factors associated with it in Aden governorate, Yemen. Four districts were randomly selected from across the governorate of Aden, 2 schools were selected at random in each district, and then 1066 pupils were randomly selected from the 8 schools. An anonymous self-administered questionnaire was used for data collection. Data were analyzed using Statistical Package for Social Sciences ver.15. Mean, standard deviation and chi square were used for descriptive statistics. Univariate and Multivariate logistic regression analysis was used to examine the associations between emotional abuse with pupils/parents characteristics. Pupils reported high rates of emotional abuse 55.2% at least once in their school lifetime. Male pupils had higher prevalence of emotional abuse 72.6% than females 26.1%. Teachers constituted the highest proportion of perpetrators 45.6%. Odds Ratio (95% confidence interval) showed statistically significant association between emotional abuse and pupils' gender, family type and father education: 9.94 (7.19-13.74), 1.40 (1.02-1.91), .58 (.39-.86) respectively. Emotional child abuse was highly prevalent in pupils in basic school education. Pupils' gender, family type and father education were the main risk factors associated with emotional abuse.

The one-child policy introduced in China in 1979 has led to far-reaching changes in socio-demographic characteristics. Under this policy regime, each household has few children. In Chapter 5, Hua and colleagues aim to describe the prevalence of child neglect in one-child families in China and to examine the correlates of child neglect. A cross-sectional study of 2044 children aged 6 to 9 years and recruited from four primary schools in Suzhou City, China was conducted. Neglect subtypes were determined using a validated indigenous measurement scale reported by parents. Child, parental and family characteristics were obtained by questionnaires and review of social security records. Linear regression analyses were performed to estimate the associations between these factors and the subtypes of child neglect. The prevalence of child any neglect was 32.0% in one child families in Suzhou City, China. Supervisory (20.3%) neglect was the most prevalent type of child neglect, followed by emotional (15.2%), physical (11.1%), and educational (6.0%) neglect After simultaneous adjustment to child and family characteristics and the school factor, boys, children with physical health issues and cognitive impairment, younger and unemployed mother, were positively associated with neglect subtypes. The authors also found that parents with higher education and three-generation families were negatively associated with neglect. The rates of child neglect subtypes vary across different regions in China probably due to the different policy implementation and socio-economic levels, with a lower level of physical and educational neglect and a higher level of emotional neglect in this study. The three-generation family structure was correlates of neglect which may be unique in one child families. This indicates that future intervention programs in one-child families should target these factors.

Understanding how parental Post-Traumatic Stress Disorder (PTSD) may or may not affect the development and mental health in the offspring is particularly important in conflict regions, where trauma-related illness is endemic. In Rwanda, organised atrocities and the genocide against the Tutsi of 1994 have left a significant fraction of the population with chronic PTSD. The aim of Chapter 6, by Roth and colleagues, was to establish whether PTSD in mothers is associated with symptoms of depression, anxiety, and aggressive and antisocial behaviour in their children. A community sample of 125 Rwandan mothers who experienced the genocide of 1994 and their 12-year-old children were interviewed. Using a structured interview, symptoms of maternal PTSD and children's depression, anxiety, and aggressive and antisocial behaviour were assessed by trained and on-site supervised local B.A. psychologists. The interview also included a detailed checklist of event types related to family violence. In showing that a maternal PTSD was not associated with child's psychopathology, the results contradict the assumption of straight "trans-generational trauma transmission". Instead, a child's exposure to maternal family violence posed a significant risk factor for a negative mental health outcome. Furthermore, it was not maternal PTSD-symptoms but mother's exposure to family violence during her own childhood that was associated with the magnitude of adversities that a child experiences at home. Contrary to a simple model of a trans-generational transmission of trauma, neither maternal PTSD nor maternal traumatic experiences were directly associated with symptoms of anxiety, depression, or antisocial and aggressive behaviour in the children. Instead, the present results suggest a relationship between parental child rearing practices and children's mental health. Furthermore, the study details the "cycle of violence", showing a significant link between maternal violence against a child and its mother's experience of childhood maltreatment.

The short- and medium-term effects of conflict on population health are reasonably well documented. Less considered are its consequences across generations and potential harms to the health of children yet to be born. Looking first at the nature and effects of exposures during conflict, and then at the potential routes through which harm may propagate within families, Chapter 7, by Devakumar and colleagues, considers the intergenerational effects of four features of conflict: violence, challenges to mental health, infection and malnutrition. Conflict-driven harms are transmitted through a complex permissive environment that includes biological, cultural and economic factors, and feedback loops between sources of harm and weaknesses in individual and societal resilience to them. The authors discuss the multiplicative effects of ongoing conflict when hostilities are prolonged. The article summarizes many instances in which the effects of war can propagate across generations. The authors hope that the evidence laid out in the article will stimulate research and—more importantly—contribute to the discussion of the costs of war; particularly in the longer-term in post-conflict situations in which interventions need to be sustained and adapted over many years.

Although the independent effects of childhood adversities and of recent negative events on suicidality have been well-documented, the combinative role of childhood and recent adversities on risk for suicidality is still underexplored, especially in the context of Chinese culture and in consideration of specific types of negative events. In Chapter 8, 5989 students, randomly sampled from six universities in central China, completed the online survey for this study by You and colleagues. Suicidal behavior, life adversity during childhood and stressful events in recent school life were assessed with designed questionnaires. Students experiencing recent stressful life events more often reported an experience of life adversity during childhood. While recent stressful life events and childhood life adversity both were associated with an increased risk for suicidal behavior, the two exposures presented conjunctively and acted interactively to increase the risk. There was noticeable variation of effects associated with specific childhood life adversities, and sexual abuse, poor parental relationship, divorce of parents and loss of a parent were among the adversities associated with the highest increased risk. Recent conflicts with classmates, poor school performance and rupture of romantic relationships were the recent school life stressors associated with the highest increased risk. Childhood adversity and recent school life stressors had a combinative role in predicting suicidality of young people studying in Chinese colleges. Unhappy family life during childhood and recent interpersonal conflicts in school were the most important predictors of suicidality in this population.

Chen and colleagues' prior study in Han Chinese women has shown that women with a history of childhood sexual abuse (CSA) are at increased risk for developing major depression (MD). Chapter 9 explores the question of whether or not this relationship could be found in their whole data set? Three levels of CSA (non-genital, genital, and intercourse) were assessed by self-report in two groups of Han Chinese women: 6017 clinically ascertained with recurrent MD and 5983 matched controls. Diagnostic and other risk factor information was assessed at personal interview. Odds ratios (ORs) were calculated by logistic regression. The authors confirmed earlier results by replicating prior analyses in 3,950 new recurrent MD cases. There were no significant differences between the two data sets. Any form of CSA was significantly associated with recurrent MD (OR 4.06, 95% confidence interval (CI) [3.19–5.24]). This association strengthened with increasing CSA severity: non-genital (OR 2.21, 95% CI 1.58–3.15), genital (OR 5.24, 95% CI 3.52–8.15) and intercourse (OR 10.65, 95% CI 5.56–23.71). Among the depressed women, those with CSA had an earlier age of onset, longer depressive episodes. Recurrent MD patients those with CSA had an increased risk for dysthymia (OR 1.60, 95%CI 1.11–2.27) and phobia (OR 1.41, 95%CI 1.09–1.80). Any form of CSA was significantly associated with suicidal ideation or attempt (OR 1.50, 95% CI 1.20–1.89) and feelings of worthlessness or guilt (OR 1.41, 95% CI 1.02–2.02). Intercourse (OR 3.47, 95%CI 1.66–8.22), use of force and threats (OR 1.95, 95%CI 1.05–3.82) and how strongly the victims were affected at the time (OR 1.39, 95%CI 1.20–1.64) were significantly associated with recurrent MD. In Chinese women CSA is strongly associated with recurrent MD and this association increases with greater severity of CSA. Depressed women with CSA have some specific clinical traits. Some features of CSA were associated with greater likelihood of developing recurrent MD.

Childhood trauma has previously been associated with adult obesity. The aim of Chapter 10, by Goedecke and colleagues, was to determine if ethnicity altered the relationship between childhood trauma and obesity in South African women. Forty-four normal-weight (BMI<25kg/m^2) and obese (BMI>30kg/m^2), black and white pre-menopausal women completed the Childhood Trauma Questionnaire (CTQ), which retrospectively assessed emotional and physical neglect, and emotional, physical and sexual abuse in childhood. Body composition did not differ by ethnicity in the normal-weight and obese groups. However,independent of BMI group, there were significant differences in socioeconomic status (SES) between black and white women (P<0.01). Total CTQ score, as well as the sub-scales, physical and emotional neglect, and physical and sexual abuse were higher in black than white women (all P<0.05), but these scores did not differ between BMI groups. Apart from the sexual abuse score, the differences in physical and emotional neglect and physical abuse scores were no longer significant after adjusting for ethnic differences in age and SES. For sexual abuse, there was a significant interaction between ethnicity and BMI group(P=0.04), with scores in normal weight women being higher in black than white women, but scores in obese women not differing by ethnicity. Ethnicity alters the association between childhood sexual abuse and BMI status. Larger studies are required to verify this finding, including measures of body image and body size satisfaction that may explain these findings.

A growing body of evidence suggests a link between early childhood trauma, post-traumatic stress disorder (PTSD) and higher risk for dementia in old age. The aim of Burri and colleagues in Chapter 11 was to investigate the association between childhood trauma exposure, PTSD and neurocognitive function in a unique cohort of former indentured Swiss child laborers in their late adulthood. To the best of the authors' knowledge this is the first study ever conducted on former indentured child laborers and the first to investigate the relationship between childhood versus adulthood trauma and cognitive function. According to PTSD symptoms and whether they experienced childhood trauma (CT) or adulthood trauma (AT), participants (n = 96) were categorized as belonging to one of four groups: CT/PTSD+, CT/PTSD-, AT/PTSD+, AT/PTSD-. Information on cognitive function was assessed using the Structured Interview for Diagnosis of Dementia of Alzheimer Type, Multi-infarct Dementia and Dementia of other Etiology according to ICD-10 and DSM-III-R, the Mini-Mental State Examination, and a vocabulary test. Depressive symptoms were investigated as a potential mediator for neurocognitive functioning. Individuals screening positively for PTSD symptoms performed worse on all cognitive tasks compared to healthy individuals, independent of whether they reported childhood or adulthood adversity. When controlling for depressive symptoms, the relationship between PTSD symptoms and poor cognitive function became stronger. Overall, results tentatively indicate that PTSD is accompanied by cognitive deficits which appear to be independent of earlier childhood adversity. The findings suggest that cognitive deficits in old age may be partly a consequence of PTSD or at least be aggravated by it. However, several study limitations need to considered. Consideration of cognitive deficits when treating PTSD patients and victims of lifespan trauma (even without a diagnosis of a psychiatric condition) is crucial. Furthermore, early intervention may prevent long-term deficits in memory function and development of dementia in adulthood.

Development policymakers and child-care service providers are committed to improving the educational opportunities of the 153 million orphans worldwide. Nevertheless, the relationship between orphanhood and education outcomes is not well understood. Varying factors associated with differential educational attainment leave policymakers uncertain where to intervene. Chapter 12, by Escueta and colleagues, examines the relationship between psychosocial well-being and cognitive development in a cohort of orphans and abandoned children (OAC) relative to non-OAC in five low and middle income countries (LMICs) to understand better what factors are associated with success in learning for these children. Positive Outcomes for Orphans (POFO) is a longitudinal study, following a cohort of single and double OAC in institutional and community-based settings in five LMICs in Southeast Asia and sub-Saharan Africa: Cambodia, Ethiopia, India, Kenya, and Tanzania. Employing two-stage random sampling survey methodology to identify representative samples of OAC in six sites, the POFO study aimed to better understand factors associated with child well-being. Using cross-sectional and child-level fixed effects regression analyses on 1,480 community based OAC and a comparison sample of non-OAC, this manuscript examines associations between emotional difficulties, cognitive development, and a variety of possible co-factors, including potentially traumatic events. The most salient finding is that increases in emotional difficulties are associated with lags in cognitive development for two separate measures of learning within and across multiple study sites. Exposure to potentially traumatic events, male gender, and lower socio-economic status are associated with more reported emotional difficultiesin some sites. Being female and having an illiterate caregiver is associated with lower performance on cognitive development tests in some sites, while greater wealth is associated with higher performance. There is no significant association between orphan status per se and cognitive development, though the negative and significant association between higher emotional difficulties and lags in cognitive development hold across all orphan subgroups. These findings suggest that interventions targeting psychosocial support for vulnerable children, especially vis a vis traumatic experiences, may ease strains inhibiting a child's learning. Family based interventions to stabilize socioeconomic conditions may help overcome psychosocial challenges that otherwise would present as barriers to the child's learning.

Armed conflicts are associated with a wide range of impacts on the mental health of children and adolescents. In Chapter 13, Tol and colleagues evaluated the effectiveness of a school-based intervention aimed at reducing symptoms of posttraumatic stress disorder, depression, and anxiety (treatment aim); and improving a sense of hope and functioning (preventive aim). The authors conducted a cluster randomized trial with 329 children in war-affected Burundi (aged 8 to 17 (mean 12.29 years, standard deviation 1.61); 48% girls). One group of children (n = 153) participated in a 15-session school-based intervention implemented by paraprofessionals, and the remaining 176 children formed a waitlist control condition. Outcomes were measured before, one week after, and three months after the intervention. No main effects of the intervention were identified. However, longitudinal growth curve analyses showed six favorable and two unfavorable differences in trajectories between study conditions in interaction with several moderators. Children in the intervention condition living in larger households showed decreases on depressive symptoms and function impairment, and those living with both parents showed decreases on posttraumatic stress disorder and depressive symptoms. The groups of children in the waitlist condition showed increases in depressive symptoms. In addition, younger children and those with low levels of exposure to traumatic events in the intervention condition showed improvements on hope. Children in the waitlist condition who lived on their original or newly bought land showed improvements in hope and function impairment, whereas children in the intervention condition showed deterioration on these outcomes. Given inconsistent effects across studies, findings do not support this school-based intervention as a treatment for posttraumatic stress disorder and depressive symptoms in conflict-affected children. The intervention appears to have more consistent preventive benefits, but these effects are contingent upon individual (for example, age, gender) and contextual (for example, family functioning, state of conflict, displacement) variables. Results suggest the potential benefit of school-based preventive interventions particularly in post-conflict settings.

Trauma-focused cognitive behavioral therapy (TF-CBT) is an evidence-based treatment approach shown to help children, adolescents, and their caregivers overcome trauma-related difficulties. It is designed to reduce negative emotional and behavioral responses following child sexual abuse, domestic violence, traumatic loss, and other traumatic events. The treatment—based on learning and cognitive theories—addresses distorted beliefs and attributions related to the abuse and provides a supportive environment in which children are encouraged to talk about their traumatic experience. TF-CBT also helps parents who were not abusive to cope effectively with their own emotional distress and develop skills that support their children. Chapter 14, originally published by the Child Welfare Information Gateway as a information brief, is intended to build a better understanding of the characteristics and benefits of TF-CBT. It was written primarily to help child welfare caseworkers and other professionals who work with at-risk families make more informed decisions about when to refer children and their parents and caregivers to TF-CBT therapists. This information also may help biological parents, foster parents, and other caregivers understand what they and their children can gain from TF-CBT and what to expect during treatment. In addition, this issue brief may be useful to others with an interest in implementing or participating in effective strategies for the treatment of children who have suffered from sexual abuse or multiple traumatic events.

PART I

AN INTERNATIONAL PROBLEM

CHAPTER 1

ACTS OF OMISSION: AN OVERVIEW OF CHILD NEGLECT

CHILD WELFARE INFORMATION GATEWAY, U.S. DEPARTMENT OF HEALTH AND HUMAN SERVICES, CHILDREN'S BUREAU

1.1 SCOPE OF THE PROBLEM

Neglect is by far the most common form of maltreatment. More than 538,000 children were neglected in 2010, accounting for about 78 percent of all unique victims of child maltreatment. In addition, neglect was either the sole cause or one of the contributors to over 68 percent of the 1,560 child maltreatment-related deaths in 2010 (U.S.Department of Health and Human Services, 2011).

These statistics include only children who came to the attention of State child protective services (CPS) agencies. The National Incidence Study (NIS) of Child Abuse and Neglect, which generates broader estimates by gathering data from multiple sources, generally shows higher numbers of maltreatment. The NIS-4, which is the most recent version,

Child Welfare Information Gateway. (2012). *Acts of omission: An overview of child neglect.* Washington, DC: U.S. Department of Health and Human Services, Children's Bureau.

uses data from 2005–2006 to show that more than 770,000 children were neglected, accounting for about 77 percent of all children harmed or endangered by maltreatment (Sedlak et al., 2010). While the incidence of other maltreatment types has declined in recent years, the persistently high rates of neglect point to the need for more effective prevention and intervention in cases of neglect.

1.2 DEFINING CHILD NEGLECT

Both Federal and State laws provide basic definitions of child abuse and neglect. The Federal Child Abuse Prevention and Treatment Act (CAPTA) (42 U.S.C.A. §5106g), as amended by the CAPTA Reauthorization Act of 2010, defines child abuse and neglect as, at minimum:

- Any recent act or failure to act on the part of a parent or caretaker which results in death, serious physical or emotional harm, sexual abuse or exploitation; or
- An act or failure to act which presents an imminent risk of serious harm.

   Neglect is commonly defined in State law as the failure of a parent or other person with responsibility for the child to provide needed food, clothing, shelter, medical care, or supervision to the degree that the child's health, safety, and well-being are threatened with harm. Some States specifically mention types of neglect in their statutes, such as educational neglect, medical neglect, and abandonment; in addition, some States include exceptions for determining neglect, such as religious exemptions for medical neglect and financial considerations for physical neglect (Child Welfare Information Gateway, 2011b).

   To see how your State addresses neglect definitions in law, see Information Gateway's State statute publication Definitions of Child Abuse and Neglect: http://www.childwelfare.gov/systemwide/laws_policies/statutes/define.cfm

   Most States publish policy or procedure manuals to help professionals apply legal definitions of child abuse and neglect in practice. Use Information Gateway's State Guides and Manuals Search to find your State's resources online: http://www.childwelfare.gov/systemwide/sgm

Neglect definitions are impacted by the accepted standards of care for children and the role of communities in families' lives. Some issues that are taken into account when defining neglect and standards of care include:

- Harm to the child
- Parent's ability or intent
- Family's concrete resources
- Community norms
- Availability of community resources (Grayson, 2001)

Difficulties in creating specific definitions of neglect contribute to the lack of consistency in research on neglect as well as CPS responses to neglect. The different ways children may be neglected, addressed below, also make it difficult to define such a complex issue.

1.3 TYPES OF NEGLECT

Although State laws vary regarding the types of neglect included in definitions, summarized below are the most commonly recognized categories of neglect:

- *Physical neglect:* Abandoning the child or refusing to accept custody; not providing for basic needs like nutrition, hygiene, or appropriate clothing
- *Medical neglect*: Delaying or denying recommended health care for the child
- *Inadequate supervision:* Leaving the child unsupervised (depending on length of time and child's age/maturity); not protecting the child from safety hazards, providing inadequate caregivers, or engaging in harmful behavior
- *Emotional neglect:* Isolating the child; not providing affection or emotional support; exposing the child to domestic violence or substance abuse
- *Educational neglect:* Failing to enroll the child in school or homeschool; ignoring special education needs; permitting chronic absenteeism from school

For more information on types of neglect, visit Information Gateway's webpage on the Identification of Neglect: http://www.childwelfare.gov/can/identifying/neglect.cfm

1.4 CONSEQUENCES OF NEGLECT

Although the initial impact may not be as obvious as physical or sexual abuse, the consequences of child neglect are just as serious. Because the effects of neglect are cumulative, long-term research like that being performed by the Longitudinal Studies of Child Abuse and Neglect (http://www.iprc. unc.edu/longscan), funded by the Children's Bureau, helps us better understand outcomes for children affected by neglect.

Research shows child neglect can have a negative impact in the following areas:

- Health and physical development—malnourishment, impaired brain development, delays in growth or failure to thrive
- Intellectual and cognitive development— poor academic performance, delayed or impaired language development
- Emotional and psychological development—deficiencies in self-esteem, attachment, or trust
- Social and behavioral development—interpersonal relationship problems, aggression, conduct disorders (DePanfilis, 2006)

The impacts in these areas are interrelated; problems in one developmental area may influence growth in another area. In addition, research indicates that experiencing neglect along with other forms of maltreatment worsens the impact (Smith & Fong, 2004). However, the impact of neglect can vary based on:

- The child's age
- The presence and strength of protective factors
- The frequency, duration, and severity of the neglect
- The relationship between the child and caregiver (Chalk, Gibbons, & Scarupa, 2002)

1.4.1 TRAUMA AND NEGLECT

While trauma is often discussed in terms of witnessing or being harmed by an intensely threatening event, one or multiple experiences of neglect can also have a traumatic effect, especially in severe cases. One recent study found that, similar to physical and sexual abuse, neglected children showed signs of posttraumatic stress disorder and other traumatic symptoms (Milot et al., 2010). Funded by the Federal Child Neglect Consortium, De Bellis (2005) summarized the results of numerous research studies that found that neglected children experienced adverse brain development and neuropsychological and psychosocial outcomes.

For more information on addressing trauma in neglected children and their families, visit the National Child Traumatic Stress Network's Child Welfare Trauma Training Toolkit (http://www.nctsn.org/ products/child-welfare-trauma-trainingtoolkit- 2008) or read Information Gateway's Supporting Brain Development in Traumatized Children and Youth (http://www.childwelfare.gov/pubs/ braindevtrauma.cfm)

1.4.2 FATAL NEGLECT

A child's death is the most tragic consequence of neglect, and neglect causes or contributes to roughly two-thirds of all child maltreatment-related deaths (U.S. Department of Health and Human Services, 2011). Victims of fatal neglect are more likely to be age 7 or younger (U.S. Government Accountability Office, 2011). The most common reasons for fatal neglect are supervision neglect, chronic physical neglect, and medical neglect (Grayson, 2001). Neglect fatalities can be difficult to identify due to lack of definitive evidence, limited investigative and training resources, and differing interpretations of child maltreatment definitions (U.S. Government Accountability Office, 2011). For more information, visit the National Center for Child Death Review website: http://www.childdeathreview.org

The next section discusses the most common family, parent, and child factors that place children at risk for neglect as well as factors that can protect children from neglect.

1.5 RISK FACTORS

While the presence of a risk factor does not mean a child will be neglected, multiple risk factors are a cause for concern. Research indicates that the following factors place children at greater risk of being harmed or endangered by neglect:

Environmental Factors
- Poverty
- Lack of social support
- Neighborhood distress

Family Factors
- Single parent households
- Family stress or negative interactions
- Domestic violence

Parent Factors
- Unemployment or low socioeconomic status
- Young maternal age
- Health, mental illness, or substance use problems
- Parenting stress

Child Factors
- Age
- Developmental delays (DePanfilis, 2006)

Ultimately, as Straus and Kaufman (2005) caution, the only certain risk is that the more often a child experiences neglect, the more likely he or she will be harmed by it—which is why prevention and early identification of neglect are critical.

1.5.1 PROTECTIVE FACTORS

Although a number of factors place children at greater risk of neglect, research shows that families with one or more of the following protective factors are less likely to experience abuse or neglect:

- Nurturing and attachment
- Knowledge of parenting and child development
- Parental resilience

- Social connections
- Concrete supports for parents
- Social and emotional competence of children

Protective factors are a key component of the Children's Bureau's national child abuse prevention initiative. For more information, see Preventing Child Maltreatment and Promoting Well-Being: A Network for Action 2012 Resource Guide (http://www.childwelfare.gov/ preventing/ preventionmonth/guide2012).

1.6 SPECIAL CONSIDERATIONS

Neglect rarely occurs in isolation; commonly related issues include poverty, substance abuse, and domestic violence. There are special considerations for addressing these issues with at-risk or neglected children and their families.

1.6.1 POVERTY

Poverty is frequently linked to child neglect, but it is important to note that most poor families do not neglect their children. Poverty likely increases the risk of neglect by interacting with and worsening related risks like "parental stress, inadequate housing and homelessness, lack of basic needs, inadequate supervision, substance abuse, and domestic violence" (Duva & Metzger, 2010).

Caseworkers must differentiate between neglectful situations and poverty; in many States, definitions of neglect include considerations for a family's financial means. For example, if a family living in poverty was not providing adequate food for their children, it would be considered neglect only if the parents were aware of but chose not to use food assistance programs. Taking poverty into consideration can prevent unnecessary removals and place the focus on providing concrete services for families to protect and provide for their children.

1.6.2 CHRONIC NEGLECT

Although some individual incidents of neglect may not appear harmful, multiple incidents of neglect occurring over time— known as chronic neglect—can have a greater negative impact on the child. Chronic neglect is "an ongoing, serious pattern of deprivation" of a child's basic needs that results in "accumulation of harm" (Gilmore & Kaplan, 2009).

Chronic neglect can be hard to identify and treat; affected families face complex problems that require specialized, often long-term, interventions and coordinated community support. For more on strategies to address chronic neglect, see Information Gateway's bulletin Chronic Neglect: The Elephant in the Room (in press; find at http://www.childwelfare. gov/catalog/index.cfm?event=catalog. viewSeriesDetail&series=1).

1.6.3 SUBSTANCE ABUSE

Parental substance abuse is more closely related to child neglect than other forms of maltreatment (DePanfilis, 2006). Parents who lose control under the influence of substances may have impaired reasoning abilities, leave the child in an unsafe situation, or neglect the child's basic needs (Children's Bureau, 2009). These parents may also have difficulty conforming to expected parenting roles and providing the child with emotional support (Children's Bureau). While treating the parent's substance abuse is a priority, treatment must be combined with services to address the child's needs and improve overall family functioning.

Substance-exposed newborns. When a woman abuses drugs or alcohol during her pregnancy, the unborn child is at greater risk for developmental delays. In addition, some substance-exposed newborns are left at the hospital by their parents; these infants, sometimes referred to as "boarder babies," usually require CPS intervention to place them in out-of-home care. Child welfare caseworkers and health-care providers must work together to identify, assess, and develop a plan to care for affected infants and their families. For more information, visit the National Abandoned Infants Assistance Center's website: http://aia. berkeley.edu/

For more information, visit the National Center on Substance Abuse and Child Welfare, which is co-sponsored by the Children's Bureau and the Substance Abuse and Mental Health Services Administration: http://www.ncsacw. samhsa.gov/

Family Reclaim, a child neglect demonstration project funded by the Children's Bureau, helped families affected by substance abuse and child neglect by involving them in the design of their service plan; key services included substance abuse treatment, intensive case management, life skills training, and respite care. Family Reclaim provided services collaboratively with the family's support network, community leaders, and other agencies; program staff found that long-term intensive services were necessary to address the family's multiple stressors (Chambers, 2002).

1.6.4 DOMESTIC VIOLENCE

Some States include exposure to domestic violence in their legal definitions of child abuse or neglect due to its potential effects on children (Child Welfare Information Gateway, 2011c). An unintended consequence of these policies is that parents who are domestic violence victims sometimes are charged with a type of neglect termed "failure to protect," despite circumstances that may have impacted the victim's ability to prevent the child's exposure to violence. Child welfare caseworkers, in collaboration with domestic violence professionals, should consider the victim's access to resources or services outside the home as well as the victim's reasonable efforts to ensure the child had basic necessities and lived in the least detrimental environment possible.

A strong relationship with the victim parent is a protective factor that can increase the child's resilience, and research indicates one of the most effective ways to protect the child is to keep the victim safe (Clarke, 2006; Bandy, Andrews, & Moore, 2012; Nicholson v. Williams, 2002). To address domestic violence cases involving children, workers should keep the victim parent and child together whenever possible; enhance the safety, stability, and well-being of all victims; and hold perpetrators of violence accountable through mechanisms such as batterer intervention programs.

For more information, visit the websites of the Greenbook Initiative (http://
www.thegreenbook.info) or the National Resource Center on Domestic
Violence: Child Protection and Custody (http://www.ncjfcj.org/our-work/
domestic-violence).

1.6.5 EDUCATIONAL NEGLECT

Many States struggle to respond efficiently to reports of educational neglect due to overlapping responsibilities and lack of coordination between
the departments of social services and education. A national review by
Kelly (2010) found that nearly half of States neither define educational
neglect in law nor hold one agency responsible for reporting it. There is
inconsistency among the remaining States regarding which agency is responsible for enforcing neglect provisions, including the court, the school
or school district, and the department of education.

Kelly (2010) recommends that the State's department of social services
be primarily responsible for addressing educational neglect because it is
better equipped to address the co-occurring problems families often face.
He also cites promising programs in Missouri and Idaho that offer coordinated and flexible services through the department of social services to
respond quickly to families in crisis and at risk of educational neglect

1.7 INVESTIGATION AND ASSESSMENT

Identifying child neglect may seem more difficult than identifying other
forms of maltreatment because neglect usually involves the absence of a
certain behavior, rather than the presence. A thorough investigation of the
child's safety and risk followed by a comprehensive family assessment can
help determine what kinds of services and supports the family may need.

Consider the possibility of neglect when the child:

- Is frequently absent from school
- Begs or steals food or money
- Lacks needed medical or dental care, immunizations, or glasses
- Is consistently dirty and has severe body odor

- Lacks sufficient clothing for the weather
- Abuses alcohol or other drugs
- States that there is no one at home to provide care

Consider the possibility of neglect when the parent or other adult caregiver:

- Appears to be indifferent to the child
- Seems apathetic or depressed
- Behaves irrationally or in a bizarre manner
- Is abusing alcohol or other drugs

Find these and other indicators in Child Welfare Information Gateway's Recognizing Child Abuse and Neglect: Signs and Symptoms (http://www.childwelfare.gov/ pubs/factsheets/signs.cfm)

1.7.1 INVESTIGATION

The initial investigation should determine if neglect occurred and examine the child's safety and risk. Two of the most important factors to consider are (1) whether the child has any unmet cognitive, physical, or emotional needs and (2) whether the child receives adequate supervision (DePanfilis, 2006).

Straus and Kaufman (2005) offer the following tips to assess neglect in families:

- Gather information from multiple sources (child and parent self-reports; caseworker and neighbor observations)
- Ensure confidentiality to collect more honest and accurate reports
- Use nonjudgmental, open-ended questions that encourage diverse viewpoints on the situation
- Probe for signs of different types of neglect
- Consider contexts like the child's age, the home environment, and community resources
- Note the severity and frequency of neglect incidents and the length of time since the last incident and between multiple incidents

Safety. Determining the child's safety is as critical in the decision-making process in cases of possible neglect as it is in physical or sexual abuse cases. The determination should consider threats of danger in the family, the child's vulnerability, and the family's protective capacity. Lund and Renne (2009) encourage caseworkers to investigate the following key threats of danger:

- No adult in the home routinely performs basic and essential parenting duties and responsibilities
- The parent lacks sufficient resources, such as food and shelter, or parenting knowledge, skills, and motivation to meet the child's basic needs
- Living arrangements seriously endanger the child's physical health
- The parent refuses and/or fails to meet the child's needs or arrange care when the child:
  - Exhibits self-destructive behavior or serious emotional symptoms requiring immediate help
  - Has exceptional needs that can result in severe consequences to the child
  - Has serious physical injuries or symptoms from maltreatment

The results of the investigation will inform whether the family requires additional assessment and intervention. A low-risk family may be referred for differential response, while the most severe cases may require placement in out-of-home care, preferably with relatives, to ensure the child's immediate safety while the family is assessed and a safety and service plan is developed.

1.7.2 DIFFERENTIAL RESPONSE

Although one report or incident of neglect may not require CPS response, many families could still benefit from services. Particularly in cases of neglect, by the time the situation becomes serious enough for the child welfare system to respond, the family's issues are likely more complex and require intensive intervention (DePanfilis, 2006).

To address this service gap, many States use differential response systems in which families with low risk are redirected to voluntary, often community-based, services to receive the supports they need. For more information:

- Read Information Gateway's Differential Response to Reports of Child Abuse and Neglect: http://www. childwelfare.gov/pubs/issue_briefs/ differential_response
- Visit the Children's Bureau's National Quality Improvement Center on Differential Response in Child Protective Services at http://www.differential-responseqic.org/

1.7.3 ASSESSMENT

A comprehensive family assessment should help uncover the potential causes of neglect and underlying factors affecting the family's ability to care for the child. Because neglected children and their families often face complex issues, it is critical to use a holistic approach that looks at the child, family, and community context to identify strengths and the most effective ways to reduce risks and to engage the family in the assessment process.

The key purposes of assessment are:

- To understand the neglect and its impact on the child and family
- To make decisions to plan for the child's safety and connect the family to services
- To engage the family and its extended support network in services (Schene, 2001)

Overarching categories for assessing child neglect include:

- The child's cognitive, physical, and emotional needs and capacities
- The parent's expectations and parenting abilities
- The family's circumstances, attitudes, and behaviors
- Family members' interactions and relationships in and outside the home (DePanfilis, 2006)

To focus on strengths during the assessment process, the Children's Bureau's *Preventing Child Maltreatment and Promoting Well- Being: A Network for Action 2012 Resource Guide* (http://www.childwelfare.gov/ preventing/preventionmonth/guide2012) emphasizes identifying and enhancing the following protective factors in at-risk families:

- Nurturing and attachment
- Knowledge of parenting and child development
- Parental resilience
- Social connections
- Concrete supports for parents
- Social and emotional competence of children

The assessment process ultimately informs the level of intervention necessary for the family. Assessment should continue throughout the family's case to ensure progress toward goals.

For assessment tools and references, see Information Gateway's webpage on Assessing Child Neglect: http://www.childwelfare.gov/ systemwide/assessment/family_assess/id_can/ neglect.cfm

1.8 PREVENTION AND INTERVENTION

The services and supports that at-risk or neglected children and their families need vary greatly depending on the type of neglect they experienced, the severity of their situation, underlying risks, strengths, and many other factors. Analyzing the information gathered during the investigation and assessment is essential to developing an effective case plan in collaboration with the family, their support network, and related service providers.

1.8.1 CHILDREN'S BUREAU PROJECTS

Many of the strategies discussed below are informed by the results of the child neglect demonstration projects funded by the Children's Bureau from 1996 to 2002 to address the prevention, intervention, and treatment needs of neglected children and their families. For more on these projects, see Information Gateway's Child Neglect Demonstration Projects: Synthesis of Lessons Learned (http://www. childwelfare.gov/pubs/candemo) and the companion piece, Program Evaluation: A Synthesis of Lessons Learned by Child Neglect Demonstration Projects (http://www.childwelfare.gov/ pubs/focus/ evaldemo).

1.8.2 BEGIN EARLY

Children are more likely to be harmed by neglect the earlier they experience it. Although it can be difficult to prevent neglect and identify it in its early stages, you can have a greater impact on families the earlier you intervene. At this stage, assess the parent's readiness to enhance their parenting abilities and help the family focus on meeting the child's developmental needs. Assume that parents want to improve the quality of their children's care—they just need support to identify and build on their strengths.

For more on early intervention with families, read Information Gateway's Addressing the Needs of Young Children in Child Welfare: Part C— Early Intervention Services (http://www.childwelfare.gov/pubs/partc).

1.8.3 CULTURAL COMPETENCE AND NEGLECT

As with all child protection practice, cultural issues must be taken into consideration both when assessing and intervening with families at risk of neglect. For example, a culture in which shared caregiving is the norm may see no problem with allowing young children to care for their siblings, perhaps in a way that does not conform to cultural norms in the United States (Smith & Fong, 2004).

When working with diverse families, maintain focus on ensuring that children's needs are met and that they are not harmed or endangered. Consult with knowledgeable staff or community members on how best to intervene in a way that is consistent with families' cultural practices. Visit the Cultural Competence section of the Information Gateway website for more information: http://www. childwelfare.gov/systemwide/cultural

1.8.4 PROVIDE CONCRETE SERVICES FIRST

Most parents cannot focus on interventions like parenting classes when they are still addressing crises in their family. In the early stages of working with a family, be sure basic needs are met before expecting parents to fulfill other aspects of their case plan. Some concrete supports to address include:

- Housing and utilities
- Food and clothing
- Safety for domestic violence victims
- Transportation
- Child care
- Health care and public benefits

1.8.5 FOCUS ON STRENGTHS

You can form better relationships with families when you encourage them to focus on positive parenting strategies and supports they already have in place. The six protective factors described earlier can serve as a framework for assessing families' strengths and helping them identify ways to build upon those strengths to protect their children from harm. The Children's Bureau's 2012 Resource Guide for child abuse prevention offers numerous tools and strategies for talking with families about their strengths and incorporating them into service systems (http://www.childwelfare.gov/preventing/preventionmonth/guide2012).

New Jersey's Strengthening Families Initiative is making child and family strengths an essential component of prevention efforts statewide. Programs are required to demonstrate that they incorporate the protective factors framework into their services, and professionals are being trained on how to identify and build upon strengths in at-risk families. Learn more on the New Jersey Department of Children and Families website: http://www.nj.gov/dcf/families/ early/strengthening/

1.8.6 OFFER CUSTOMIZED, COORDINATED SERVICES

Be flexible; there is no "one size fits all" solution to addressing neglect. Offer or refer families to a broad array of services and collaborate with other services providers to ensure the family's needs are met. Some of the most common services provided by the Federal child neglect demonstration project grantees included:

- Parent education and support
- Home visits
- Referrals or links to community resources
- Mental health services
- Concrete assistance and crisis intervention (Child Welfare Information Gateway, 2004)

Home visiting programs, which provide in-home services to families with young children, show promise in engaging parents to reduce risks related to child abuse and neglect. Professional or paraprofessional home visitors can build relationships with parents and tailor their visits to address the family's needs and strengths. Some of the topics home visitors may address include:

- The mother's personal health and life choices
- Child health and development
- Environmental concerns such as income, housing, and domestic or community violence
- Family functioning, including adult and child relationships
- Access to services (Child Welfare Information Gateway, 2011a)

Supporting Evidence-Based Home Visiting is a Federal initiative to generate knowledge of home visiting practices and models; find more information on the initiative's website: http:// www.supportingebhv.org

1.8.7 ENCOURAGE INCREMENTAL CHANGE

Most changes don't happen overnight. Especially with families that are stressed by the demands of caring for their child, parents may feel overwhelmed if you expect them to accomplish too many goals too quickly. In collaboration with the family, establish a contract with a timeline for accomplishing specific goals as well as obligations for both you and the parents to meet (McSherry, 2007).

Remember to start with the most basic needs (e.g., food, housing, safety), then address critical underlying issues (e.g., substance abuse, mental health). Once those supports are in place, there will be fewer obstacles to improving higher family functioning. Many programs have found that working with families affected by neglect requires intensive, long-term services to help them achieve changes over time.

The Family Connections (FC) program in Baltimore, MD, began as a demonstration project, funded by the Children's Bureau, to prevent neglect in at-risk families. Core program components include emergency assistance, home-visiting family intervention, advocacy and service coordination, and multifamily supportive and recreational activities. FC results were so promising in reducing risk factors and increasing protective factors that replication demonstration grants at eight additional sites were funded by the Children's Bureau. For more information about the program and its replication, visit the Family Connections website: http:// www.family.umaryland.edu/ryc_best_ practice_services/family_connections.htm

Intensive family preservation services provide short-term crisis support to high-risk families to prevent unnecessary child placement in out-of-home care. Children and families experiencing severe neglect may benefit from these kinds of services to address urgent issues, like housing or financial assistance, followed by ongoing family preservation and support to target underlying risk factors. For more information, visit Information Gateway's web section on Family Preservation Services: http://www.childwelfare.gov/supporting/ preservation

1.8.8 ADDRESS THE SOCIAL SUPPORT NETWORK.

Because your time with the family is limited, a strong social support network for the family can reinforce lessons learned and address needs as they arise. Seek out relatives, friends, community members, and other service providers who will help the family practice and build new skills over time. Positive relationships with other caring adults can help support the child's healthy development and serve as a source of respite for parents if they face future crises.

Help the family find a local parent support group through Circle of Parents® (http://www. circleofparents.org) or Parents Anonymous® (http://www.parentsanonymous.org), or connect them to a respite program using the ARCH National Respite Network and Resource Center's locator service (http://archrespite.org/ respitelocator).

1.8.9 PUT AFTERCARE SERVICES IN PLACE

As the family begins achieving major goals, develop a roadmap for services and supports after more intensive interventions end. An aftercare services plan will ensure opportunities for follow-up and help families maintain improvements over time.

1.9 TRAINING

Effective training is important for caseworkers addressing the often complex issues faced by at-risk or neglected children and their families. Training on child neglect should emphasize the following strategies:

- Address definitions of different types of neglect as well as the importance of cultural competence in understanding how neglect is perceived in different cultures.
- Describe long-term consequences to counteract the common but inaccurate belief that neglect is not as harmful as physical or sexual abuse.
- Help caseworkers learn how to develop a positive helping relationship with families—a key contributor to success when providing long-term, intensive services.
- Use case studies to demonstrate the complex interaction of issues that can impact the effectiveness of intervention (McSherry, 2007).

Because neglect is still misunderstood by many professionals serving children and families, ongoing training can help caseworkers remain aware of the latest research and refresh skills over time.

To locate sources of training on child neglect in your State, refer to Information Gateway's related organizations list of State Child Welfare Training Resources (http://www.childwelfare. gov/pubs/reslist/rl_dsp_ scwt. cfm?typeID=144&rate_chno=19-00082)

For additional practice tips and an in-depth exploration of the topics addressed in this bulletin, read the Children's Bureau's User Manual, Child

Neglect: A Guide for Prevention, Assessment, and Intervention (http://www.childwelfare.gov/pubs/ usermanuals/neglect)

1.10 CONCLUSION

Child neglect is the most prevalent type of child maltreatment but has historically received the least attention from researchers and others. While there appears to be growing interest, child neglect continues to be a complex problem that is difficult to define, prevent, identify, and treat.

Neglect is a term used to encompass many situations, but their commonality is a lack of action—an act of omission—regarding a child's needs. Neglect most commonly involves physical, medical, educational, or emotional neglect or inadequate supervision. Neglect can range from a caregiver's momentary inattention to chronic or willful deprivation. Single incidents can have no harmful effects or, in some cases, they can result in trauma or death.

Investigating and assessing neglect involves a thorough examination of the child's safety and risk as well as the larger family and community context. To understand neglect, caseworkers should know how to address related problems such as poverty, substance abuse, and domestic violence. Interventions for children and families affected by neglect require customized and coordinated services. Defining, preventing, identifying, and treating child neglect is a significant challenge but one that researchers, professionals, communities, and families must face together if they are to protect children from its harmful consequences.

REFERENCES

1. Bandy, T., Andrews, K. M., & Moore, K. A. (2012). Disadvantaged families and child outcomes: The importance of emotional support for mothers. Child Trends Researchto-Results Brief, 2012-05. Retrieved May 2012 from http://www.childtrends.org/Files/Child_Trends-2012_03_21_RB_MaternalSupport.pdf
2. Chalk, R., Gibbons, A., & Scarupa, H. J. (2002). The multiple dimensions of child abuse and neglect: New insights into an old problem. Child Trends Research Brief. Retrieved February 2012 from http://www.childtrends.org/files/ChildAbuseRB.pdf

3. Chambers, P. (2002). Family reclaim: A community-based collaborative to strength-
    en families with substance abuse and neglect issues. Oakland, CA: Family Support
    Services of the Bay Area.
4. Child Welfare Information Gateway. (2004). Child neglect demonstration projects:
    Synthesis of lessons learned. Washington, DC: U.S. Department of Health and
    Human Services, Children's Bureau. Retrieved February 2012 from http://www.
    childwelfare.gov/pubs/candemo
5. Child Welfare Information Gateway. (2011a). Child maltreatment prevention: Past,
6. present, and future. Washington, DC: U.S. Department of Health and Human Ser-
    vices, Children's Bureau. Retrieved February 2012 from http://www.childwelfare.
    gov/pubs/issue_briefs/cm_prevention.cfm
7. Child Welfare Information Gateway. (2011b). Definitions of child abuse and ne-
    glect. Washington, DC: U.S. Department of Health and Human Services, Children's
    Bureau. Retrieved February 2012 from http://www.childwelfare.gov/systemwide/
    laws_policies/statutes/define.cfm
8. Child Welfare Information Gateway. (2011c). Definitions of domestic violence.
    Washington, DC: U.S. Department of Health and Human Services, Children's Bu-
    reau. Retrieved February 2012 from http://www.childwelfare.gov/systemwide/
    laws_policies/statutes/defdomvio.cfm
9. Children's Bureau, Office on Child Abuse and Neglect. (2009). Protecting children
    in families affected by substance use disorders. Washington, DC: U.S. Department
    of Health and Human Services, Administration for Children and Families, Adminis-
    tration on Children, Youth and Families, Children's Bureau, Office on Child Abuse
    and Neglect. Retrieved February 2012 from the Child Welfare Information Gateway
    website: http://www.childwelfare.gov/pubs/usermanuals/substanceuse
10. Clarke, S. N. (2006). Strictly liable: Governmental use of the parent-child relation-
    ship as a basis for holding victims liable for their child's witness to domestic vio-
    lence. Family Court Review, 44(1), 149-163.
11. De Bellis, M. D. (2005). The psychobiology of neglect. Child Maltreatment, 10(2),
    150-172.
12. DePanfilis, D. (2006). Child neglect: A guide for prevention, assessment, and inter-
    vention. Washington, DC: U.S. Department of Health and Human Services, Admin-
    istration for Children and Families, Administration on Children, Youth and Families,
    Children's Bureau, Office on Child Abuse and Neglect. Retrieved February 2012
    from the Child Welfare Information Gateway website: http://www.childwelfare.gov/
    pubs/usermanuals/neglect
13. Duva, J., & Metzger, S. (2010). Addressing poverty as a major risk factor in child
    neglect: Promising policy and practice. Protecting Children, 25(1), 63-74. Retrieved
    February 2012 from http://aia.berkeley. edu/media/2011_teleconferences/poverty/
    Protecting%20Children%20Article%20 on%20Poverty%20and%20Neglect.pdf
14. Gilmore, D., & Kaplan, C. (2009). Chronic families, chronic neglect [PowerPoint
    slides]. Retrieved February 2012 from the American Humane Association website:
    http://www.americanhumane.org/assets/pdfs/children/pc-chronic-families-chronic-
    neglect.pdf
15. Grayson, J. (2001). The state of child neglect. In T. D. Morton & B. Salovitz (Eds.),
    The CPS response to child neglect: An administrator's guide to theory, policy, pro-

gram design and case practice (pp. 1-36). Retrieved February 2012 from the National Resource Center for Child Protective Services website: http://www.nrccps.org/PDF/ CPSResponsetoChildNeglect.pdf

16. Kelly, P. (2010). Where are the children?: Educational neglect across the fifty states. The Researcher, 23(1), 41-58. Retrieved February 2012 from http://www.nrmera.org/ PDF/Researcher/Researcherv23n1Kelly.pdf

17. Lund, T. R. & Renne, J. (2009). Child safety: A guide for judges and attorneys. Retrieved March 2012 from the National Resource Center for Child Protective Services website: http://nrccps.org/documents/2009/pdf/ The_Guide.pdf

18. McSherry, D. (2007). Understanding and addressing the "neglect of neglect": Why are we making a mole-hill out of a mountain? Child Abuse & Neglect: The International Journal, 31(6), 607-614. Milot, T., St-Laurent, D., Éthier, L. S., & Provost,

19. M. A. (2010). Trauma-related symptoms in neglected preschoolers and affective quality of mother-child communication. Child Maltreatment, 15(4), 293-304. Nicholson v. Williams, 203 F. Supp. 2d 153, 169 (E.D.N.Y. 2002).

20. Schene, P. (2001). CPS responsibility for child neglect. In T. D. Morton & B. Salovitz (Eds.), The CPS response to child neglect: An administrator's guide to theory, policy, program design and case practice (pp. 60-74). Retrieved February 2012 from the National Resource Center for Child Protective Services website: http://www.nrccps.org/PDF/ CPSResponsetoChildNeglect.pdf

21. Sedlak, A. J., Mettenburg, J., Basena, M., Petta, I., McPherson, K., Greene, A., & Li, S. (2010). Fourth national incidence study of child abuse and neglect (NIS–4): Report to congress. Washington, DC: U.S. Department of Health and Human Services, Administration for Children and Families. Retrieved February 2012 from http:// www. acf.hhs.gov/programs/opre/abuse_neglect/ natl_incid

22. Smith, M. G., & Fong, R. (2004). The children of neglect: When no one cares. New York, NY: Brunner-Routledge.

23. Straus, M. A., & Kaufman, G. K. (2005). Definition and measurement of neglectful behavior: Some principles and guidelines. Child Abuse and Neglect: The International Journal, 29(1), 19-29.

24. U.S. Department of Health and Human Services, Administration for Children and Families, Administration on Children, Youth and Families, Children's Bureau. (2011). Child maltreatment 2010. Retrieved February 2012 from http://www.acf.hhs.gov/ programs/cb/pubs/cm10

25. U.S. Government Accountability Office. (2011). Child maltreatment: Strengthening national data on child fatalities could aid in prevention. Retrieved February 2012 from http://www.gao.gov/assets/330/320774.pdf

CHAPTER 2

FREQUENCY OF CHILD MALTREATMENT IN A REPRESENTATIVE SAMPLE OF THE GERMAN POPULATION

BENJAMIN IFFLAND, ELMAR BRÄHLER, FRANK NEUNER, WINFRIED HÄUSER, AND HEIDE GLAESMER

2.1 BACKGROUND

Child maltreatment refers to all forms of abusive and neglectful behavior involving emotional, physical and sexual transgressions, resulting in actual or potential harm to the child's health, survival or development [1,2]. Although child maltreatment is one of the most important social challenges worldwide and is associated with substantial impairments of social wellbeing and health [3-6], information about the frequency of child maltreatment in high-income societies is still scarce and inconsistent.

For example, there are hardly any studies that have reported rates of child maltreatment in the German population. As an exception Wetzels [7] has included an instrument for the assessment of sexual and physical abuse in a representative survey of 3,289 subjects in the age range

Frequency of Child Maltreatment in a Representative Sample of the German Population. © *Iffland B, Brähler E, Neuner F, Häuser W, and Glaesmer H.; licensee BioMed Central Ltd. BMC Public Health, 13,980 (2013). doi:10.1186/1471-2458-13-980 Licensed under Creative Commons Attribution 2.0 Generic License, http://creativecommons.org/licenses/by/2.0/.*

of 16 to 59. Sexual abuse was reported by 8.6% of the women and 2.8% of the men and prevalence rate of physical abuse was 10.6%. However, this study is limited by the fact that the assessment of child maltreatment was not comprehensive. Although consensus definitions of child maltreatment include five types, i.e. physical abuse, physical neglect, emotional abuse, emotional neglect and sexual abuse [8-10], and the emotional types of maltreatment seem to have similar detrimental health effects as sexual and physical abuse [11], the emotional forms of maltreatment have commonly been excluded from large-scale representative surveys in different countries [12-15]. In addition, similar to the other studies Wetzels [7] concentrated on the assessment of physical and sexual abuse using an ad-hoc developed scale that does not allow a comparison of results with other surveys or data from clinical populations that used different questionnaires.

Recently, Haeuser et al. [16] reported the frequency of child maltreatment from a representative survey in Germany. This study is outstanding since data on child maltreatment was collected using the standard and well validated child maltreatment instrument Childhood Trauma Questionnaire (CTQ) [17] that allows the assessment of all common types of child maltreatment. The strength of this instrument is that it allows a severity rating of sexual abuse, physical abuse, physical neglect, emotional abuse and emotional neglect, which reflects the fact that the different forms of child maltreatment may be continuous phenomena ranging from small to severe transgressions rather than clearly delimitable entities [18,19]. However, a dichotomous categorization of the forms of child maltreatment using a severity cut-off is indicated to allow the comparison of rates of child maltreatment from studies that applied different instruments based on similar definition. While the authors of the CTQ do not provide thresholds to determine the presence of the different types of maltreatment on a dichotomous basis, Haeuser et al. [16] reported frequency rates based on severity ratings above the severity range labeled as "low to moderate". The resulting prevalence rates were as high as for emotional (49.5%) and physical neglect (48.4%), with 12% for physical abuse, 15% for emotional abuse and 12,6% for sexual abuse.

The present article presents a re-analysis of the German general survey data which had also been used by the Haeuser et al. [16] study. In contrast to the previous analysis, this analysis did not rely on cut-off scores based on the original severity ratings, but on empirically determined and validated threshold values for the different types of child maltreatment as reported by Walker et al. [20]. These cut-off criteria had been ascertained by relating CTQ subscale scores to ratings of experts blind for the CTQ scores who administered detailed clinical interviews. Based on the fulfillment of consensus child abuse and neglect criteria [20], experts determined whether participants had a history of clinically significant abuse or neglect. Walker et al. [20] used the same definitions of child abuse and neglect the items of the five subscales of the CTQ were derived from. Emotional abuse was defined as "verbal assaults on a child's sense of worth or well-being or any humiliating or demeaning behavior directed toward a child by an adult or older person". Emotional neglect was defined as "the failure of caretakers to meet children's basic emotional and psychological needs, including love, belonging, nurturance, and support". Physical abuse was defined as "bodily assaults on a child by an adult or older person that posed a risk of, or resulted in, injury". Physical neglect was defined as "the failure of caretakers to provide for a child's basic physical needs, including food, shelter, clothing, safety, and health care" (poor parental supervision was also included if it placed a child's safety in jeopardy). Sexual abuse was defined as "sexual contact or conduct between a child younger than 17 years of age and an adult or older person (at least 5 years older than the child)". Receiver operating characteristic (ROC) methods had been employed to determine threshold scores for each subscale. Resulting threshold scores showed good to excellent sensitivity and specificity. Maltreatment is assumed when threshold scores for emotional abuse (10), emotional neglect (15), physical abuse (8), physical neglect (8), and sexual abuse (8) are met. In contrast threshold scores that were established by Bernstein et al. [18] and used in the Haeuser et al. [16] study were 9 for emotional abuse, 10 for emotional neglect, 8 for physical abuse, 8 for physical neglect, and 6 for sexual abuse. With this procedure we aim to provide the first comprehensive and representative prevalence data on different types of child maltreatment based on empirically derived cut-off criteria for the German population. Empirically derived and externally validated cut-off criteria allow for a more accurate and clinically significant evaluation of the presence of a history of abuse and neglect while clinical relevance of the cut-off scores used in previous studies remain uncertain. In addition, inter-correlations and co-occurrence of different kinds of maltreatment as well as their association to age and sex were examined.

2.2 METHODS

2.2.1 SUBJECTS

A representative sample of the German general population was selected with the assistance of a demographic consulting company (USUMA, Berlin, Germany). The area of Germany was separated into 258 sample areas representing the different regions of the country. Households of the respective area and one member of this household fulfilling the inclusion criteria (age at or above 14, able to read and understand the German language) were selected randomly through the Kish-selection-grid technique. The Kish-selection-grid technique aims to sample individuals on the doorstep. The system is devised so that all individuals in a household have an equal chance of selection. The sample was designed to be representative in terms of age, gender, and education. A first attempt was made for 4,455 persons. If not at home, a maximum of three attempts were made to contact the selected person. All subjects were visited by a study assistant, informed about the investigation (covering several research questions), and self-rating questionnaires were presented. All participants signed an informed consent. When under the age of 18, the parents were asked to sign a written consent. The assistant waited until participants answered all questionnaires and offered help if persons did not understand the meaning of questions. A total of 2,500 people between the ages of 14 and 90 years agreed to participate and completed a questionnaire on physical and mental health which included socio-demographic information as well as the German version of the CTQ. Data was collected in April 2010. The response rate reached 56%. All relevant international guidelines and ethical standards relating to the collection of personal data from human beings have been abided. Participants were recruited by a professional demographic consulting company (USUMA, Berlin, Germany) that abides to the ICC/ESOMAR International Code on Market and Social Research regarding ethics in social sciences research [21]. This code embodies the highest professional and ethical standards relating to market and social research, and guarantees informed consent and the anonymous processing of personal data. Additionally, the company conducting data sampling is a member of a group with general ethical approval from the German government to conduct these types of surveys. According to the Federal Data Protection Act (Bundesdatenschutzgesetz BDSG, § 30a), the need for consent from a specific ethics commitee is waived for USUMA surveys.

The German version of the CTQ [22] is a 28-item self-rating scale consisting of five subscales. The items are rated from 1 (never true) to 5 (very often true) with a possible range of subscale scores of 5 to 25. The German version of the CTQ has been shown to be a reliable and valid screening tool for childhood maltreatment in clinical samples [22,23]. However, in a recent validation study from the general population [24], the five factor structure of the original version showed only a moderate fit. The subscale "physical neglect" was highly correlated with the other subscales and presented a weak internal consistency in comparison to other subscales. The fit of a four factor structure excluding the physical neglect items was superior to the five factor model, suggesting that the CTQ would benefit from disregarding the physical neglect subscale [24]. Nevertheless, prevalence rates for the physical neglect subscale will be presented here, since it is widely used in clinical research.

In the present study, threshold scores suggested by Walker et al. [20] were applied to determine presence of the different types of child maltreatment. In addition, three of the items of the CTQ are used as a minimization/denial scale to identify cases with problematic validity. In this scale, only extreme scorings (score 5) are counted. Three such extreme scorings should be regarded as an indication of probable minimization, unrealistic statements and severe psychological defences [17]. In the following analyses, participants were categorized as minimizing if they score "very often true" on all of the three items of this scale.

2.2.2 STATISTICAL ANALYSES

The population was divided into groups according to fulfillment of the different types of maltreatment. For each type of maltreatment, these groups were compared pair-wise using the Student t test for independent groups for continuous normally distributed dependent variables. The Mann–Whitney U test was used for ordinally scaled data or data from skewed distributions. Statistical associations among categorical variables were analyzed using Pearson's chi-square test and the Fisher exact test. Associations among ordinally scaled variables were estimated using the Spearman rank order correlation.

2.3 RESULTS

2.3.1 DEMOGRAPHICS

The CTQ and the other baseline assessment instruments were fully completed by 2,500 subjects. The average age of the respondents was M = 50.66 (SD = 18.56). Table 1 presents participants' demographics and means on the assessments.

TABLE 1: Subject characteristics and mean values on psychopathology (N = 2,500)

Age, M (SD, range)	50.66 (18.56, 14–90)
Gender, % male (n)	46.90 (1172)
Family status, % single (n)	39.40 (986)
Childhood Trauma Questionnaire, M (SD)	35.99 (10.48)[a]
Emotional Abuse, M (SD)	6.51 (2.60)
Emotional Neglect, M (SD)	10.09 (4.23)
Physical Abuse, M (SD)	5.88 (2.17)
Physical Neglect, M (SD)	8.15 (3.02)
Sexual Abuse, M (SD)	5.45 (1.66)
Minimization/Denial, M (SD)	10.73 (2.78)

Note: [a]CTQ sum score for the 28-item version.

TABLE 2: Prevalence of child abuse by trauma type and comparison of childhood abuse type by mean age (N = 2,500)

| | Sex | | | | | | Age | | | |
| | Total | | Male | | Female | | | Abused | | Non-abused | |
	n	%	n	%	n	%	p	Mean age	SD	Mean age	SD	p
Emotional Abuse	254	10.2	109	9.3	145	10.9	.184a	50.60	18.65	50.67	18.56	.954b
Emotional Neglect	348	13.9	171	14.6	177	13.4	.374a	51.50	17.46	50.51	18.72	.444c
Physical Abuse	301	12.0	149	12.7	152	11.5	.335a	54.09	18.88	50.18	18.48	.001b
Physical Neglect	1210	48.4	580	49.5	630	47.5	.305a	55.76	18.21	45.81	17.54	.000c
Sexual Abuse	156	6.2	44	3.8	112	8.4	.000a	52.03	17.68	50.56	18.62	.339b
								Minimizing		Non-minimizing		
Minimization/Denial	214	8.6	94	8.0	120	9.0	.365a	44.27	18.34	51.25	18.47	.000b

Test statistic: [a]Pearson chi square, [b]two sample t test, [c]Mann–Whitney U test.

We found that 13.9% of the subjects went beyond the pre-established threshold for emotional neglect, 10.2% for emotional abuse, 12.0% for physical abuse, 48.4% for physical neglect, and 6.2% for sexual abuse (Table 2). Sexual abuse was significantly more prevalent among women. No differences between sexes were found for the other types of abuse (Table 2). Cumulative frequencies of the different types of child maltreatment are presented in Table 3. In our sample, 33.9% reported experience of at least one type of abuse. All subtypes of maltreatment were significantly inter-correlated. Emotional and physical abuse showed a moderate correlation, whereas the other correlations were rather small (Table 4).

TABLE 3: Frequency of total number of abuse types

Numbers of types of abuse reported	n	%
0	1133	45.4
1	847	33.9
2	295	11.8
3	94	3.8
4	82	3.3
5	42	1.7

Test statistic: Pearson chi square, p < .001.

TABLE 4: Correlation coefficients of abuse types

	Emotional abuse	Emotional neglect	Physical abuse	Physical neglect	Sexual abuse
Emotional Abuse	1.00				
Emotional Neglect	.364	1.00			
Physical Abuse	.461	.293	1.00		
Physical Neglect	.218	.328	.232	1.00	
Sexual Abuse	.353	.196	.338	.154	1.00

Spearman rank order correlation matrix. All correlations were significant, p < .001.

For each trauma type, mean ages of subjects meeting the threshold were compared to the mean ages of those who did not. Significant differences were found for physical abuse and physical neglect. Respectively, subjects who met the thresholds were significantly older than subjects who did not (Table 2).

On the minimization/denial scale, 8.6% of the participants endorsed all items. No sex differences could be found on this scale, while participants who were minimizing were significantly younger than participants who did not minimize (Table 2).

TABLE 5: Survey of prevalence rates reported in previous studies (in %)

	Emotional abuse	Emotional neglect	Physical abuse	Physical neglect	Sexual abuse
Present Study	10.2	13.9	12.0	48.4	6.2
Glaesmer et al. [25]	-	-	8.5	-	1.0
Green et al. [27]	-	-	8.4	5.6a	6.0
Haeuser et al. [16]	15.0	49.5	12.0	48.4	12.6
Hauffa et al. [26]	-	-	3.9	-	1.2
Thombs et al. [28]	30.6	-	16.5	-	10.3
von Sydow [29]	-	-	-	-	18-21
Wetzels [7]	-	-	10.6	-	5.7

Note: aIn this study, there was no distinction made between emotional and physical neglect. Neglect presented here was the frequency of not having adequate food, clothing, or medical care, having inadequate supervision, and having to do age-inappropriate chores.

2.4 DISCUSSION

In this study, we presented prevalence rates of child abuse in a representative sample of the German population based on empirically derived cutoff scores. The frequency of emotional neglect was 13.9%, 10.2% of the subjects reported emotional abuse, 12.0% met criteria for physical abuse, 48.4% for physical neglect, and 6.2% for sexual abuse.

Unsurprisingly, as all of the cut-off values used in our analysis were lower than those applied in the previous analysis of this dataset reported by Haeuser et al. [16], frequencies reported here were lower on all subscales except for the physical abuse and the physical neglect scale (a survey of prevalence rates presented in previous studies is given in Table 5). In particular, our cut-off resulted in considerably lower frequencies for emotional neglect. Previous representative surveys in Germany [7,25,26] were restricted to the assessment of physical or sexual abuse. While the magnitudes of physical abuse in the studies by Wetzels [7] as well as Glaesmer et al. [25] were tentatively comparable, Hauffa et al. [26] reported an exceptionally low rate of physical violence. Since regional or temporal factors as well as the use of different assessments are not sufficient to explain these differences, the authors suggested that the answering patterns of subjects may account for the discrepancy in reported frequencies [26].

Frequencies of sexual abuse reported in previous representative surveys showed a wide range. While Wetzels [7] reported a rate that was comparable to our findings, frequencies of sexual abuse in the studies of Glaesmer et al. [25] and Hauffa et al. [26] were rather small. Comparison of prevalence rates for sexual abuse is limited by the fact that Glaesmer et al. [25] as well as Hauffa et al. [26] reported frequencies of subjects being raped. Criteria for sexual abuse used in our study embodied a wide range of sexual assaults including rape. The wide range of criteria for sexual abuse may account for higher prevalence rates for both sexes in our study compared to previous findings.

In a survey of 91 women born in the years 1895 to 1936, von Sydow [29] reported much higher prevalence rates for sexual abuse. Experiences of sexual abuse under the age of 12 were reported by 18% of the women, 21% reported sexual abuse between the age of 13 and 21.

A recent validation study of the German translation of the CTQ has indicated that the scale for physical neglect has weak psychometric properties, is highly correlated with the other subscales and presented with a weak internal consistency in comparison to the other subscales [24]. These factors may have contributed to the uncommon and possibly excessive rates of physical neglect found in this study. As a consequence, findings based on this subscale from our study as well as from other studies should be interpreted with caution.

In our study, sex differences in the frequencies of child abuse were only found for sexual abuse. Prevalence rates of physical and sexual abuse reported for both sexes were comparable to frequencies reported by Wetzels [7]. In their sample, 11.8% of the men and 9.9% of the women experienced a history of physical maltreatment in childhood. A history of sexual abuse was reported for 2.8% of the men and 8.6% of the women. In contrast to the findings of Glaesmer et al. [25], prevalence rates of physical abuse in women were higher. While Glaesmer et al. [25] reported a frequency of 5.1%, 11.5% of the women in our sample met criteria for physical abuse.

In a population-based study in the US, the CTQ short form was administered in a randomized telephone interview survey with adults aged 18 to 65 [28]. Respondents were classified as having been abused if they either explicitly labeled themselves as having been abused or rated anything other than "never" to the single item of the various CTQ subscales that explicitly used the term "abused". Prevalence rates for the subscales physical, emotional and sexual abuse were presented. Findings from our German sample were lower on all subscales. However, these differences might be attributed to differences in sampling as well as in the applied cut-off values. It is noteworthy that, despite the differences in measurement, the replication of the National Comorbidity Survey (NCS-R) presented prevalence rates for child adversities similar to the rates reported in our study [27].

The intercorrelations and co-occurrence of maltreatment types presented in this study were consistent with previous reports [7,16,20,30]. All types of maltreatment were significantly inter-correlated. In line with findings of Haeuser et al. [16], the smallest relationship was found for emotional neglect and sexual abuse. In our study, fulfillment of multiple types of maltreatment was reported for 20.6%. In the sample of Walker et al. [20] 23% of the subjects met criteria for more than one type of abuse. Reports of Haeuser et al. [16] were even higher. In their study, 40.3% of the participants reported at least two kinds of maltreatment. When the physical neglect subscale is excluded, in our study merely 9.6% of the subjects fulfill criteria for multiple types of maltreatment. This rather small frequency suggests that high frequencies of co-occurrence in prior studies result from the inclusion of the CTQ physical neglect subscale and the use of cut-off values that were based on severity ratings.

Limitations of our study include the fact that the assessment of childhood maltreatment is based on retrospective accounts and self-report, which is subject to recall biases [16]. However, the analysis of that recall bias indicates that these distortions are not sufficiently large to invalidate retrospective reports in general [31]. In addition, the present study is limited by a response rate of 56%. Prior surveys conducting a similar technique to recruit subjects reached higher response rates (62.1%) [32]. Due to data protection, differences between responders and non-responders on clinical and socio-demographical data could not be analyzed. Therefore, frequencies may have been affected by participation bias. Particularly, assessment of trauma associated experiences might have caused avoidance and refusal to participate.

2.5 CONCLUSION

In summary, findings from our study confirmed that methodological details, in particular the definition of maltreatment types and cut-off values, have a substantial impact on the frequency rates determined in surveys. However, a validation of the cut-off scores used in the present study in a German sample would be desirable in order to achieve more accurate assessments of prevalence rates. Furthermore, the present study is to our knowledge the first to present prevalence rates for the minimization/denial scale in a representative sample. In general, our analysis based on empirically derived cut-off values resulted in lower rates of child maltreatment than in previous reports that used less well validated criteria. However, still as many as 33.9% (Table 3) reported experience of a type of maltreatment, which demonstrates that child maltreatment is a significant social problem in Germany like in other countries world-wide. Commonly, prevention efforts are restricted to targeting the reduction of sexual or physical abuse. Our findings show that emotional types of abuse and neglect are at least as common and that new and more comprehensive forms of child protection may be indicated. Prevalence rates reported in our study allow for more thorough evaluation of data found for child maltreatment in clinical samples and in future research.

REFERENCES

1. Krug EG, Dahlberg L, Mercy J, Zwi A, Lozano R: World report on violence and health. Geneva: World Health Organization; 2002.
2. World Health Organization: Report of the consultation on child abuse prevention. Geneva: World Health Organization; 1999.
3. Arnow BA: Relationships between childhood maltreatment, adult health and psychiatric outcomes, and medical utilization. J Clin Psychiatry 2004, 65(Suppl 12):10-15.
4. Dubowitz H, Bennett S: Physical abuse and neglect of children. Lancet 2007, 369(9576):1891-1899.
5. Egle UT, Hoffmann SO, Joraschky P: Sexueller Missbrauch, Misshandlung, Vernachlässigung : Erkennung, Therapie und Prävention der Folgen früher Stresserfahrungen [Sexual abuse, physical abuse, neglect. Diagnosis, therapy, and prevention of the effects of early stress experiences]. Stuttgart: Schattauer; 2005.
6. Kessler RC, McLaughlin KA, Green JG, Gruber MJ, Sampson NA, Zaslavsky AM, Williams DR: Childhood adversities and adult psychopathology in the WHO World Mental Health Surveys. Br J Psychiatry 2010, 197(5):378-385.
7. Wetzels P: Zur Epidemiologie physischer und sexueller Gewalterfahrungen in der Kindheit: Ergebnisse einer repräsentativen retrospektiven Prävalenzstudie für die BRD [Epidemiology of physical and sexual violence experiences in childhood: Results of a representative prevalence study in Germany]. Hannover: Kriminologisches Forschungsinstitut Niedersachsen; 1997.
8. Engfer A: Formen der Misshandlung von Kindern – Definitionen, Häufigkeiten, Erklärungsansätze. In Sexueller Missbrauch, Misshandlung, Vernachlässigung: Erkennung, Therapie und Prävention der Folgen früher Stresserfahrungen (pp. 3–19). Edited by Egle U, Hoffmann SO, Joraschky P. Stuttgart: Schattauer; 2005.
9. Herrenkohl RC: The definition of child maltreatment: from case study to construct. Child Abuse Neglect 2005, 29(5):413-424.
10. Manly JT: Advances in research definitions of child maltreatment. Child Abuse Neglect 2005, 29(5):425-439.
11. Egeland B: Taking stock: childhood emotional maltreatment and developmental psychopathology. Child Abuse Neglect 2009, 33(1):22-26.
12. Banyard VL: Childhood maltreatment and the mental health of low-income women. Am J Orthopsychiatry 1999, 69(2):161-171.
13. Bensley LS, Van Eenwyk J, Spieker SJ, Schoder J: Self-reported abuse history and adolescent problem behaviors. I. Antisocial and suicidal behaviors. J Adolesc Health 1999, 24(3):163-172.
14. Riggs S, Alario AJ, McHorney C: Health risk behaviors and attempted suicide in adolescents who report prior maltreatment. J Pediatr 1990, 116(5):815-821.
15. Swett C, Halpert M: Reported history of physical and sexual abuse in relation to dissociation and other symptomatology in women psychiatric inpatients. J Interpers Violence 1993, 8(4):545-555.
16. Haeuser W, Schmutzer G, Braehler E, Glaesmer H: Maltreatment in childhood and adolescence. [Results from a survey of a representative sample of the German population]. Dtsch Arztebl Int 2011, 108(17):287-294.

17. Bernstein DP, Fink L: Childhood Trauma Questionnaire: A retrospective self-report. Manual.. Childhood Trauma Questionnaire: A retrospective self-report. Manual; 1998.
18. Bernstein DP, Stein JA, Newcomb MD, Walker E, Pogge D, Ahluvalia T, Zule W: Development and validation of a brief screening version of the Childhood Trauma Questionnaire. Child Abuse Neglect 2003, 27(2):169-190.
19. Lipschitz DS, Bernstein DP, Winegar RK, Southwick SM: Hospitalized adolescents' reports of sexual and physical abuse: A comparison of two self-report measures. J Trauma Stress 1999, 12(4):641-654.
20. Walker EA, Gelfand A, Katon WJ, Koss MP, Von Korff M, Bernstein D, Russo J: Adult health status of women with histories of childhood abuse and neglect. Am J Med 1999, 107(4):332-339.
21. ICC/ESOMAR: International Code on market and social research. Amsterdam: ESOMAR; 2008. http://www.esomar.org/index.php/codes-guidelines.html webcite
22. Wingenfeld K, Spitzer C, Mensebach C, Grabe HJ, Hill A, Gast U, Driessen M: Die deutsche Version des Childhood Trauma Questionnaire (CTQ): Erste befunde zu den psychometrischen Kennwerten [The German version of the Childhood Trauma Questionnaire (CTQ): Preliminary psychometric properties]. Psychother Psychosom Med Psychol 2010, 60(11):442-450.
23. Bader K, Haenny C, Schaefer V, Neuckel A, Kuhl C: Childhood Trauma Question- naire - Psychometrische Eigenschaften einer deutschsprachigen Version. [Childhood Trauma Questionnaire - Psychometric properties of a German version]. Z Klin Psy- chol Psychother 2009, 38(4):223-230.
24. Klinitzke G, Romppel M, Haeuser W, Braehler E, Glaesmer H: Die deutsche Ver- sion des Childhood Trauma Questionnaire (CTQ)-psychometrische Eigenschaften in einer bevölkerungsrepräsentativen Stichprobe [The German Version of the Child- hood Trauma Questionnaire (CTQ): psychometric characteristics in a representative sample of the general population]. [Validation Studies]. Psychotherapie, Psychoso- matik, medizinische Psychologie 2012, 62(2):47-51.
25. Glaesmer H, Gunzelmann T, Braehler E, Forstmeier S, Maercker A: Traumatic expe- riences and post-traumatic stress disorder among elderly Germans: results of a rep- resentative population-based survey. Int Psychogeriatrics/IPA 2010, 22(4):661-670.
26. Hauffa R, Rief W, Braehler E, Martin A, Mewes R, Glaesmer H: Lifetime traumatic experiences and posttraumatic stress disorder in the German population: Results of a representative population survey. J Nerv Mental Dis 2011, 199(12):934.
27. Green JG, McLaughlin KA, Berglund PA, Gruber MJ, Sampson NA, Zaslavsky AM, Kessler RC: Childhood adversities and adult psychiatric disorders in the national comorbidity survey replication I: associations with first onset of DSM-IV disorders. Arch Gen Psychiatry 2010, 67(2):113.
28. Thombs BD, Bernstein DP, Ziegelstein RC, Scher CD, Forde DR, Walker EA, Stein MB: An evaluation of screening questions for childhood abuse in 2 community sam- ples: implications for clinical practice. Arch Intern Med 2006, 166(18):2020-2026.
29. von Sydow K: Psychosexuelle Entwicklung im Lebenslauf: Eine biographische Studie bei Frauen der Geburtsjahrgänge 1895 bis 1936 [Psychosexual development in the life span. A biographical analysis with women born between 1895 and 1936]. Regensburg: Roderer; 1991.

30. Edwards VJ, Holden GW, Felitti VJ, Anda RF: Relationship between multiple forms of childhood maltreatment and adult mental health in community respondents: results from the adverse childhood experiences study. Am J Psychiatry 2003, 160(8):1453-1460.

31. Hardt J, Rutter M: Validity of adult retrospective reports of adverse childhood experiences: review of the evidence. J Child Psychol Psychiatry Allied Discip 2004, 45(2):260-273.

32. Haeuser W, Schmutzer G, Glaesmer H, Braehler E: Prävalenz und Prädiktoren von Schmerzen in mehreren Körperregionen: Ergebnisse einer repräsentativen deutschen Bevölkerungsstichprobe [Prevalence and predictors of pain in several body regions: Results of a representative German population survey]. Schmerz 2009, 23(5):461-470.

CHAPTER 3

SETTING THE STAGE FOR CHRONIC HEALTH PROBLEMS: CUMULATIVE CHILDHOOD ADVERSITY AMONG HOMELESS ADULTS WITH MENTAL ILLNESS IN VANCOUVER, BRITISH COLUMBIA

MICHELLE L. PATTERSON, AKM MONIRUZZAMAN, AND JULIAN M. SOMERS

3.1 BACKGROUND

Research into the causes of homelessness suggests complex interactions between structural and individual factors, both of which are often present long before the onset of first homelessness [1,2]. The childhoods of homeless adults are disproportionately characterized by persistent poverty, residential mobility, school problems, and other stressful and/or traumatic experiences [3-5] particularly among homeless individuals with mental illness [2]. In fact, the childhoods of homeless people with mental illness have been described as a "double dose" of disadvantage in the form of poverty as well as violence and family instability [2].

A large body of evidence suggests that adverse childhood experiences, which typically include physical, sexual, and emotional abuse, neglect, dysfunctional family environments, and unstable family structure, are linked to later psychological functioning and may affect multiple domains of health and well-being [6-8]. Moreover, it appears that adverse childhood experiences tend to cluster together [9,10] and the number of adverse experiences may be more predictive of negative adult outcomes than particular categories of events. Using a sample of adults served by a large health maintenance organization in California, a growing body of research has established a strong dose–response relationship between the number of adverse childhood experiences and poor health outcomes in adulthood including alcohol and drug use, mental health, physical illness, and a variety of risk behaviours [6-8]. However, this sample includes individuals with private health insurance and, therefore, is not generalizable to people with histories of chronic homelessness and mental illness.

Few studies to date have looked at the accumulation of adverse childhood experiences and their effect on the adult lives of individuals who are homeless. Recently, Tsai, Edens and Rosenheck [11] examined the childhood profiles of 738 homeless adults and found three clusters: numerous childhood problems (21%); disrupted family structure (44%); and few childhood problems (35%). Participants with numerous childhood problems were significantly younger when first homeless and engaged in more severe drug use than other participants. Tam, Zlotnick and Robertson [12] examined the long-term effects of adverse childhood experiences on adult substance use, social service use, and employment among 397 homeless adults in Oakland. Adverse childhood experiences were positively correlated with consistent substance use over 15 months of follow-up as well as social service use. Further, consistent substance use was negatively associated with employment and social service use.

No studies to our knowledge have examined the cumulative impact of adverse childhood events on the adult lives of homeless people with mental illness. However, evidence suggests that adults with mental disorders report greater exposure to adverse childhood experiences compared to the general population [13] and that exposure may be related to symptom severity and course of illness [14,15]. Furthermore, studies have found that cumulative exposure to adverse childhood events was related to homelessness in the past 6 months among adults with severe mood disorders [14] and with psychotic disorders [15].

How are adverse childhood experiences linked to health risk behaviors and illness in adulthood? Research to date has focused on behaviors such as alcohol or drug use, smoking, or other behaviors that have immediate psychological or pharmacological benefit as coping strategies in the face of consistently high levels of stress [6-8]. However, few studies have examined the use of alcohol and other drugs in detail; for example, what frequency and type of substance use is associated with chains of risk? The current study further examines the relationship between adverse childhood events and a variety of adult health outcomes among a sample of homeless adults with mental illness in Vancouver, British Columbia. More specifically, we aim to explore the relationship between adverse childhood events, substance use disorders (including frequency, severity and type of substance), mental illness, duration of homelessness, and vocational functioning. In identifying early indicators for problematic substance use and/or homelessness, we are posing a larger question about how we might prevent or attenuate a myriad of negative health and social outcomes in adulthood.

3.2 METHODS

The Vancouver At Home Study is a randomized controlled trial involving homeless adults with mental illness in Vancouver, British Columbia. Study design and sample size were determined by the At Home/Chez Soi National Research Team which monitored activities at five different study sites [16]. Details related to the trial protocol such as CONSORT have been reported elsewhere [16,17]. The current study focuses on baseline data from one study site (Vancouver) prior to randomization and does not incorporate any longitudinal findings.

Eligibility criteria included legal adult status (19 years and older), current mental disorder on the MINI International Neuropsychiatric Interview (MINI) [18], and being absolutely homeless or precariously housed. Absolute homelessness was defined as living on the streets or in an emergency shelter for at least the past seven nights with little likelihood of obtaining secure accommodation in the upcoming month. Precariously housed was defined as living in a rooming house, hotel or other transitional housing; in addition, individuals must have experienced at least two episodes of absolute homelessness in the past year, or one episode lasting for at least four weeks in the past year.

Participants were recruited through referral from over 40 agencies available to homeless adults in Vancouver; the majority was recruited from homeless shelters, drop-in centres, homeless outreach teams, hospitals, community mental health teams, and criminal justice programs. We specifically targeted organizations that serve women, youth, aboriginal peoples, and gay/lesbian individuals in order to obtain as diverse and representative a sample as possible. Referral was typically initiated by service providers and a preliminary screening for eligibility (e.g., duration of homelessness, mental health and substance use problems), was conducted via telephone with the referral agent. All participants met face-to-face with a trained research interviewer who explained procedures, obtained informed consent, and confirmed study eligibility. A cash honorarium of $5 was provided to the participant for the screening process. Institutional ethics board approval was obtained through Simon Fraser University and the University of British Columbia.

If the individual met all study criteria, they were enrolled as a participant and the baseline interview commenced, consisting of a series of interviewer-administered questionnaires including socio-demographic characteristics, psychiatric symptoms, substance use, physical health, service use, and quality of life [17]. Participants received a further cash honorarium of $30 upon completion of the baseline interview which typically took 90 minutes to complete. The following analyses are based upon data from the baseline questionnaires of 497 participants recruited from October 2009 to June 2011 and data from the Adverse Childhood Experiences scale [19], which was administered 18 months after baseline.

3.2.1 VARIABLES OF INTEREST

Childhood events were assessed 18 months after the baseline interview using the Adverse Childhood Experiences (ACE) scale [19], which consists of 17 questions pertaining to age 18 or younger. The ACE includes three categories of childhood abuse: psychological abuse (2 questions), physical abuse (2 questions), contact sexual abuse (2 questions); and two categories of neglect: emotional (2 questions) and physical (2 questions). In addition, the ACE inquires about four categories of exposure to household dysfunction during childhood: parental separation or divorce (1 question), exposure to substance abuse (1 question), mental illness (1 question), violent treatment of mother or stepmother (3 questions), and incarceration (1 question) in the household. Participants received a positive score for a category if they responded "yes" to one or more of the questions in a particular category, for a maximum score of 10. Response options included Yes, No, Don't know or Decline. Only a response of "yes" was recorded as a positive endorsement of items on the ACE. The response "don't know" was recorded as a negative response and declining to respond was considered as missing data.

With regard to mental disorders, Severe Cluster includes at least one of current Psychosis, Mood Disorder with Psychotic Features, and Hypomanic or Manic Episode, as identified through the MINI or documented physician diagnosis. Less Severe Cluster includes at least one of current Major Depressive Episode, Panic Disorder, and Post-traumatic Stress Disorder. Suicidality, Alcohol Dependence, and Substance Dependence were also identified using the MINI. Frequency and type of substance use over the past month were recorded using the Maudsley Addiction Profile (MAP) [20]. Physical illness was assessed by self-report using a checklist of 30 chronic health conditions (lasting longer than six months). Blood-borne infectious disease consisted of positive self-report diagnosis of HIV, Hepatitis B or Hepatitis C. Vocational functioning included two variables: (1) have you ever had a job that lasted for at least one year? (yes/no) and (2) are you currently employed in paid work? (yes/no) Psychometric properties for all measures are provided in previous manuscripts [16,17].

3.2.3 STATISTICAL ANALYSES

Comparisons of categorical data between participants who completed or did not complete the ACE were conducted using Pearson's chi-square or

Fisher's exact test. Comparisons of numeric variables (e.g., age at enrolment) between groups were conducted using the Student t test and Wilcoxon's rank-sum test. Univariate and multivariable logistic regression analyses were used to model the independent associations between ACE total score and a series of a priori outcome variables. Each outcome variable was modeled in both univariate and multivariate settings using ACE total score as an independent risk factor. Outcome variables that were significant at the $p \leq 0.10$ level were considered for the multivariable logistic regression analyses using the same set of controlling variables (age at enrolment, gender, ethnicity, educational attainment, and level of need) chosen based on previous literature [7,8,11,12]. Both unadjusted and adjusted odds ratios and 95% confidence intervals (CI) are reported as effect sizes and all p-values are two-sided. SPSS-21 was used to conduct these analyses. Missing values ranging from zero to 2% for all outcome and controlling variables in the regression analysis were excluded.

3.3 RESULTS

In total, 497 participants completed the baseline questionnaire. Of the total sample, 413 participants (83%) were located for the 18 month follow-up interview and 364 of these participants (88%) provided a valid response on all ACE items. Declined items ranged from 9.2% (physical abuse) to 10.9% (maternal violence) and "don't know" responses ranged from 2.2% (psychological and physical abuse) to 9.7% (household mental illness). Table 1 presents the baseline characteristics for the full baseline sample (n=497) and for participants who completed the ACE (n=364). At baseline, the majority of participants who responded to the ACE was male (71%) and White (55%); the mean age at enrollment was 41.0 (SD=10.6) years; and the mean age when first homeless was 29.0 (SD=13.1) years. The median duration of lifetime homelessness was 36 months (IQR: 12–84 months). Compared to the baseline sample, participants who completed the ACE were more likely to be categorized as "moderate" than "high" needs ($p \leq 0.05$), based on an algorithm that considered type of mental disorder, history of psychiatric hospitalization, substance dependence and/ or criminal justice involvement, and community functioning [17]. Otherwise, there were no significant differences at baseline between the full sample and participants who completed the ACE.

TABLE 1: Socio-demographic, mental disorder, and substance use-related characteristics for Vancouver At Home study participants (n=497)

Variable	Total sample (n=497)	Participants with valid ACE total score (n=364)	Participants with missing or declined responses (n=133)	P value
	N (%)	N (%)	N (%)	
Need level (High)	297 (60)	208 (57)	89 (67)	0.049*
Gender (Male)	359 (73)	255 (71)	104 (78)	0.103
Age at enrolment visit				
Youth	36 (7)	24 (7)	12 (9)	0.344
25-44 years	281 (57)	202 (56)	76 (59)	
> 44 years	180 (36)	138 (38)	42 (32)	
Ethnicity				
Aboriginal	77 (15)	62 (14)	15 (11)	0.251
White	280 (56)	199 (55)	81 (61)	
Other	140 (28)	103 (28)	37 (28)	
Incomplete high school	280 (57)	210 (58)	70 (53)	0.270
Marital status (Single)	343 (70)	250 (69)	93 (72)	0.570
Precariously housed	109 (22)	76 (21)	33 (25)	0.544
Duration of homelessness				
Lifetime (>36 months)1	234 (48)	173 (48)	61 (46)	0.697
Longest single period (>1 yr)2	245 (50)	184 (51)	61 (47)	0.373
First homeless prior to age 25 yrs	214 (44)	152 (42)	62 (47)	0.313
Overall health (Poor)	67 (13)	53 (14)	14 (10)	0.240
Type of mental disorder				
Less severe	264 (53)	202 (56)	62 (47)	0.079+

TABLE 1: *Cont.*

Variable	Total sample (n=497)	Participants with valid ACE total score (n=364)	Participants with missing or declined responses (n=133)	P value
	N (%)	N (%)	N (%)	
Severe	363 (73)	258 (71)	105 (79)	0.073+
Multiple (≥2) mental disorders	240 (48)	180 (49)	60 (45)	0.392
Alcohol dependence	121 (24)	91 (25)	30 (23)	0.574
Substance dependence	288 (58)	218 (60)	70 (53)	0.126
High suicidality	87 (17)	69 (19)	18 (13)	0.159
Blood-borne infectious disease	157 (32)	118 (33)	39 (30)	0.540
Multiple (≥3) physical illness	344 (69)	253 (70)	91 (68)	0.817
Age first drunk (≤13 yrs)	164 (47)	51 (40)	215 (46)	0.153
Age of first drug use (≤13 yrs)	140 (42)	43 (35)	183 (40)	0.178
Daily substance use	143 (29)	105 (29)	38 (29)	0.952
Daily drug use	93 (25)	33 (25)	126 (25)	0.867
Injection drug use	88 (18)	64 (18)	24 (19)	0.834
Poly-substance use				
Two or more	257 (52)	193 (53)	64 (49)	0.397
Three or more	148 (30)	113 (31)	35 (27)	0.345
Poly-drug use				
Two or more	188 (38)	145 (40)	43 (33)	0.150
Three or more	108 (22)	84 (23)	24 (18)	0.253
Weekly alcohol use	111 (22)	85 (23)	26 (20)	0.394
Daily alcohol use	26 (5)	20 (5)	6 (5)	0.678
Daily marijuana use	70 (14)	49 (13)	21 (16)	0.509

1Dichotomized based on median score (3 years). 2Dichotomized based on median score (1 year). *p≤0.05. +p≤0.10.

The proportion of positive responses for the ten categories included in the ACE ranged from 20% for a household member being incarcerated to 54% for psychological abuse (often experiencing an adult in the household swear, insult or humiliate the participant, or act in a way that made the participant afraid that they might be physically hurt; see Table 2). Only 12% of participants did not endorse any of the ACE items and 42% positively endorsed five or more items. The mean ACE total score was 3.9 (SD=2.8) (see Table 2).

TABLE 2: Prevalence of adverse childhood experiences (ACE) among Vancouver At Home study participants

Overall score (n=364)	N (%)
0	43 (12)
1	45 (12)
2	50 (14)
3	41 (11)
4	33 (9)
5-10	152 (42)
Mean (SD)	3.9 (2.8)
Median (range)	4 (0–10)
Child abuse	
Emotional abuse (n=374)[1]	203 (54)
Physical abuse (n=375)	186 (50)
Sexual abuse (n=370)	104 (28)
Emotional neglect (n=369)	168 (45)
Physical neglect (n=371)	106 (29)
Household dysfunction	
Parental separation or divorce (n=371)	197 (53)
Mother treated violently (n=368)	90 (24)
Substance abuse (n=373)	196 (53)
Mental illness (n=370)	134 (36)
Incarceration (n=370)	76 (20)

[1]*Number of participants who provided a valid response to each item on the ACE.*

Bivariate comparisons by ACE total score are summarized in Table 3. Participants with higher ACE scores were significantly more likely to share certain socio-demographic characteristics (i.e., Aboriginal ethnicity, incomplete high school, having children under age 18), and were significantly more likely to report a number of negative health outcomes related to physical health (i.e., blood-born infectious diseases, rating overall health as "poor"), mental health (i.e., less severe cluster of mental disorders, multiple mental disorders) and substance use (i.e., alcohol and/or substance dependence, early initiation of alcohol and/or drug use, daily alcohol and/or drug use).

TABLE 3: ACE total score by socio-demographic, physical health, mental disorder and substance use variables (n=364)

Variable	Mean (SD)	P value
Socio-demographic variables		
Need Level		
High	3.8 (2.8)	0.423
Moderate	4.0 (2.8)	
Gender		
Male	3.7 (2.8)	0.071+
Female	4.3 (2.8)	
Age at enrolment		
19-24 years	3.5 (2.7)	0.672
25-44 years	4.0 (2.8)	
> 44 years	3.8 (2.8)	
Ethnicity		
Aboriginal	4.8 (3.0)	0.004**
White	3.9 (2.7)	
Other	3.4 (2.7)	
Education		
Completed high school	3.3 (2.6)	0.001***
Incomplete high school	4.3 (2.8)	
Marital status		
Single (never married)	3.8 (2.6)	0.204
Other	4.2 (3.1)	

TABLE 3: *Cont.*

Variable	Mean (SD)	P value
Housing status		
Precariously housed	3.9 (2.8)	0.570
Absolutely homeless	3.7 (2.8)	
Duration of homelessness (lifetime)		
> 36 months	3.8 (2.7)	0.711
≤ 36 months	3.9 (2.8)	
Duration of homelessness (longest single episode)		
> 12 months	3.6 (2.7)	0.032*
≤ 12 months	4.2 (2.8)	
Age of first homelessness		
< 25 years	3.8 (2.8)	0.413
≥ 25 years	4.0 (2.8)	
Physical health		
Blood-borne infectious disease		
No	3.6 (2.7)	0.008**
Yes	4.5 (2.9)	
Multiple (≥3) physical illness		
No	3.1 (2.7)	<0.001***
Yes	4.2 (2.8)	
Overall health		
Fair/good/excellent	3.7 (2.7)	0.029*
Poor	4.6 (3.1)	
Mental disorders (past month)		
Less severe cluster		
No	3.4 (2.6)	0.001**
Yes	4.3 (2.9)	
Severe cluster		
No	4.1 (2.6)	0.314
Yes	3.8 (2.9)	
Multiple (≥2) mental disorders		
No	3.4 (2.6)	<0.001***
Yes	4.4 (2.9)	
Alcohol dependence		
No	3.7 (2.7)	0.005**

TABLE 3: *Cont.*

Variable	Mean (SD)	P value
Yes	4.6 (2.8)	
Substance dependence		
No	3.7 (2.7)	0.005**
Yes	4.6 (2.8)	
Suicidality		
High	3.7 (2.7)	0.038*
No/low/moderate	4.5 (2.9)	
Substance use (past month)		
Age first drunk		
Before 14 years	4.6 (2.7)	<0.001***
14 years or after	3.3 (2.7)	
Age first used drugs		
Before 14 years	4.8 (2.7)	<0.001***
14 years or after	3.5 (2.7)	
Frequency of substance use (including alcohol)		
Less than daily/none	3.6 (2.7)	0.006**
Daily	4.5 (2.9)	
Frequency of drug use		
Less than daily/none	3.6 (2.7)	0.001***
Daily	4.7 (2.9)	
Frequency of marijuana use		
Less than daily/none	3.8 (2.7)	0.015*
Daily	4.8 (3.0)	
Frequency of alcohol use		
Less than weekly/none	3.8 (2.8)	0.089+
Weekly or more	4.3 (2.8)	
Injection drug use		
No	3.8 (2.8)	0.148
Yes	4.3 (2.8)	
Poly-substance use		
Two or less	3.7 (2.8)	0.056+

TABLE 3: *Cont.*

Variable	Mean (SD)	P value
Three or more	4.3 (2.7)	
Poly-drug use		
Two or less	3.8 (2.8)	0.122
Three or more	4.3 (2.6)	

*p≤0.05. + p≤0.10. **p≤0.01. ***p≤0.001.*

Unadjusted (UOR) and adjusted odds ratios (AOR) and 95% CI for variables included in the univariate and multivariable analyses are presented in Table 4. Results from the multivariable logistic regression analyses indicate that ACE total score independently predicted meeting criteria for the less severe cluster of mental disorder(s) (AOR: 1.13), Alcohol Dependence (AOR: 1.11), Substance Dependence (AOR: 1.09), high risk of suicidality (AOR: 1.11), and two or more mental disorders (AOR: 1.15); positive self-report of infectious disease (AOR: 1.09), three or more chronic physical illnesses (AOR: 1.15), and "poor" overall health (AOR: 1.12); early initiation (prior to age 14 years) of alcohol (AOR: 1.17) and/ or drugs (AOR: 1.20), current daily substance use (AOR: 1.10), daily drug use (AOR: 1.14), and daily marijuana use (AOR: 1.16). Further, a significant positive trend was observed between ACE total score and a longest single episode of homelessness of one year or more (AOR: 1.07) and past month use of three or more substances (AOR: 1.07).

3.4 DISCUSSION

Among our sample of homeless adults with mental illness, we found a strong relationship between the breadth of exposure to abuse or household dysfunction during childhood (ACE total score) and a number of indicators of poor mental and physical health as well as problematic substance use in adulthood. ACE total score independently predicted meeting criteria for a current mental disorder in the less severe cluster (i.e., major depressive episode, panic disorder or post-traumatic stress disorder), multiple mental disorders, and high risk of suicide; infectious disease, three or more chronic physical conditions, and poor self-rated health; alcohol and/ or substance dependence, early initiation of alcohol and/or drug use, and daily use of any substance, illicit drugs, and marijuana. These findings suggest that the impact of adverse childhood experiences on adult health and social functioning is strong and cumulative among homeless individuals with mental illness.

Of concern was the very high rate of adverse events reported by our sample: 65% reported personally experiencing abuse, 53% reported experiencing neglect, and 79% reported household dysfunction. The mean number of adverse childhood experiences reported was 4. Only 24% of participants reported 1 or zero adverse childhood experiences, 34% reported 2 to 4 events, and 42% reported 5 to 10 events. Rates of adverse childhood experiences in our study were two to nine times higher than those reported by Dube et al. [7] using a large HMO sample. Our findings are similar to those reported by Wu et al. [21] who administered the Life Stressor Checklist-Revised to adults with concurrent mental illness and substance dependence in a residential drug treatment program: 16% of participants reported 1 or zero adverse childhood experiences, 49% reported 2 to 4 events, and 34% reported 5 or more events. Sullivan et al. [2] reported that about one-quarter of their sample of homeless adults with mental illness experienced residential instability as children and over one-third witnessed violence in the home or personally experienced abuse. These authors concluded that homeless people with mental illness appear to receive a "double dose" of disadvantage in the form of poverty as well as family instability and violence. Our findings suggest that childhood adversity among homeless adults with mental illness is much more pervasive and cumulative, and likely contributes to a number of chronic health problems in adulthood.

Consistent with other studies, multiple adverse childhood experiences predicted a variety of adult health problems including physical illness [22,23], mental illness [24] and substance use problems [12,25,26]. As expected, ACE score is predictive of depressive and anxiety disorders, including post-traumatic stress disorder, rather than disorders that are typically characterized as "severe" such as psychotic and bipolar disorders. However, the relationship between ACE score and physical illness and substance abuse suggests a complex syndrome that can be very severe in terms of its impact and duration. ACE total score independently predicted a range of substance use problems in our adult sample, including early initiation of drug and/or alcohol use (before age 14). Along with other studies, our findings suggest that daily drug use is a common mediator for a range of early risk factors [27]. Thus, it appears that abuse of alcohol and other drugs places an individual at greater risk of homelessness, but is not a direct causal factor [28]. Previous research using our sample of homeless adults with mental disorders found that daily drug use significantly predicts the duration of homelessness [29] as well as the severity of mental health symptoms [30].

Cross-sectional, retrospective data cannot disentangle the unique predictors of homelessness and mental illness, but it is likely that negative childhood experiences have both direct and indirect effects on participants' history of homelessness. Documentation of these underlying common factors points to a broad range of vulnerabilities for homelessness and mental illness. These common factors increase the complexity of personal problems as well as the duration of homelessness [29]. Therefore, substance dependence, especially when concurrent with mental illness among homeless populations, is not only a clinical problem but also a critical indicator for a range of other social and psychological problems that may need to be addressed before homelessness can be resolved.

According to Briere's [31] self-trauma model, beyond its initial negative effects, early and cumulative childhood trauma interrupts normal child development, conditions negative affect to abuse-related stimuli, and interferes with the usual acquisition of self-capacities such as affect regulation skills. Reduced affect regulation places an individual at risk for being more easily overwhelmed by emotional distress associated with memories of trauma, and increases the likelihood of using dissociation and other avoidant coping strategies in adolescence and adulthood. In this way, impaired affect regulation leads to reliance on avoidance strategies which, in turn, further prevent the development of self-regulation capacities. This negative cycle is exacerbated by the individual's tendency to repetitively re-experience cognitive-emotional memories of the traumatic event in an effort to process conditioned emotional responses and distorted cognitive schema—a process that can further overwhelm self-regulation and produce distress. Therefore, in addressing the long-term impact of adverse child-hood experiences, the role of family context and environment (e.g., par-enting and attachment) must be considered alongside avoidance strategies such as substance use.

3.4.1 IMPLICATIONS

Children who have experienced trauma are more likely to experience trau-ma and abuse in the future [32]. Furthermore, victims of childhood trauma often engage in post-victimization behavior in the form of violence against self or others and poor personal and occupational functioning [33]. The experience of homelessness increases the likelihood that an individual will witness or experience trauma, and homelessness itself is considered as a traumatic experience that interrupts routines and damages social networks [34]. Among homeless populations, having a mental illness and bearing witness to multiple violent events are predictive of increased severity of trauma symptoms [35], placing the individual at higher risk for social and functional difficulties including reduced social support and impaired work performance [12].

Research on early indicators of risk for homelessness has important implications for the prevention of homelessness as well as intervention and service provision. Given the high prevalence and long-term negative consequences associated with adverse childhood experiences (in general as well as homeless populations), increased attention to primary, second-ary and tertiary prevention strategies is needed. Primary prevention of adverse events will ultimately require societal changes that improve the quality of family and household environments during childhood, particu-larly for poor households. Longitudinal evaluations of early intervention programs (secondary prevention) such as Head Start [36] and the Nurse Family Partnership [37] have documented the prevention of a range of health, social and justice related problems with vulnerable groups (e.g., low income children and first-time mothers).

Prevention also requires increased recognition of the effects of child-hood trauma as well as a better understanding of the behavioral coping strategies that are commonly adopted to reduce the emotional impact of these experiences. However, psychological assessment and treatment for children and adolescents is often grossly inadequate. Where psychosocial interventions are available, improved coordination between mental health professionals, general practitioners, child protection and public health workers, and families is greatly needed in order to better understand how social, emotional, and medical problems are linked throughout the lifespan.

3.4.2 LIMITATIONS

A potential weakness of studies with retrospective reporting of childhood experiences is recall bias. Longitudinal follow-up of adults whose childhood abuse was documented has shown that their retrospective reports of such abuse are likely to underestimate actual occurrence [38]. Therefore, difficulty recalling childhood events likely results in misclassification (classifying people who truly were exposed to ACEs as unexposed) that would bias our results toward the null hypothesis. Also, substance use is likely under-reported by participants particularly given that the baseline questionnaires were administered prior to randomization to supported housing or usual care. In addition, the number of participants who declined to respond to items on the ACE was relatively high, and suggests an attempt to avoid thinking about distressing past events. If this is the case, it would result in further under-reporting of adverse events in our sample. Other than level of need, we found no significant differences between participants who completed vs. those who did not complete the ACE. Finally, there may be mediators of the relationship between childhood experiences and adult health status other than the risk factors we examined such as childhood conduct problems or foster care placement.

The retrospective and cross-sectional nature of our data preclude the kind of modeling required to identify the primary adult outcomes related to adverse childhood events. Further longitudinal research is required to more fully understand the developmental and social sequelae related to childhood adverse events. Further research is also needed to understand how social factors regulate behaviours or distribute individuals into risk groups and how those social factors push individual trajectories towards or way from adverse outcomes.

TABLE 4: Logistic regression analysis for socio-demographic, mental illness, and substance use-related outcomes based on ACE total score (n=364)

Outcome1	Unadjusted OR (95% CI)	p value	Adjusted OR (95% CI)2	p value
Duration of homelessness				
Cumulative lifetime (>3 years)	1.10 (0.94, 1.09)	0.710		
Longest single episode (>1 year)	1.09 (1.01, 1.17)	0.032*	1.07 (0.99, 1.16)	0.108+
Age first homeless (<25 years)	1.03 (0.96, 1.11)	0.412		
Mental disorder				
Less severe cluster	1.14 (1.05, 1.23)	0.001**	1.13 (1.04, 1.23)	0.004**
Severe cluster	0.96 (0.88, 1.04)	0.313		
Alcohol dependence	1.13 (1.04, 1.23)	0.006**	1.11 (1.01, 1.21)	0.030*
Substance dependence	1.11 (1.02, 1.19)	0.012*	1.09 (1.00, 1.19)	0.040*
High suicidality	1.10 (1.01, 1.21)	0.039*	1.11 (1.01, 1.23)	0.032*
Multiple (≥2) mental disorders	1.15 (1.07, 1.24)	<0.001***	1.15 (1.06, 1.24)	0.001**
Physical health				
Blood-borne infectious diseases (HIV/HCV/HBV)	1.11 (1.03, 1.21)	0.008**	1.09 (1.01, 1.19)	0.039*
Multiple (≥3) physical illness	1.17 (1.07, 1.27)	0.001**	1.15 (1.05, 1.26)	0.015*
Overall health (poor)	1.12 (1.01, 1.25)	0.030*	1.12 (1.00, 1.25)	0.047*
Substance use				
Age first drunk (<14 years)	1.19 (1.10, 1.29)	<0.001***	1.17 (1.08, 1.28)	<0.001***
Age of first drug use (<14 years)	1.20 (1.10, 1.30)	<0.001***	1.20 (1.10, 1.31)	<0.001***
IV drug use	1.07 (0.98, 1.18)	0.149		
Daily substance use	1.12 (1.03, 1.22)	0.007**	1.10 (1.01, 1.20)	0.027*
Daily illicit drug use	1.15 (1.06, 1.25)	0.001**	1.14 (1.04, 1.25)	0.005**
Daily hard drug use (no marijuana)	1.09 (0.98, 1.20)	0.104+	1.05 (0.95, 1.17)	0.349
Weekly alcohol use	1.08 (0.99, 1.18)	0.089+	1.06 (0.97, 1.16)	0.191
Daily marijuana use	1.14 (1.02, 1.27)	0.017*	1.16 (1.04, 1.31)	0.010*
Poly-substance (≥3) use	1.08 (1.00, 1.17)	0.057+	1.07 (0.99, 1.17)	0.099+
Poly-drug (≥3) use	1.07 (0.98, 1.17)	0.123		
Poly-drug (≥2) use	1.05 (0.97, 1.13)	0.257		

*p≤0.05 **p≤0.01 ***p≤0.001 +p≤0.10. 1Separate binary logistic regression analyses (univariate and multivariable) were conducted for each outcome using ACE total score (continuous measure) as an independent variable. 2Each multivariable model was controlled for age (continuous), gender (male vs. female), ethnicity (Aboriginal, Caucasian, Other), need level (High vs. Moderate), and education (completed vs. incomplete high school).

3.5 CONCLUSIONS

Our research, along with others', shows that the problems experienced by the majority of homeless adults with mental illness have longstanding histories dating back to childhood. Poverty, family instability, damaging psychological experiences, and general household distress are all disproportionately present in the childhood backgrounds of our participants. These early experiences likely work both directly and indirectly to produce risk for homelessness in various ways, shaping, influencing and constraining the intra- and interpersonal resources that children can draw from adults [4].

REFERENCES

1. Shinn M: International homelessness: policy, socio-cultural, and individual perspectives. J Soc Issues 2007, 63(3):657-677.
2. Sullivan G, Burnam A, Koegel P: Pathways to homelessness among the mentally ill. Soc Psychiatry Epidemiol 2000, 35:444-450.
3. Herman D, Susser ES, Struening EL, Link BL: Adverse childhood experiences: are they risk factors for adult homelessness? Am J Pub Health 1997, 87(2):249-255.
4. Koegel P, Malamid E, Burnam MA: Childhood risk factors for homelessness among homeless adults. Am J Pub Health 1995, 85(12):1642-1649.
5. Lehmann ER, Kass PH, Drake CM, Nichols SB: Risk factors for first-time homelessness in low-income women. Am J Orthopsychiatry 2007, 77:20-28.
6. Corso PS, Edwards VJ, Fang X, Mercy J: Health-related quality of life among adults who experienced maltreatment during childhood. Am J Pub Health 2008, 98:1094-1100.
7. Dube S, Felitti VJ, Dong M, Chapman D, Giles W, Anda R: Childhood abuse, neglect and household dysfunction and the risk of illicit drug use: the adverse childhood experience study. Pediatr 2003, 111:564-572.
8. Edwards VJ, Anda RF, Nordenberg DF, Felitti VJ, Williamson DF: Factors affecting probability of response to a survey about childhood abuse. Child Abuse Negl 2001, 25:307-312.
9. McLaughlin K, Green J, Gruber MJ, Sampson N, Zaslavsky A, Kessler R: Childhood adversities and adult psychiatric disorders in the national comorbidity survey replication II: associations with persistence of DSM-IV disorders. Arch Gen Psychiatry 2010, 67:124-132.
10. Green J, McLaughlin K, Berglund P, Gruber M, Sampson N, Zaslavsky A, Kessler R: Childhood adversities and adult psychiatric disorders in the national comorbidity survey replication I: associations with the onset of DSM-IV disorders. Arch Gen Psychiatry 2010, 67:113-123.

11. Tsai J, Edens E, Rosenheck R: A typology of childhood problems among chronically homeless adults and its association with housing and clinical outcomes. J Health Care Poor Underserved 2011, 22:853-870.

12. Tam T, Zlotnick C, Robertson M: Longitudinal perspective: adverse childhood events, substance use, and labor force participant among homeless adults. Am J Drug Alcohol Abuse 2003, 29:829-846.

13. Kessler RC, Davis CG, Kendler KS: Childhood adversity and adult psychiatric disor- der in the United States national comorbidity survey. Psych Med 1997, 27:1101-1119.

14. Lu W, Mueser K, Rosenberg S, Jankowski M: Correlates of adverse childhood experiences among adults with severe mood disorders. Psych Serv 2008, 59:1018-1026.

15. Rosenberg SD, Lu W, Mueser KT, Jankowski M, Cournos F: Correlates of adverse childhood events among adults with schizophrenia spectrum disorders. Psych Serv 2007, 58:245-253.

16. Goering PN, Streiner DL, Adair C, Aubry T, Barker J, Distasio J, Hwang S, Komaroff J, Latimer E, Somers J, Zabkiewicz D: The at home/Chez Soi trial protocol: a pragmatic, multi-site, randomised controlled trial of a housing first intervention for homeless individuals with mental illness in five Canadian cities. BMJ Open 2011, 1(2):e000323.

17. Somers J, Patterson M, Moniruzzaman A, Currie L, Rezansoff S, Palepu A, Fryer K: Vancouver at home: pragmatic randomized trials investigating housing first for homeless and mentally ill adults. Trials 2013, 14:365. http://www.trialsjournal.com/content/14/1/365

18. Sheehan DV, Lecrubier Y, Sheehan KH, Amorim P, Janavs J, Weiller E, Herguta T, Baker R, Dunbar G: The Mini-International Neuropsychiatric Interview (M.I.N.I.): the development and validation of a structured diagnostic psychiatric interview for DSM-IV and ICD-10. J Clin Psychiatry 1998, 59(Suppl 20):22-33.

19. Felitti VJ, Anda RF, Nordenberg D, Williamson DF, Spitz AM, Edwards V, Koss MP, Marks JS: Relationship of childhood abuse and household dysfunction to many of the leading causes of death in adults. Am J Prev Med 1998, 14:245-258.

20. Marsden J, Gossop M, Stewart D, Best D, Farrell M, Strang J: The Maudsley Addiction Profile (MAP): a brief instrument for treatment outcome research. Development and User Manual. London UK: National Addiction Centre/Institute of Psychiatry; 1998. Available at: http://proveandimprove.org.uk/documents/Map.pdf

21. Wu N, Schairer L, Dellor E, Grella C: Childhood trauma and health outcomes in adults with comorbid substance abuse and mental health disorders. Addictive Behav 2010, 35:68-71.

22. Anda R, Felitti V, Bremmer J, Walker J, Whitfield C, Perry B, Dube S, Giles W: The enduring effects of abuse and related adverse experiences in childhood: a convergence of evidence from neurobiology and epidemiology. Euro Arch Psychiatr Clin Neurosci 2006, 256:174-186.

23. Felitti V, Anda R, Nordenberg D, Williamson D, Spitz A, Edwards V, Koss M, Marks J: Relationship of childhood abuse and household dysfunction to many of the leading causes of death in adults: the adverse childhood experiences (ACE) study. Am J Prev Med 1998, 14:245-258.

24. Turner RJ, Lloyd DA: Stress burden and the lifetime incidence of psychiatric disorder in young adults: racial and ethnic contrasts. Arch Gen Psychiatry 2004, 61:481-488.
25. Wilsnack S, Vogeltanz ND, Klassen A, Harris TR: Childhood sexual abuse and women's substance abuse: national survey findings. J Studies Alc 1997, 58:264-271.
26. Zlotnick C, Tam T, Robertson MJ: Disaffiliation, substance abuse and exiting homelessness. Subst Use Misuse 2004, 38:577-599.
27. Sosin MR, Bruni M: Homelessness and vulnerability among adults with and without alcohol problems. Subst Use Misuse 1997, 32(7–8):939-968.
28. Brook DW, Brook JS, Zhang C, Cohen P, Whiteman M: Drug use and the risk of major depressive disorder, alcohol dependence, and substance use disorder. Arch Gen Psychiatry 2002, 59(11):1039-1044.
29. Patterson M, Somers JM, Moniruzzaman A: Prolonged and persistent homelessness: multivariable analyses in a cohort experiencing current homelessness and mental illness in Vancouver, British Columbia. Ment Health Subst Use 2012, 5:85-101.
30. Palepu A, Patterson M, Strehlau V, Moniruzzaman A, Tan De Bibiana J, Frankish C, Krausz M, Somers J: Daily substance use and mental health symptoms among a cohort of homeless adults in Vancouver, British Columbia. J Urban Health 2013, 90:740-746.
31. Briere J, et al.: A self trauma model for treating adult survivors of severe child abuse. In The APSAC handbook on child maltreatment. Edited by Briere J, Berliner L, Bulkley C. Thousand Oaks, CA: Sage; 1996:140-157.
32. Mullen PE, Martin J, Anderson J, Romans S, Herbison G: The long-term impact of the physical, emotional, and sexual abuse of children: a community study. Child Abuse Negl 1996, 20:7-21.
33. Briere J, Elliott D: Prevalence and psychological sequelae of self-reported childhood physical and sexual abuse in a general population sample of men and women. Child Abuse Negl 2003, 27:1205-1222.
34. Goodman LA, Saxe L, Harvey M: Homelessness as psychological trauma: broadening perspectives. Am Psychol 1991, 46:1219-1225.
35. Kim M, Arnold E: Stressful live events and trauma among substance-abusing homeless men. J Soc Work Pract Addict 2004, 4:3-19.
36. Garces E, Thomas D, Currie J: Longer-term effects of head start. Am Econ Rev 2002, 92:999-1012.
37. Olds DL, Sadler L, Kitzman H: Programs for parents of infants and toddlers: recent evidence from randomized trials. J Child Psychol Psychiatr 2007, 48:355-391.
38. Della Femina D, Yeager CA, Lewis DO: Child abuse: adolescent records vs. adult recall. Child Abuse Negl 1990, 14:227-231.

CHAPTER 4

EMOTIONAL ABUSE TOWARDS CHILDREN BY SCHOOLTEACHERS IN ADEN GOVERNORATE, YEMEN: A CROSS-SECTIONAL STUDY

AMAL S. S. BA-SADDIK AND ABDULLAH S. HATTAB

4.1 BACKGROUND

Emotional abuse may be the most prevalent type of child abuse; however, it is also the most hidden, under-reported, and least studied type of abuse [1,2]. Literature on emotional abuse is limited, which could be attributed to the fact that it is the most difficult form of abuse to research, because of lack of a consistent definition, detect, assess, and substantiate [2].

A growing body of research highlights the harmful effects of emotional maltreatment in children. As such, victims experience difficulties in terms of physical health and neurophysiological, emotional, behavioral, and cognitive development [3]. Also, it is significantly related to subsequent delinquent behavior and academic difficulties in early adolescence [4].

Many psychologists assert that emotional abuse is the most devastating form of child abuse, because of its traumatic effects in the development of school pupils [2,5,6], and it underlies all types of child abuse as a perpetrator of emotional abuse can abuse many victims at one particular moment [7].

To date, studies on pupils' abuse by teachers are relatively limited and those that exist mainly focus on corporal punishment [8-10]. Nevertheless, high prevalence of emotional child abuse was reported from India, United States, Zimbabwe, Nigeria and Cyprus [11-15]. The study from India found that 47.9% of surveyed boys and 52.1% of girls had experienced emotional abuse in schools [11].

It is important to explore the issue of pupils abused by educators in educational settings in the Eastern Mediterranean regions, since only two studies [16,17] have indicated that pupils' abuse in schools was enormous. In Bahrain, Al-Mahrous in 1997 found that emotional abuse was very frequently reported by girls 78% [16], while a study from Iran showed that emotional abuse among schoolgirls was 49.8% [17].

In Yemen, documented studies on child abuse are very scarce. Nevertheless, literature search revealed two important studies that addressed the problem of child abuse in family setting [18,19]. The third one [20] was more comprehensive covering the problem of child abuse in family, community and school setting and showed that 42.3% of the school pupils experienced humiliating as an undesirable emotional behavior by their teachers.

This study aimed to assess the prevalence of emotional abuse among schoolchildren in Aden schools and associated factors. Also, we expect that it will contribute to better understanding of emotional abuse in school setting in a developing country.

4.2 METHODS

4.2.1 STUDY DESIGN AND SETTING

This study is a part of a more comprehensive cross-sectional survey of different types of abuse among schoolchildren of basic education in Aden Governorate in Yemen that was conducted during the school year 2009–2010.

4.2.2 STUDY POPULATION

Pupils of grades 7, 8 and 9 were targeted in the survey. Children, at the age of 12–17 years, usually are capable of perceiving what is and is not abuse within the school context, they also could provide reliable information, and are capable of answering the questionnaire [10,21].

4.2.3 SAMPLE SIZE

The sample size was calculated using the assumed proportion of 0.5 in order to obtain the maximum possible sample size, with a level of confidence 95%, and 0.03, as maximum allowable error. Accordingly, the calculated sample size was 1066 pupils who were proportionally distributed according to pupils' gender (667 males and 399 females).

4.2.4 SAMPLING METHOD

A multi-stage stratified random sampling was performed. In the first stage, four districts were randomly selected. In the second stage, two schools from each district also were randomly selected. In the third stage, the sample size (1066) was proportionally distributed according to the proportion of students in the selected grades for each school by gender. The sample frame for this study was the pupils' list in the selected grades of the schools incorporated in this study. Systematic random sampling was applied to select the number of pupils assigned for each grade in the selected schools.

4.2.5 INSTRUMENT

An anonymous self-administered questionnaire adapted from the Arabic version of Child Abuse Screening Tool Children's Institutional Version [21], was used for data collection.

The first part of the instrument covers questions about pupil's variables: gender, age, school grade, residence, in addition to parent's socio-demographic variables: family type, parent's education and parent's marital status.

The second part includes 10 items including acts such as humiliating, shouting, calling names, embarrassing them of being orphan, poor, having health problems, threatening with giving them bad marks, or expelling from school, isolating them from other children and destroying their belongings.

Experts in child abuse from Yemeni Universities judged the questionnaire, to find out if it is socially acceptable. Accordingly, some items were rephrased, and other items were dropped out. The final modified version of the questionnaire used in this study included the following questions:

Have you ever been exposed to any of these acts at school?

Humiliating, shouting, calling names, embarrassing of being orphan, embarrassing of being poor, threatening with bad marks, threatening to expelling from school, embarrassing for having health problems, isolating from children, destroying belongings. Pupils who answered with "Yes" were asked to report the frequency of the abuse acts by indicating 1-2 times, 3-4 times, ≥ 5 times. In addition they were asked to mention who did it: a teacher or a school administrator? [21].

4.2.6 PILOT STUDY

A pilot study was conducted among 60 pupils (30 males and 30 females) from two schools not included in the main study, to ensure that the questionnaire items were clear, understandable and culturally acceptable. Chronbach alpha was used to test the internal consistency reliability, which was found to be 0.78.

We explained the questionnaire in detail to the pupils, and asked them to answer "yes" or "no" to each item and how many times they have experienced abusive acts during scholastic years. Those who responded affirmatively were asked to identify the perpetrators: teacher or school administrative staff. The rate of physical abuse was calculated by recoding the acts into dichotomous categories, with 0 = never and 1 = once or more [22]. A 4- point scale (0 = none; 1 = 1-2 times; 2 = 3–4 times; 3 = 5 times and more) was used to indicate how often they had experienced each abuse act [23].

4.2.7 OPERATIONAL DEFINITION

Emotional abuse in this study refers to pupils' reports of any undesirable or unpleasant emotional act inflicted on them by teachers or other school administrators (school principal, vice principal or other workers) which could potentially make them feel embarrassed while in school. Emotionally abused pupils were defined as those who answered positively to one or more of the emotional abuse acts.

4.2.8 ETHICAL CONSIDERATIONS

1. The research protocol was approved by the Committee of Research and Postgraduate Studies in the Faculty of Medicine and Health Sciences, Aden University. Several levels of permission were granted before the study could proceed, including official approval from the authority of Aden Education Office. In addition, permission was sought from the Districts Directors of Education, as well as from school principals.

2. A written informed consent was sent to the pupils' parents describing the nature of the study, its importance, and its objectives. The consent also stated that the data's confidentiality would be assured, that the participation in the study was voluntary and those who refused participation will not lose any rights or privilege. Parents were asked to put their signature if they agree to have their child participate in the survey. The response rate was 85% of the targeted parents. For those who declined to consent, equal number was substituted following the same methodology.

3. The pupils' informed assent was obtained orally during which detailed explanation of the objectives and the importance of the

research was provided. Potential participants were assured that all information obtained will be handled confidentially. Pupils were informed that they have the right to decline answering any question and/or to withdraw from the study at any time. All pupils whose parents gave consent to their participation have assented to participate in the study.

4.2.9 DATA ANALYSIS

The Statistical Package for Social Science—SPSS—version 15 was used for data analysis. Quantitative variables were normally distributed after testing for normality using Kolmogorove-Smirnov test. Percentage was calculated as summary measure for the qualitative variables. Arithmetic mean, standard deviation and chi square test were used for the descriptive statistics. The statistical significant level was set at p-value < 0.05.

Binary logistic regressions were conducted to describe the bivariate association between emotional abuse and the pupils and parents variables. Multivariate analysis was performed to identify risk factors associated with emotional abuse. The results were discussed in terms of the odds ratio (OR) with 95% Confidence Interval (CI). The OR of the reference category is equal to "1". If an OR is greater than "1" this indicates an increase likelihood of the event (emotional abuse in this research) occurrence, while an OR less than "1" indicates a decreased likelihood of its occurrence.

4.3 RESULTS

4.3.1 SOCIODEMOGRAPHIC CHARACTERISTICS OF THE STUDY POPULATION

Table 1 shows the socioeconomic characteristics of the study population. Male pupils constituted the highest proportion 62.6%. The mean age was 14.03 ± 1.13 years. Most of the pupils lived in nuclear families. More than 50% of the mothers were illiterates or could only read and write.

TABLE 1: Distribution of pupils and their families by socio- demographic characteristics

Pupils characteristicsllr	No.	%
Gender		
Male	667	62.6
Female	399	37.4
Age group (years)		
12-13	363	34.0
14-15	618	58.0
16-17	85	8.0
Mean age = 14.03 ± 1.13 years		
School grade		
Grade 7	322	30.2
Grade 8	366	34.3
Grade 9	378	35.5
Family socio-demographic characteristics		
Family type		
Nuclear	747	70.1
Extended	319	29.9
Parents marital status		
Married	952	89.3
Separated	21	2.0
Divorced	33	3.1
Widow	60	5.6
Father education		
Illiterate	74	6.9
Read and write	281	26.4
Basic	103	9.7
Secondary	202	18.9
University	406	38.1
Mother education		
Illiterate	264	24.8
Read and write	324	30.4
Basic	177	16.6
Secondary	162	15.2
University	139	13.0

4.3.2 PREVALENCE OF EMOTIONAL ABUSE

The study sample included 1066 pupils: 588 of them reported one or more emotional abuse acts, before the age of 18 years. The prevalence of emotional abuse in the surveyed sample was 55.2% (95% CI: 52.1 - 58.2). Teachers occupied the higher proportion of being responsible for emotional abuse 45.6%, followed distantly by the administrative staff 5.0%. As summarized in Table 2. The most common emotional abuse act reported by pupils was shouting 48.1%, the next most common emotional abuse acts were calling names 36.1% and threatening to give bad marks 31.9%. The lowest emotional abuse acts the pupils experienced was being embarrassed by teachers and school administrators for being an orphan 1.7% and 2.0% reported being threatened that their belongings will be destroyed. However, it is important to note that there are gender statistically significant differences: Males had higher prevalence rates than females on almost all of the acts of abuse.

TABLE 2: Distribution of emotional abuse acts by gender

Emotional abuse acts	Gender						P-value
	Male		Female		Total		
	(n = 667)		(n = 399)		1066		
Humiliating	221	33.1	82	20.5	303	28.4	0.000
Shouting	351	52.6	162	40.6	513	48.1	0.022
Calling names	290	43.5	95	23.8	385	36.1	0.000
Embarrassed of being orphan	17	2.54	1	0.3	18	1.7	0.005
Embarrass of being poor	51	7.6	6	1.5	57	5.3	0.000
Threaten with bad marks	242	36.3	98	24.6	340	31.9	0.003
Threaten to drop out school	268	40.2	65	16.3	333	31.2	0.000
Embarrass by having health problems	38	5.7	14	3.5	52	4.8	0.125
Isolated from children	59	8.8	15	3.8	74	6.9	0.002
Destroying belongings	19	2.8	2	0.5	21	2.0	0.008

The frequency of emotional abuse acts is presented in Table 3. Abuse acts that were experienced 1–2 times were shouting 20.7%, threaten to drop out school 16.9% and calling names 15.0%. On the other hand, those acts that were experienced 3–4 times were shouting 12.1%, calling names 8.3%, and threaten with bad marks 8.2%. While those acts that were experienced five times or more were shouting 15.3%, calling names 12.8% and humiliating 9.6%.

TABLE 3: frequency of emotional abuse acts

Emotional abuse acts	Never		1-2 times		3-4 times		≥ 5 times	
	No.	%	No.	%	No.	%	No.	%
Humiliating	763	71.6	134	12.6	66	6.2	103	9.6
Shouting	553	51.9	221	20.7	129	12.1	163	15.3
Calling names	681	63.9	160	15.0	88	8.3	137	12.8
Embarrassed of being orphan	1048	98.3	12	1.1	3	0.3	3	0.3
Embarrass of being poor	1009	94.7	28	2.6	14	1.3	15	1.4
Threaten with bad marks	726	68.1	156	14.6	87	8.2	97	9.1
Threaten to drop out school	733	68.8	180	16.9	68	6.4	85	7.9
Embarrass by having health problems	1014	95.1	26	2.4	17	1.6	9	0.8
Isolated from children	992	93.1	32	3.0	27	2.5	15	1.4
Destroying belongings	1045	98.0	8	0.8	2	0.2	11	1.0

4.3.3 ASSOCIATION ANALYSIS

4.3.3.1 UNIVARIATE ANALYSIS

Table 4 shows the association of the pupils' socio-demographic factors with emotional abuse. Gender and age group have a significant association with emotional abuse. Male had a significantly higher odd of experiencing emotional abuse (OR = 7.50; CI: 5.66 - 9.93) than females. With respect to the age group, emotional abuse significantly increases at the age group 16–17 years (OR = 1.91; 95%CI: 1.17-3.11). The univariate analysis does not show any significant association between school grade and emotional abuse.

TABLE 4: Univariate analysis for pupils' variables and emotional abuse

Variables	Emotional abuse				
	No	%	OR	(95 % CI)	P-value
Gender					
Female*	104	26.1	1.00		
Male	484	72.6	7.50	5.66 - 9.93	.000
Age group					
12-13*	173	47.7	1.00		
14-15	361	58.4	1.54	1.18 –2.00	.001
16-17	54	63.5	1.91	1.17 – 3.11	.009
School grade					
Grade 7*	171	53.1	1.00		
Grade 8	212	57.9	1.21	.89 – 1.64	.205
Grade 9	205	54.2	1.04	.77– 1.41	.766

* Reference category.

Table 5 illustrates that pupils living in extended families were more likely to experience emotional abuse (OR = 1.55; 95%CI: 1.18-2.03). Concerning parents' marital status, only pupils with divorced parents were significantly more likely to experienced emotional abuse (OR = 2.20; CI: 1.01-4.79). On the other hand, the high education levels of fathers play a protective role against pupils' emotional abuse (OR = .64; 95%CI: .46-.90).

4.3.3.2 MULTIVARIATE ANALYSIS OF PREDICTORS OF EMOTIONAL ABUSE

All the variables that were significant in the univariate models with a p value < 0.05 were entered into the backward logistic regression. The final multivariate logistic regression models included all variables retaining significant after adjusting for each other. As can be seen in Table 6 the significant predictors were male gender, family type and father education. Male pupils had about ten times greater risk of experiencing emotional abuse (OR = 9.94; CI: 7.19–13.74) than female. On the other hand, a protective association was found among pupils belonging to highly educated fathers (OR = .58; CI: .39–.86).

TABLE 5: Univariate analysis for parent's variables and emotional abuse

Variables	Emotional abuse				
	No	%	OR	(95 % CI)	P-value
Family type					
Nuclear*	388	51.9	1.00		
Extended	200	62.7	1.55	1.18- 2.03	.001
Father education					
Illiterate*	46	62.2	1.00		
Read/write	162	57.7	1.28	.77-2.13	.338
Basic	61	59.2	1.06	.78-1.44	.698
Secondary	91	45.0	1.13	.73-1.75	.575
University	228	56.2	.64	.45-.89	.010
Mother education					
Illiterate*	151	57.2	1.00		
Read/write	190	58.6	1.28	.84-1.93	.241
Basic	95	53.7	1.35	.91-2.02	.133
Secondary	81	50.0	1.11	.71-1.73	.647
University	71	51.1	.95	.60-1.50	.852
Parents Marital Status					
Married*	521	54.7	1.00		
Separated	13	61.9	1.34	.55-3.27	.515
Divorced	24	72.7	2.20	1.01-4.79	.046
Widow	30	50.0	.82	.49-1.39	.476

* *Reference category.*

4.4 DISCUSSION

This study is the first in Aden to explore the issues related to pupils' reports of emotional abuse in the school context. This study was conducted to describe the prevalence of emotional abuse by teachers and administration staff in schools. In addition, it provides empirical evidence on how pupils and parents socio-demographic characteristics were associated with pupils' victimization by school staff in Aden governorate.

TABLE 6: Multivariate analysis for pupils and parents variables with emotional abuse

Variables	Emotional abuse				
	No.	%	OR	(95.0 % CI)	P-value
Gender					
Female*	104	26.1	1.00		
Male	484	72.6	9.94	7.19-13.74	.000
Family type					
Nuclear*	388	51.9	1.00		
Extended	200	62.7	1.40	1.02-1.90	.056
Father education					
Illiterate*	46	62.2	1.00		
Read/write	162	57.7	.84	.46-1.51	.549
Basic	61	59.2	.73	.50-1.06	.094
Secondary	91	45.0	.99	.60-1.65	.967
University	228	56.2	.58	.39-.86	.007

* *Reference category.*

It is often assumed that the consequences of emotional abuse are not as severe as those of more obvious forms of abuse [24], but in fact, relatively little is known about the magnitude of the problem of child emotional abuse worldwide. The prevalence of emotional abuse in the current study was 55.2%; it was relatively lower than that found in Iran 59.9% [17], but higher than that reported in Cyprus 33.1% [15] and Taiwan 11.6% [23]. Prevalence rates of emotional abuse are difficult to ascertain because they capture a wide range of teaching behaviors, and there is little, or no consensus across studies as to what phenomena should be included. The observed differences between countries could be examined from several perspectives. First, it might be that the overall teacher behavior in the various countries is genuinely different, and emotional abuse of pupils was frequently noted as a means of controlling the classroom [25]. Second, emotional abuse might be conceptualized differently in these countries, and what "falls outside the range of acceptability" is variously defined [26]. Third, the methodology used, the study population, and the timing frame are not the same for all studies. Finally, cultural context could differently influence the perception of the abuse acts, where a lot of acts might be culturally accepted ways of disciplining pupils and are therefore not perceived to be abuse acts by a teacher or school administrators [11,27].

In our study, the relatively high frequency of teachers' emotionally abusive behavior could be explained by different social, cultural, and organization factors. For example, some abusive behaviors might be culturally acceptable, such as "shouting and calling names". On the other hand, teachers might not be fully aware about child rights in addition to lack of comprehensive disciplinary rules concerning the appropriate management of pupils.

The current study indicates that males had significantly higher odds of experiencing emotional abuse than females, which is consistence with previous studies [15,17,28]. This could be interpreted by the fact that boys are more likely to have a conflicting relationship with their teachers than their female counterparts [29,30]. Interestingly, inattention seemed to provoke the teacher's scorn, especially for boys but not for girls. One possible explanation may be that, in girls, a lack of attention may be considered a temporary lapse and thus, be more readily excused or ignored than in boys. In line with this notion, low-achieving boys have been shown to have been treated more negatively by teachers than their female counterparts [4]. On the other hand, it has been noticed that male pupils are more involved in disruptive behaviors in the classroom, such as noise, shouting, fighting and throwing up, to get attention compared to girls. This may prompt teachers to emotionally abuse boys more than girls. Moreover, it was concluded that, compliance, following rules and being neat and orderly, is valued and reinforced in many classrooms. In addition, they stressed that these are behaviors, which are typically associated with girls rather than boys, and this may account for the reason why boys experience emotional abuse more often than girls from their teachers [31]. Furthermore, it was reported that poor academic performance of male pupils might explain the higher prevalence of emotional abuse among boys. They found that low achieving boys have been more emotionally abused by both male and female teachers compared to girls [29]. Accordingly, we can conclude that gender is a strong predictor of emotional abuse.

With respect to pupils' age group, the findings indicated that the risk of emotional abuse in schools increase when pupils grow up. This result is consistent to what was found in Iran [17]. Pupils aged 16–17 years are typically those who have failed school years and are thus prone to experience emotional abuse, being threatened with school expulsion [17]. Another explanation is that teachers of older pupils use scolding and grades deduction more [25]. Insulting pupils in our study was 28.4% very much lower than what was reported in an earlier study from Yemen where 42.3% of the pupils aged 6–15 years old claimed that they were insulted at school when they make a mistake [20].

Emotional abuse is prevalent in 7th, 8th, and 9th grades; however, there was no statistical significant association with school grade, though findings show relatively higher odds among 8th graders. This could be explained by the increasing conflict situations between teachers and the 8th grade pupils because of their higher claims for autonomy. Furthermore, it is well known that early adolescence is often a time of increased emotional sensitivity, and even relatively benign comments by teachers can at times be interpreted by adolescent pupils as offending [26]. Further studies are required to examine more closely the characteristics of abusive teachers' behaviors in relation to the pupils' school grade and age groups.

For the assessment of the prevalence of emotional abuse, it is also important to analyze how the family structure and parent's socio-demographic characteristics may be related to pupil's abuse in schools. In our study, we examined the relationship between the prevalence of emotional abuse in a school and the educational level, family type, and marital status of the pupil's parents.

The study findings showed that pupils living in extended families have higher odd of reporting being emotionally abused at school. This could be interpreted according to the social learning theory, where pupils from extended families live in crowded homes and witness family violence. In addition, children remain outdoors long hours observing and imitating aggressive behaviors that affects their relationship with teachers and make them at higher risks of emotional abuse [32]. The study findings revealed that pupils whose parents have low education level, exhibited higher odds of emotional abuse but was not statistically significant.

Parents with low education level may be less able to avail themselves of resources for coping with family problems, avoiding abusive relationships, and for that, they solve their problems aggressively [33]. Children of those families usually witness violence at home, which negatively influence their behavior at school and make them at higher risks of abuse. The findings of our study indicate that the higher education level of fathers play a protective role against child abuse at school.

4.5 CONCLUSION

Emotional abuse of schoolchildren is a highly prevalent problem with social, cultural and health dimensions. Child gender, family type, and father's education level were the main predictors for emotional abuse. Accordingly, appropriate social, legislative and administrative interventions at the family, school and community levels are essential to deal with the problem of schoolchildren emotional abuse by their teachers. Further studies at a national level are required for better understanding the different dimensions of this problem.

REFERENCES

1. McEachern A, Aluede O, Kenny M: Emotional abuse in the classroom: Implications and interventions for counselors. J Couns Dev 2008, 86:3-10.
2. Aluede O: Psychological Maltreatment of Students: A Form of Child Abuse and School Violence. J Hum Ecol 2004, 16:265-270.
3. Yates TM: The developmental consequences of child emotional abuse: A neurodevelopmental perspective. J Emo Abuse 2007, 7:9-34.
4. Brendgen M, Wanner B, Vitaro F: Verbal Abuse by the Teacher and Child Adjustment from Kindergarten through Grade 6. Pediatrics 2006, 117:1585-1598.
5. Shaffer A, Yates TM, Egeland BR: The relation of emotional maltreatment to early adolescent competence: Developmental processes in a prospective study. Child Abuse Negl 2009, 33:36-44.

6.   Hart SN, Brassard MR, Binggeli NJ, Davidson HA: Psychological maltreatment. In The APSAC handbook on child maltreatment. 2nd edition. Edited by Myers JE, Berliner L, Briere J, Hendrix CT, Jenny C, Reid TA. Thousand Oaks: Sage Publications; 2002:79-104.

7.   Brassard MR, Donovan KL: Defining psychological maltreatment. In Child abuse and neglect: Definitions, classifications, and a framework for research. Edited by Freerick MM, Knutson JF, Trickett PK, Flanzer SM. Baltimore: Brookes Publishing; 2006:151-197.

8.   Chianu E: Two deaths, one blind eye, one imprisonment: Child abuse in the guise of corporal punishment in Nigerian schools. Child Abuse Negl 2000, 24:1005-1009.

9.   Dupper DR, Dingus AEM: Corporal punishment in U.S. public schools: A continuing challenge for school social workers. Child Sch 2008, 30:243-250.

10. Youssef RM, Attia MS, Kamel MI: Children experiencing violence II: prevalence and determinants of corporal punishment in schools. Child Abuse Negl 1998, 22:975-985.

11. Kacker L, Varadan S, Kumar PK: Study on Child Abuse – India 2007. New Delhi: Kiriti; 2007.

12. Whitted KS, Dupper DR: Do Teachers Bully Students? Findings from a survey of students in an alternative education setting. Educ Urb Soc 2008, 40:329-341.

13. Shumba A: The nature, extent and effects of emotional abuse on primary school pupils by teachers in Zimbabwe. Child Abuse Negl 2002, 26:783-791.

14. Okoza J, Aluede O, Ojugo A: Sex and Class of Secondary School Students in Experiencing Emotional Abuse by Teachers in Edo State, Nigeria. J Soc Sci Hum 2011, 19:385-392.

15. Theoklitou D, Kabitsis N, Kabitsi A: Physical and emotional abuse of primary school children by teachers. Child Abuse Negl 2012, 36:64-70.

16. Al Mahroos F: Corporal punishment and psychological maltreatment among schoolgirls in Bahrain. Bahrain Med Bull 1997, 19(Suppl 3):70-73.

17. Sheikhattari P, Stephenson R, Assasi N, Eftekhar H, Zamani Q, Maleki B, Kiabayan H: Child maltreatment among school children in the Kurdistan Province, Iran. Child Abuse Negl 2006, 30:231-245.

18. Alyahri A, Goodman R: Harsh corporal punishment of Yemeni children: Occurrence, type and associations. Child Abuse Negl 2008, 32:766-773.

19. Basaddik A: Prevalence of child abuse in Aden governorate. Aden University: Social Medicine and Public Health Department; 2007. MD thesis

20. Al-Dabhani N: Violence against children in selected areas of Yemen. Sana'a: Graphics International Press; 2005.

21. International Society for prevention of child abuse and neglect. Child Abuse Screening Tool-Children's Institutional Version (ICAST-CT); 2007. www.ispcan.org/

22. Straus MA: New scoring methods for violence and new norms for the Conflict Tactics Scale. In Physical violence in American families. Edited by Straus MA, Gelles RJ. New Brunswick: Transaction Publishers; 1992:529-559.

23. Chen J, Wei H: Student victimization by teachers in Taiwan: Prevalence and associations. Child Abuse Negl 2011, 35:382-390.

24. Egeland B: Taking stock: Childhood emotional maltreatment and developmental psychopathology. Child Abuse Negl 2009, 33:22-26.

25. Plan Philippines: Toward a Child-Friendly Education Environment: A Baseline Study on Violence against Children in Public Schools. 2009. http://plan-international.org/learnwithoutfear/resources/publications/philippines-report].
26. Sebre S, Sprugevica L, Novotni A, Bonevski D, Pakalniskiene V, Popescu D, Turchina T, Friedrich W, Lewis O: Cross-cultural comparisons of child-reported emotional and physical abuse: rates, risk factors and psychosocial symptoms. Child Abuse Negl 2004, 28:113-127.
27. Kim D, Kim K, Park Y, Zhang LD, Lu MK, Li D: Children's experience of violence in Chin and Korea: A Transcultural study. Child Abuse Negl 2000, 24:1163-1173.
28. Delfabbro P, Winefield T, Trainor S, Dollard M, Anderson S, Metzer J, Hammarstrom A: Peer and teacher Bullying/Victimization of south Australian secondary school students: Prevalence and psychosocial profiles. Br J Educ Psychol 2006, 76:71-90.
29. Hughes JN, Cavell TA, Willson V: Further support for the developmental significance of the quality of the teacher-student relationship. J Sch Psychol 2001, 39:288-301.
30. Kesner JE: Teacher characteristics and the quality of child-teacher relationship. J Sch Psychol 2000, 38:133-149.
31. De Zolt DM, Hull SH: Classroom and school climate. In Encyclopedia of women and gender. Edited by Worrell J. San Diego: Academic Press; 2000.
32. Newberger EH: Child abuse. In Public Health & Preventive Medicine. 14th edition. Edited by Wallace RB, Doebbeling BN. US: Appeleton & Lang; 1998:1241-1260.
33. Cox CE, Kotch JB, Everson MD: A longitudinal study of modifying influences in the relationship between domestic violence and child maltreatment. J Fam Violence 2003, 18:5-17.

CHAPTER 5

CHILD NEGLECT IN ONE-CHILD FAMILIES FROM SUZHOU CITY OF MAINLAND CHINA

JING HUA, ZHE MU, BRIGHT I. NWARU, GUIXIONG GU, WEI MENG, AND ZHUOCHUN WU

5.1 BACKGROUND

Child neglect is the failure of a parent or a caregiver in a parenting role to meet the basic needs of the child, which poses a major threat to the child's healthy growth and well-being [1]. The National Incidence Study of Child Abuse and Neglect [2,3] in the United States defined neglect as encompassing physical neglect, child abandonment and expulsion, inadequate supervisory neglect, emotional neglect, and educational neglect by parents, parent substitutes, or other adult caregivers of children. The prevalence of child neglect varies across countries. The rates of neglectful behavior of parents recalled by university students in 17 nations ranged from 3.2% to 36% [4]. The prevalence of supervisory and physical neglect reported by a national sample of adolescents in the United States were 42% and 12%, respectively [5]. In the United Kingdom, 6% and 5% of young adults reported the absence of care and supervision, respectively [6].

There is evidence that children's and familial characteristics are the main determinants of child neglect, including maternal education [7], maternal age [8], family structure [9], and employment instability and poverty [10]. Other studies have also shown that prematurity, prolonged hospitalization during childhood, mental impairments and developmental disabilities [11] of children were positively associated with child neglect.

Despite its negative effects and accordingly, warranting active research, studies on child neglect in China are scarce. One reason for the limited studies may be the lack of appropriate validated instruments because cultural norms concerning neglectful behaviors could vary from society to society. Recently, Pan et al have developed and validated the Scale on Child Neglect in Urban China (SCNUC) [12-14]. The instrument's cultural appropriateness was examined through focused (semi-structured) interview with China-born mothers. The results showed that SCNUC is culturally sensitive, although there would be no assurance that the instruments would be useful for cross-cultural comparisons [12,14]. Researches using SCNUC have reported the rates of neglect vary across different regions from 11.6% in Guangzhou City (among children aged 3-6 years old in South China) to 50.0% in Yinchuan City (among children aged 6-8 years old in western China) in Chinese language literature [15-20]. The correlates of childhood neglect such as low parental education, young maternal age, and children with physical and cognitive problems were also reported in these studies [15-20].

Additionally, the Chinese State Council launched the one child policy in 1979 [21], which is almost unique globally. Under this policy regime, each household has few children. As a result, each child, often described as the 'little emperor' or 'little sun' [22], has increasingly become the center of attention in the household and has become more precious to parents than ever. Recently, Zhang et al [19] have found that the one-child and multiple-child families differ in their level of neglect in preschool children based on a relatively small sample in Guangzhou city of China. The one-child families were characterized by lower prevalence of neglect, although the levels of specific neglect subtypes were not reported in that study. Because only 17% of Chinese elders currently have some form of pension and more than 70% rely only on the support of their children [23], the child in one-child families was regarded as the "only hope" of giving their parents support when they become old [23]. Parents from one-child families attach high value to their children, hence may take steps to protect them from physical harm and foster in them socially desirable and culturally approved values. In addition, by the end of 1992, employed females have made up more than 70 percent of all women over 15 years old in China [24]. Mothers spent limited time to take care of their children although most of them were still the primary caregivers under the influence of the traditional Chinese culture. Under the socio-cultural regime, mothers in one-child families may pay great attention to children's education and physical needs possibly at the cost of providing them with adequate emotional environment.

To understand the patterns of child neglect in one-child families in China, we therefore conducted a pilot study in Suzhou City in Yangtze River Delta, one of the most developed areas in China with rigorous operation of the 'one-child' policy. We hypothesized that the prevalence of child neglect in one-child families may be lower than that in multi-child families. There are cross-region difference in child neglect due to the different policy implementation and socio-economic levels in China. We also hypothesized that there would be a lower level of physical and educational neglect and a higher level of emotional neglect in our sample. Moreover, we expected that the correlates of neglect found in this sample would be similar to those reported in other studies. However, unique factors in one-child families associated with child neglect may also exist. For example, three generation families under one-child policy are structured as 4-2-1(four grandparents, two parents and one child), and this structured may decrease the likelihood of child neglect with more adult family members taking care of their "only one" child [25]. We aimed: (1) to describe the prevalence of child neglect and its subtypes among children from one-child families in Suzhou City, China, and (2) to examine the correlates of child neglect in one-child families in this context. Because the measurement for child neglect is different in each age group and its determinants may vary across age groups [13], the focus of the current study is on child neglect in children aged 6-9 years old. Child neglect in other age groups will be reported in another parallel study.

5.2 METHODS

5.2.1 STUDY DESIGN AND PARTICIPANTS

Of the three districts (Pingjiang, Canglang, Jinchang) in Suzhou Ancient City (urban area of Suzhou), Canglang district was randomly sampled for the study. Of the 19 public primary schools in this district, five were randomly selected in the study using stratified random sampling. The size of the sample in each stratum is taken in proportion to the size of the stratums (of these schools, 40% were key primary schools, and 60% were general primary schools). Only one school refused to participate in the study because the study period coincided with the school sports meetings. Therefore, a total of 2230 children's caregivers in four primary schools were recruited, which involved filling out a self-administered questionnaire. The survey was conducted from October to November 2006. Teachers of the participating schools handed out the questionnaires to the children's primary caregivers (biological mothers 89%, biological fathers 6%, and grandparents 5%) at the parent-teacher meeting. The primary caregivers were asked to fill out the questionnaire individually in half an hour at end of the conference according to the attached illustration, then place it in a sealed envelope and return to the children's teachers. Only the researchers involved in the study could open the envelope when it was returned. The questionnaire comprised of 91 question items which asked information related to child neglect. Of the 2230 questionnaires distributed, 2166 (97.1%) were returned. Of the returned 2166 questionnaires, 117 (5.6%) were excluded from the analysis due to missing values, and five subjects were excluded because their families had more than one child. The final sample used for the analysis comprised 2044 children. All of these children belong to Han ethnic group (the majority of the population in the Yangtze Triangle Delta) and come from one child families. The study was approved by the local Education Board and Ethics Committee of Children's Hospital of Suzhou University. Participation in the study was voluntary. Oral parental/guardian consent and students' assent were obtained before the commencement of the study. All the information acquired was kept confidential and was only accessible to the researchers.

5.2.2 MEASURES

In this study, the child neglect was measured by SCNUC [12-14]. The internal consistency (Cronbach's alpha and split-half coefficients were 0.94 and 0.88 respectively), test-retest reliability (Pearson correlation coefficient were 0.93), and construct validity of SCNUC (Item-total correlation were above 0.93) were good. Four subtests of SCNUC were used in this study, which contained physical neglect (12 items), emotional neglect (11 items), educational neglect (16 items), and supervisory neglect (11 items). Physical neglect refers to caregivers not taking care of child's basic needs (such as "Neglect to provide breakfast for child", and "Neglect to provide the individual-used toiletries for children" and the reversed item of "Buy fruit and vegetables for child every day"). Educational neglect refers for the caregiver's failure to provide educational opportunity to the child (such as "Neglect the child's schooling", and the reversed item of "Pay attention to the child's performance during school time"). Emotional neglect refers to the caregiver's failure to provide the child with an emotional environment that allows adequate psychological, cognitive and physical development (such as "Break child's toy or other things when feel angry", "Scold and hit the child before others", and the reversed "Embrace or kiss the child"). Supervisory neglect describes caregiver's failure to protect the child from physical harm or danger (such as the reversed items of "Teach the child how to protect against fire, power line and gas" and "Teach child how to cross the road"). Caregivers were asked to indicate how often they had conducted the listed neglectful behavior with a 4-point Likert scale (1 = never, 2 = occasional, 3 = usual, 4 = constant) in the past one year. The scores of the subscales represented the sum of their corresponding items (the reversed items were reversely scored). A child was identified as being neglected when the scores of the subscales were above the cut-off scores (25 for physical neglect, 25 for emotional neglect, 35 for educational neglect, 25 for supervisory neglect) which were 90 percentile of the national norms based on the data from 8001 children in 28 cities of China [12-14]. The more sever the neglectful behavior, the higher the score. Additionally, we also tested the reliability and validity of the four SCNUC subscales in this sample. The results showed that the Cronbach's alpha coefficients of the physical, emotional, educational, supervisory neglect subscales (internal reliability) were 0.87, 0.82, 0.91 and 0.85, respectively. Split-half coefficients of the four subscales were 0.83, 0.85, 0.89 and 0.81, respectively. The item-total correlations of the four subscales (construct validity) were all above 0.85. For assessment of the criteria-related validity, 200 families (10% of the total sample) were randomly selected to take part in semi-structured interviews for identifying neglectful behaviors a week after filling out the SCNUC. Correlation coefficients of four SCNUC subscales between the results of interview and results determined by cut-off scores were 0.81,0.83,0.89 and 0.79, respectively, indicating the criteria-related validity of the subscales were fair. These results showed that the four subscales of SCNUC could be applied in our study.

We obtained the information about children's and families' characteristics from the questionnaires, including the child's and mother's age; child's sex; mother's employment (whether or not the mother was employed in the past two years); maternal health issues (whether or not the mother had a physical or psychological illness in the past two years); parental education (whether or not the parents obtained a degree of higher education); family structure (families with three generations, nuclear family, single mother or father); and domestic per-capita disposable income of every month in the past year. Great importance was attached to maternal features in this study because mothers are typically the primary caregivers of children in Chinese society and primarily responsible for failures to provide adequate care. "Family with three generations" refers to the child living with his/her biological parents and grandparents, and it was usual among Chinese families due to the traditional family culture. The Families with three generations are structured as 4-2-1(four grandparents, two parents and one child) in one-child families. "Nuclear family" indicates that the child was living with his/her biological parents, and "single mother or father" refers to the child living with one of his/her biological parents.

Because almost all school-aged children and their parents took part in the municipal medical insurance in Suzhou City, the information about children and their parents' history of diseases could be obtained from the medical records provided from the local medical insurance department of social security bureau. In this study, based on children and their parents' basic information including name, gender, and date of birth (obtained from the questionnaires), their medical records were found in the medical information system of local medical insurance department of social security bureau. The children or parent's health issues (whether or not they had stayed in the hospital in the past two years) and whether there was any cognitive impairment (a variety of impaired cognitive functions such as Attention Deficit Hyperactivity Disorder, Autism Spectrum and Developmental coordination disease) were measured according to their medical records.

5.2.3 STATISTICAL ANALYSIS

One-way ANOVA and independent sample t-test were used to compare the means of neglect sub-scores. And the Least Significant Difference (LSD) analysis was used for post-hoc tests of the significant ANOVAS. Linear regression analysis was used as the main statistical technique to investigate the associations between the independent variables (child's and family characteristics) and the dependent variable (scores of subscales for neglect subtypes). All the studied independent variables (child's and family characteristics) were simultaneously included in the linear regression model. Because the Variance Inflation Factor (VIF) of each independent variable in the model was less than 10, the multicolinearity was not statistically significant. Therefore, the colinearity was not considered in the model. The analysis was carried out using SPSS for Windows Version 17.0. A p-value of <0.05 was considered statistically significant.

5.3 RESULTS

5.3.1 THE RATES OF NEGLECT SUBTYPES

Mean score of physical neglect was 23.351 (range from 15 to 46) with a Standard Deviation (SD) of 4.915. Mean score of emotional neglect, educational neglect, and supervisory neglect were 23.124 (SD=3.905, rang=14 to 42), 30.513 (SD =7.636, rang=18 to 61), and 31.232 (SD=6.150, rang from 19 to 44) respectively. Table 1 shows the mean scores of subscales for neglect subtypes by children and family characteristic. According to the scores of neglect subtypes, of 2044 children, 20.3% were identified as the supervisory (95% CI 19.2% to 22.5%) neglect, followed by emotional (15.2%, 95% CI 14.1% to 17.4%), physical (11.1%, 95% CI 9.7% to 12.0%), and educational (6.0%, 95% CI 5.0% to 7.0%) neglect in one child families of Suzhou. The prevalence of any neglect (the child had experienced at least one type of neglect) was 32.0% (95% CI 30.1% to 34.0%). Moreover, 8.3% (95% CI 7.1% to 9.5%) had experienced 2 neglect subtypes, while 4.3% (95% CI 3.4% to 5.2%) had experienced ~3 subtypes of neglect.

TABLE 1: The scores of subscales for neglect subtypes according to child and family characteristics (n=2044)

Char-acteris-tic	N	Physical neglect	Emotional neglect	Educational neglect	Supervisory neglect
		Mean (SD)	Mean (SD)	Mean (SD)	Mean (SD)
Schoola					
1	263	24.008(5.115)	23.388(3.76)**	31.183(7.529)***	31.065(5.973)
2	194	24.18(5.378)	23.392(3.88)	32.263(7.86)	31.773(6.347)
3	547	23.602(4.837)	23.395(3.757)	31.554(7.118)	31.066(6.217)
4	1040	22.829(4.765)	22.785(4.002)†	29.469(7.741)††	30.707(6.114)
Children's agea					
6	417	22.736(4.659)*	23.103(3.878)	30.755(7.799)	30.633(5.862)
7	789	23.238(4.869)	22.976(3.833)	30.624(7.608)	30.932(6.131)
8	736	23.597(5.045)	23.14(4.008)	30.107(7.479)	31.035(6.257)
9	102	24.255(5.12)	23.422(3.834)	31.588(8.229)	31.775(6.636)
Genderb					
Girls	977	23.413(4.925)**	23.317(3.953)*	30.443(7.848)	30.728(6.051)
Boys	1067	22.227(4.908)	22.828(3.837)	30.576(7.44)	31.154(6.234)
Physical health issuesb					
No	1374	23.274(4.862)	22.929(3.787)*	30.432(7.575)	30.818(6.033)c
Yes	670	23.400(5.025)	23.399(4.120)	30.678(7.765)	31.221(6.379)
Cognitive impairmentb					
No	1557	23.141(4.953)**	22.704(3.812)***	30.083(7.643)***	30.719(6.103)**
Yes	487	23.873(4.757)	24.296(3.953)	31.887(7.459)	31.688(6.246)

TABLE 1: *Cont.*

Characteristic	N	Physical neglect	Emotional neglect	Educational neglect	Supervisory neglect
		Mean (SD)	Mean (SD)	Mean (SD)	Mean (SD)
Mother's employmentb					
Employed	1869	23.181(4.836)***	23.014(3.889)**	30.311(7.575)***	30.844(6.134)**
Unemployed	175	24.754(5.512)	23.817(4.010)	32.663(7.978)	32.08(6.22)
Mother's health problemsb					
No	1107	22.956(4.861)**	23.026(3.863)	29.778(7.354)***	30.668(6.041)
Yes	937	23.62(4.943)	23.132(3.941)	31.135(7.817)	31.189(6.233)
Higher education of motherb					
No	1129	23.905(4.972)***	23.524(3.828)***	31.975(7.649)***	31.281(6.278)**
Yes	915	22.588(4.747)	22.539(3.932)	28.708(7.228)	30.542(5.966)
Higher education of fatherb					
No	973	23.94(5.012)***	23.562(3.983)***	31.786(7.735)***	31.292(6.213)*
Yes	1071	22.748(4.757)	22.648(3.782)	29.356(7.361)	30.64(6.078)
Family structurea					
Nuclear family	1483	23.469(4.947)***	23.161(3.868)	30.353(7.640)	30.811(6.142)
Single family	16	21.063(5.053)	22.250(3.550)	28.563(7.090)	28.938(5.053)
Family with three generation	545	22.963(4.800)†	22.895(4.010)	31.006(7.628)	31.389(6.180)

aOne-way ANOVA. bIndependent-samples t test. *p < 0.05, **p < 0.01, ***p < 0.001.
†p < 0.05 , ††p < 0.01 (post-hoc test and compare the factor with the first one).

5.3.2 THE CORRELATES OF NEGLECT SUBTYPES

Table 2 shows the association between the studied factors and neglect subtypes. After simultaneous adjustment for the child's and family characteristics and the school factor, the results show that boys experienced less physical neglect than girls (B=-0.437; 95% CI -0.704 to -0.171; p=0.001). Children with physical health issues experience more emotional (B=0.713; 95% CI 0.339 to 1.086; p<0.001) and educational (B=1.152; 95% CI 0.423 to 1.882; p=0.002) neglect. On the other hand, children with cognitive impairment suffered from more severe physical (B=0.628; 95% CI 0.130 to 1.125; p=0.013), emotional (B=1.454; 95% CI 1.062,1.847; p<0.001), educational (B=1.393; 95% CI 0.628,2.159; p=0.001) and supervisory (B=0.865; 95% CI 0.234,1.496; p=0.007) neglect. Younger mothers (B=-0.014; 95% CI -0.133,-0.001; p=0.049) and unemployed mothers (B=0.857; 95% CI 0.079 to 1.636; p=0.031) were likely to have children with more severe educational neglect. Children of mothers with college education experience less physical (B=-0.642; 95% CI -1.197,-0.087; p=0.024), emotional (B=-0.589; 95% CI -1.027,-0.151; p=0.008), and educational neglect (B=-2.456; 95% CI-3.31,-1.601; p<0.001). At the same time, those whose fathers were college graduates experienced less emotional neglect (B=-0.531; 95% CI -0.962,-0.100; p=0.016). Additionally, children in families with three generations suffered from less physical neglect (B=0.055; 95% CI -1.039 to -0.135; p=0.023) when compared families with the nuclear family.

5.4 DISCUSSION

The present study sheds light on the regional situation of child neglect in China. Noteworthy contributions of the study include the provision of a regional data on the prevalence of neglect subtypes in one-child families of China for first time in English. The rates of child neglect subtypes vary across different regions in China probably due to the different policy implementation and socio-economic levels, with a lower level of physical and educational neglect and a higher level of emotional neglect in this study. In addition to child's gender, physical health issues, cognitive impairment, maternal age, employment, health problems, and parental education levels were associated with child neglect, which are similar to factors reported in other studies [10,26-31]. We also found that the 4-2-1 three-generation family structure was correlates of neglect which is unique in one child families of China.

TABLE 2: Associations between child and family characteristics and neglect subtypes (n=2044)

Characteristica	Physical neglect Estimates (95% CI)	Emotional neglect Estimates (95% CI)	Educational neglect Estimates (95% CI)	Supervisory neglect Estimates (95% CI)
Children's age	0.322(-0.101,0.745)	-0.007(-0.217,0.204)	0.206(-0.132,0.544)	
Gender				
Girls	Ref	Ref	Ref	Ref
Boys	-0.437(-0.704, -0.171)**	0.312(-0.021,0.646)	-0.142(-0.793,0.508)	0.288(-0.248,0.824)
Physical health issues				
No	Ref	Ref	Ref	Ref
Yes	0.339(-0.135,0.813)	0.713(0.339,1.086)***	1.152(0.423,1.882)**	0.555(-0.046,1.157)
Cognitive impairment				
No	Ref	Ref	Ref	Ref
Yes	0.628(1.125,0.130)*	1.454(1.062, 1.847)***	1.393(0.628,2.159)***	0.865(0.234,1.496)**
Mother's age	0.002(-0.075,0.079)	0.01(-0.051,0.07)	-0.014(-0.133,-0.001,)*	-0.015(-0.113,0.083)
Mother's employment				
Empolyed	Ref	Ref	Ref	Ref
Unemployed	1.028(-0.169,2.225)	0.411(-0.203,1.025)	0.857(0.079,1.636)*	0.97(-0.018,1.957)
Mother's health problems				
No	Ref	Ref	Ref	Ref
Yes	0.213(-0.232,0.658)	-0.168(-0.519,0.183)	0.559(-0.126,1.244)	0.336(-0.229,0.901)
Higher education of mother				
No	Ref	Ref	Ref	Ref
Yes	-0.642(-1.197,-0.087)*	-0.589(-1.027,-0.151)**	-2.456(-3.31,-1.601)***	-0.392(-1.096,0.313)

Childhood Adversity and Developmental Effects

TABLE 2: *Cont.*

Characteristica	Physical neglect Estimates (95% CI)	Emotional neglect Estimates (95% CI)	Educational neglect Estimates (95% CI)	Supervisory neglect Estimates (95% CI)
Higher education of father				
No	Ref	Ref	Ref	Ref
Yes	-0.509(-1.055,0.037)	-0.531(-0.962,-0.100)*	-0.688(-1.528,0.152)	-0.272(-0.965,0.420)
Family structure				
Nuclear family	Ref	Ref	Ref	Ref
Single family	-0.046(-4.932,0.002)	-0.387(-3.337,0.436)	-0.029(-6.203,1.159)	-0.031(-0.110,0.087)
Family with three generations	-0.055(-1.093,-0.135)*	-0.040(-0.732,0.023)	-0.022(-0.350,1.123)	0.038(-5.176,0.893)
Family per-capita income of every month	0.001(-0001,0.002)	0.011(-0.005,0.021)	0.012(-0.003,0.025)	0.009(-0.002,0.010)

aAdjusted for children's school and other variables in the table using linear regression model (method for variable entry and removal: "enter").
*p < 0.05, **p < 0.01, ***p < 0.001.

Our study showed a lower prevalence of child any neglect (32.2%) than that of Yinchuan City in western China (50.0%) using the same age bands of SCNUC [20]. However, it is difficult to compare the rates of neglect with those from other studies in China, because most of these studies were conducted in different age groups [15-19]. Supervisory neglect (20.3%) was the most prevalent type of child neglect, followed by emotional (15.2%), physical (11.1%), and educational (6.0%) neglect in one child family of Suzhou City using SCNUC. The study in Yinchuan City [20] also showed that the prevalence of educational neglect (18.1%) was much higher than that of Suzhou City. However, emotional neglect (8.8%) in that study was lower than that of the present study. Yinchuan city is located in ethnic minority autonomous regions (the one-child policy has not been implemented in minority population). Yinchuan city is located in ethnic minority autonomous regions (the one-child families policy has not been implemented in the minority population). The results confirm our expectation that the prevalence of neglect in one-child families were lower than that in multi-child families which is similar to the Zhang's finding in Guangzhou [19]. Child neglect subtypes may vary across different regions due to the different policy implementation and socio-economic levels in China. The results also partly confirm our hypothesis that parents in one-child families would pay greater attention to their child's education at the cost of providing them with inadequate emotional environment.

Making a cross-country comparison of neglect prevalence is difficult, because different cultures may have standard and definition of parental behaviors and practices [22], which may directly influence the type of child neglect prevalent in a particular society. In the US, educational neglect of children was reported as the most frequent child neglect subtype, followed by physical and emotional neglect [2,3]. In the current study, educational neglect was the least child neglect subtype, while emotional neglect were the second most common child neglect subtype.

Demographic characteristics that are frequently found to be associated with child neglect, such as children's sex, parental education, family economic status and structure, were also observed to be associated with child neglect in the present study. A study from Israel found that male children were more commonly involved in all types of maltreatment (including the neglect and abuse) [26]. However, the data from 50 states in United

States in 1999 showed no difference between boys and girls with regards to child neglect [32]. In the current study however, we observed that that boys were less likely to experience physical neglect than girls. Our finding may indicate that the traditional culture in which boys tend to be more valued than girls seems to be still operating in Chinese one-child families. Additionally, our results show that children with physical problems were more likely to suffer emotional neglect. Another study reveals that 68% of children with body dysmorphic disorder were emotionally neglected [27]. Our finding that the child's cognitive impairment is associated with all neglect subtypes might imply that parents from one-child families consider the child as their "only hope", thereby putting greater expectations to make them culturally desirable. A previous study has indicates that children with physical and cognitive disabilities were 3.4 times more likely to be maltreated than their nondisabled peers [28].

Our results also indicate that children of younger mothers experienced more educational neglect. Maternal age was a strong determinant of all types of child's maltreatment in a previous study [29]. This may be related to the level of experience and maturity of younger mothers, resulting in the failure to provide adequate education for their child. Furthermore, the association between maternal education and physical, emotional and educational neglect corroborates previous findings [29], which suggest that less educated mothers may more likely neglect their children than those with higher education. Mothers with limited educational background may inadequately meet their child's basic needs in proper manners. Our results also show that maternal unemployment was associated with educational neglect. It has also been reported that neglectful mothers were less likely to report ever having been employed [30]. Fathers with higher education were only associated with emotional neglect in this study. Recently, studies from western countries emphasize the importance of paternal characteristics in the care of children, showing that father's characteristics are of significance to childhood neglect [10]. However, in Chinese culture, it is the mother who is responsible more for taking care of her child, including providing emotional and educational support, and our results suggest that maternal factors are associated with more neglect subtypes than those of fathers.

Finally, we did not observe any association between family income and any neglect subtype. This is consistent with other studies [10,31], in which poverty was not associated with physical neglect. Children in 4-2-1 three-generation family experience less physical neglect than those in families with three generations. The 4-2-1 three-generation families with only one child is common (26.7% of this sample) in China according to Chinese culture and under the one-child policy. Compared with the nuclear family, there are much more adults (two parents and four grandparents) who may take care of their "only child", making child experience less physical neglect.

5.5 CONCLUSION

In conclusion, child supervisory and emotional neglect were the most common, while educational neglect was the least common among these neglect subtypes in one-child families in China. The rates of child neglect vary across the different regions of China, with a lower level of physical and educational neglect and a higher level of emotional neglect in this study. This deserves greater attention. In support of previous reports, a child's gender, physical health status, maternal age, employment, parental education level are important correlates of different subtypes of child neglect in China. The family structure which is unique in one-child family was also associated with neglect. As one of the studies in this Chinese context, this study provides a good platform for future intervention programs in one-child families in preventing child neglect, by taking into account the observed family socio-demographic characteristics as potential factors of child neglect. Further studies are also required to investigate whether intervention programs that target improving these elements would improve the childhood neglect and its subtypes.

However, in the present study, the majority of children (above 99.9%) were the "only child" in their family under the rigorous birth control policy in urban area of Mainland China. Therefore, it is impossible to make the comparison between the one-child families and families with more than one child. It is also difficult to compare the neglect prevalence between different nations because there would be no assurance that the instruments we used in this sample would be useful for cross-cultural comparisons. Moreover, the unwillingness to disclose neglectful behavior on the part of the parents may cause the social desirability response bias and underreport children's experiences of neglect.

REFERENCES

1. Hildyard KL, Wolfe DA: Child neglect: developmental issues and outcomes. Child Abuse Negl 2002, 26(6–7):679-695.
2. Sedlak AJ, Broadhurst DD: The Third National Incidence Study of Child Abuse and Neglect. Report to Congress. Washington, DC: US Department of Health and Human Services, Administration for Children and Families; 1996.
3. Sedlak AJ, Mettenburg J, Basena M, Petta I, McPherson K, Greene A, Li S: Fourth National Incidence Study of Child Abuse and Neglect. Report to Congress. Washington, DC: Administration for Children and Families, US Department of Health and Human Services; 2010.
4. Straus MA, Savage SA: Neglectful behavior by parents in the life history of university students in 17 countries and its relation to violence against dating partners. Child Maltreat 2005, 10:124-135.
5. Hussey JM, Chang JJ, Kotch JB: Child maltreatment in the United States: prevalence, risk factors, and adolescent health consequences. Pediatrics 2006, 118:933-942.
6. May-Chahal C, Cawson P: Measuring child maltreatment in the United Kingdom: a study of the prevalence of child abuse and neglect. Child Abuse Negl 2005, 29:969-984.
7. Zuravin SJ: Unplanned pregnancies, family planning problems, and child maltreatment. Fam Relat 1987, 36:135-139.
8. Lee BJ, George RM: Poverty, early childbearing, and child maltreatment: a multinomial analysis. Child Youth Serv Rev 1999, 21:755-780.
9. Chaffin M, Kelleher K, Hollenberg J: Onset of physical abuse and neglect: psychiatric, substance abuse, and social risk factors from prospective community data. Child Abuse Negl 1996, 20:191-203.
10. Carter V, Myers MR: Exploring the risks of substantiated physical neglect related to poverty and parental characteristics: a national sample. Child Youth Serv Rev 2007, 29:110-121.
11. Crosse S, Kaye E, Ratnofsky A: A Report on the Maltreatment of Children with Disabilities. National Center on Child Abuse and Neglect: Washington, DC; 1993.
12. Yang ZN, Pan JP: Collaborative Group for Survey of Neglect in 3–6 Years Old Urban Children. Investigation and analysis of child neglect in 1163 urban children aged 3–6 years. Zhonghua Er Ke Za Zhi 2003, 41:501-507. (in Chinese)

13. Liu CY, Zhong ZO, Pan JP, Wang YX, Yang B, Diao J, Zhang M, Zhong Y: Status of neglect among urban primary and secondary school students in western China. Chin J Public Health 2012, 28:734-736. (in Chinese)

14. Pan JP, Wand F, Zhang H, Zhang SJ, Yang ZN, Wang WQ, Cao CH, Luo SS, Li M: The status of child neglect for children aged 3-17 years in China. Chin J Prev Med 2012, 46:28-32. (in Chinese)

15. Hua J, Wu Y, Gu GY, Chen J, Zhu LL: An investigation of 370 cases of child neglect. Chin J Clin Rehabil 2006, 10:172-175. (in Chinese)

16. Liu CX, Luo XB, Jiang XJ, Chen GX, Zhang DN, Xiang GY, Zhao YF, Zhang XM, Wu QL, Chao X, Jing Z: Investigation and analysis of neglect of children aged 3-6 years in urban areas, Wuhan. Matern Child Health Care of China 2009, 24:65-67. (in Chinese)

17. Liu CX, Jiang XJ, luo XB, Chen GX, Zhang DN, Xiang GY, Zhao YF, Zhang XM, Wu QL, Chao X, Zhang J: Analysis of the influencing factors of child neglect in Wuhan. Chin J Sch Health 2010, 31:307-308. (in Chinese)

18. Pan JP, Yang ZN, Ren XH, Wang GX, Wang HS, Xi WP, Pan YQ, Ma BJ, Shi SH, Yi HN, Fu P, Gu GX, Jing J, Yu H, Li QZ, Li W, Yu GQ, Ma X, Wu YL, Li HQ: Study on the current situation and influential factors of child neglect. Zhonghua Liu Xing Bing Xue Za Zhi 2005, 26(4):258-264. (in Chinese)

19. Zhang DM, Zheng HY, Zou YH: Cross-sectional study on the influencing factors of neglect among children aged 3-6 in Guangzhou City. Chin J Sch Health 2006, 27:947-948.

20. Duan ZX: Analysis of the Current Situation and Influential Factors of Elementary and High School Students Neglect in the Urban Disticts of Yinchuan City. Ningxia Medical University; 2010. Thesis for application of master's degree

21. Kane P, Choi CY: China's one child family policy. BMJ 1999, 319:992-994.

22. Jing J (Ed): Feeding China's Little Emperors: Food, Children, and Social Change. Stanford: Stanford University Press; 2000. in Chinese

23. Festini F, de Martino M: Twenty five years of the one-child families policy in China. J Epidemiol Community Health 2004, 58:358-359.

24. Wei Y: Women's Education in China. Higher Education Press; 1995. In Chinese

25. Yi M: Study on education of children from one-child families Academy of Sciences. 2009. http://www.psychinese.com/Study/Html/2009/07/2007.html, The Institute of Psychology Chinese

26. Benbenishty R, Zeira A, Astor RA: Children's reports of emotional, physical and sexual maltreatment by educational staff in Israel. Child Abuse Negl 2002, 26:763-782.

27. Didie ER, Tortolani CC, Pope CG, Menard W, Fay C, Phillips KA, Tortolani A: Childhood abuse and neglect in body dysmorphic disorder. Child Abuse Negl 2006, 30:1105-1115.

28. Sullivan PM, Knutson JF: Maltreatment and disabilities: a population-based epidemiological study. Child Abuse Negl 2000, 24:1257-1273.

29. Lee BJ, George RM: Poverty, early childbearing, and child maltreatment: a multinomial analysis. Child Youth Serv Rev 1999, 21:755-780.

　　　　　　　　　　　　　　Childhood Adversity and Developmental Effects

30. Zuravin S, Starr RH: Psychosocial characteristics of mothers of physically abused and neglected children: do they differ by race? In Black Family Violence: Current Research and Theory Edited by Hampton RL. 1991, 37-71.
31. Drake B, Pandey S: Understanding the relationship between neighborhood poverty and child maltreatment. Child Abuse Negl 1996, 20:1003-1018.
32. U.S. Department of Health and Human Services, Administration for Children and Families, Administration on Children, Youth and Families, Children's Bureau: Child Maltreatment 2011. 2012. http://www.acf.hhs.gov/programs/cb/research-data-technology/statistics-research/child-maltreatment

PART II

CHILDREN AND WAR

CHAPTER 6

TRANSGENERATIONAL CONSEQUENCES OF PTSD: RISK FACTORS FOR THE MENTAL HEALTH OF CHILDREN WHOSE MOTHERS HAVE BEEN EXPOSED TO THE RWANDAN GENOCIDE

MARIA ROTH, FRANK NEUNER, AND THOMAS ELBERT

6.1 BACKGROUND

An association between parental exposure to traumatic stress and children's psychological mental health has been suggested by studies that examined families of veterans. Children of fathers suffering from PTSD showed significantly greater internalized and externalized behavioural problems [1,2], somatic complaints [3] and higher scores of depression [3,4] and anxiety [5] compared to children of veterans who did not present with a mental disorder. An increased level of behavioural disorders, anxiety and depressive symptoms, as well as posttraumatic stress were also confirmed in offspring of tortured refugee parents suffering from PTSD compared to children with non-traumatized parents [6,7]. Although chil-

Transgenerational Consequences of Ptsd: Risk Factors for the Mental Health of Children Whose Mothers Have Been Exposed to the Rwandan Genocide. © Roth M, Neuner F, and Elbert T. ; licensee BioMed Central Ltd. International Journal of Mental Health Systems, 8,12 (2014), doi:10.1186/1752-4458-8-12. Licensed under Creative Commons Attribution 2.0 Generic License, http://creativecommons.org/licenses/by/2.0/.

dren whose mothers and fathers both had PTSD show significantly higher scores of psychopathology such as anxiety and depression, the mother's anxiety was identified as the most frequent and important predictor of children's mental health status [4].

While systematic studies assessing the association of children's mental health status and parental traumatization are rare, a number of examinations focused on changes and impairments in the family system that stem from parental PTSD and trauma exposure. Several studies have found general impairments of child rearing capacities, such as inadequate emotional reaction [8], impaired parent–child relationship [9,10], disrupted communication styles [11] or physical punishment [12-15]. Physical punishment was often explained by hyperarousal symptoms or substance abuse in the parents [16] and was associated with combat experiences in veteran fathers and behavioural problems in the offspring [17]. Similar to the dose effect for vulnerability to PTSD [18,19], a dose effect for the consequences of family violence was found: children who experienced more maltreatment in childhood demonstrated more severe behavioural problems and higher rates of delinquency [20,21].

The possibility of trans-generational consequences of parental PTSD arises specifically in populations with a high prevalence of PTSD. Rwanda represents a nation with a history of numerous massacres, most devastating the genocide from 1994, killing 10% of Rwanda's almost 8 million inhabitants, mostly Tutsi and oppositional Hutu [22]. Consequently, even more than a decade after this massive violent event, the prevalence of PTSD has remained exceptionally high in Rwanda [23-26]. Additionally, the Rwandan population has to cope with experiences of massive bereavement and extensive social disruption [27]. Furthermore, Rwandans still remain in a state of hyper-vigilance and trepidation, worrying that genocidal hostilities between the two ethnic groups might occur again [23]. We suppose that existing parental psychopathology resulting from past traumatic experiences and current worries about reoccurrence of the slaughters have a substantial psychological impact on the mental health of the offspring generation. Therefore, the examination of trans-generational consequences of parental PTSD in Rwanda may help to better understand the long-term impact of parental PTSD for children's mental health, and to detect individual, familial and social needs in order to support a psychological healing process in Rwandan society.

The goal of the present study was to investigate the consequences of maternal traumatization for their children in a non-clinical setting. There is an on-going debate about trans-generational trauma transmission due to methodological flaws in studies investigating this phenomenon, such as the use of non-random samples, the lack of a control group, small sample sizes, unclear definition of "traumatized parent" or the use of non-valid instruments for assessment [28,29]. In this study, we defined a mother as being "traumatized" when she fulfilled the DSM-IV diagnosis of PTSD. This definition is one possibility for specification of the psychological state in the maternal generation and will allow comparison of the mental health of children according to the PTSD diagnosis of the mother. We aimed to examine the effects of maternal PTSD on the mental health of their school-aged children (born two years after the genocide) in the Rwandan context, including symptoms of depression, anxiety, and aggressive and antisocial behaviour. We focused our assessment on the mothers and not the fathers as studies support an increased impact of maternal anxiety on the children's mental health status compared to the father's mental wellbeing. In line with previous theory on transmission mechanisms we assumed that family violence constitutes an important impact on children's mental health. We predicted that (1) children's psychopathology is associated with the number of maternal traumatic experiences; (2) children's psychopathology is associated with maternal PTSD; (3) children's psychopathology is associated with the experiences of maternal violence at home; (4) children's experiences of maternal violence at home are associated with maternal PTSD; and (5) children's experiences of maternal violence at home are associated with maternal experiences of family violence during her childhood. See Figure 1 for a diagram, which visualizes our hypothesis.

6.1 METHODS

6.1.1 SAMPLE

From April to May 2008 we conducted a community-based survey in Rwanda in order to examine trans-generational consequences of PTSD in mothers who experienced the genocide in 1994 and their 12-year-old children who were born two years after the genocide.

The recruitment took place in three different public schools in Butare in southern Rwanda. In order to achieve a wide range of socio-economic status in the examined families, recruitment took place at two rural, and one urban schools. These schools were chosen according to logistical aspects. Participants were recruited according to the following criteria: (1) children were 12 years old, (2) children lived together with the biological mother, and (3) the mothers had lived in Rwanda during the time of the genocide in 1994. We have focused on biological mothers in order to exclude additional confounding variables, which may derive from the experienced stress in the children with the change of the most important caretaker. Approval for the survey was obtained from the National Institute of Statistics of Rwanda and the Ethical Review Board of the University of Konstanz, Germany.

6.1.1.1 SAMPLE CHARACTERISTICS

A convenient sample of 125 women and their 12-year old children (41 boys and 84 girls) were interviewed. The mothers were on average 42 years old (range=24 – 59), 52% (n=65) were married, 36% (n=45) were widows, 10% (n=13) divorced or separated, and 3 mothers (2%) were single. The children reported having on average 3 to 4 siblings (mean=3.87; range=0 – 10; SD=2.04) and attended the second (9%, n=11), third (31%, n=28), forth (40%, n=50) and fifth grade (20%, n=25). The majority of the households owned a house/hut (81%, n=101), 72% (n=90) possessed a vegetable garden and 8% (n=10) grew crops in order to sell them. A global index of the household's economical status was created in order to test its association with children's psychopathology. The index was calculated by adding up the z-standardized scores of family possession, such as furniture (table, beds, carpets), books, cooking pots, bikes, motorbikes, television, radio, property (house, garden), farm animals, children's possession (number of toys and cloths), as well as the family's average monthly income and the number of meals per day of mothers and children. This indicator ranged from -15 to 27.

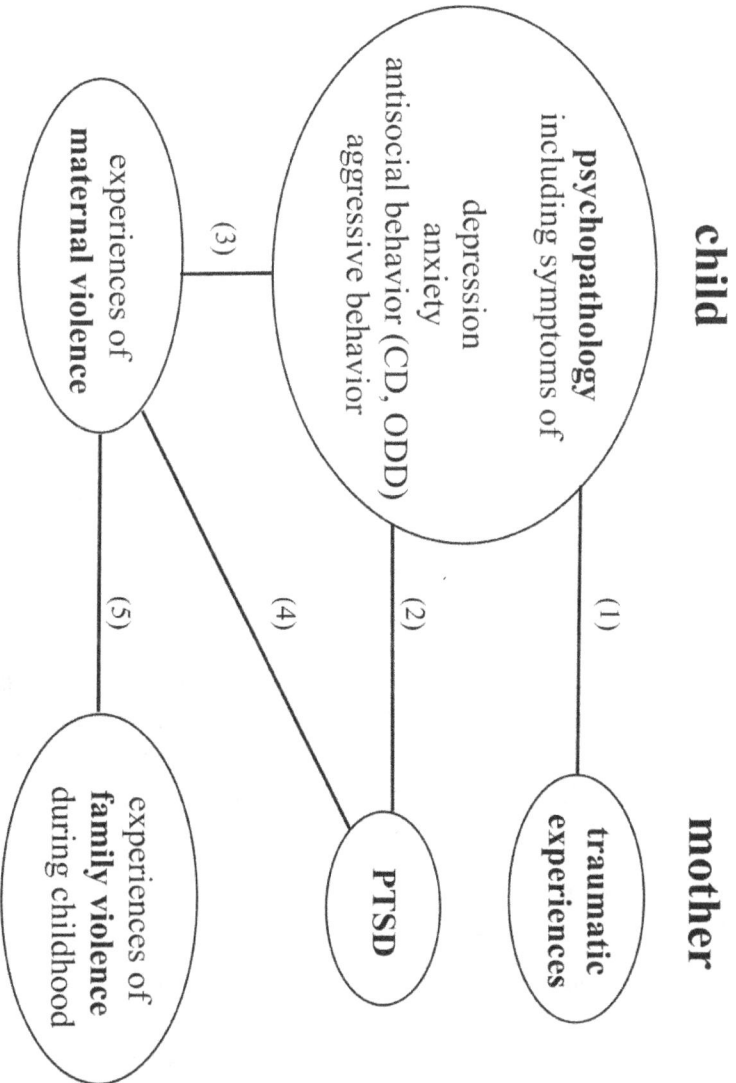

FIGURE 1: Diagram illustrating the causal pathways of the tested hypothesis.

6.1.2 PROCEDURE

The children were selected by the directors and teachers of the schools according to the inclusion criteria. The teachers first informed the children to ask their mother to come to the school on the following day, where they were informed about the investigation by the interviewers. After the mothers have agreed to take part in the study, the interviewers accompanied them to their home, where the interview took place. None of the mothers refused to participate in the study. At home in a confidential setting a more detailed explanation of the study was given. If the mother still agreed to participate, she signed a written informed consent for herself and for her child. Each mother was interviewed at her home and subsequently the child was investigated at the school. Six of the originally-recruited 131 mother-child pairs were excluded since the interviewed caregiver turned out not to be the biological mother of the child. The interviews were conducted by a group of six Rwandan B.A.-level psychologists recruited from the National University of Rwanda in Butare. The interviewers had been previously trained by colleagues from the University of Konstanz in conducting interviews in order to assess PTSD, depression, anxiety and suicidal tendencies [30]. The interviewers attended an additional training for this study. The training lasted eight days and included theoretical sessions on the purpose of the study, concepts of trauma, the questionnaires, and role-plays conducting the survey. The project coordinator closely supervised the interviewers during the whole period of data collection.

6.1.3 INSTRUMENTS

All instruments were available in their original English version. A professional translator created a Kinyarwanda language version of all questionnaires. The translated version was back-translated and discussed with the local interviewers in the training and corrected where necessary. All diagnostic instruments were administered as clinical interviews.

6.1.3.1 ASSESSMENT OF TRAUMATIC EXPERIENCES AND PTSD IN MOTHERS

An extensive list of 25 items adapted to the Rwandan genocide was used to assess traumatic experiences and included items such as "Have you seen dead or mutilated bodies?" or "Were you forced to hide under dead bodies?" [26]. The Posttraumatic Symptom Scale – Interview Version (PSS-I) [31] was chosen to assess symptoms of PTSD in the mothers. The severity of a symptom is rated on the basis of its frequency, intensity/severity, or both. The diagnosis for PTSD was created regarding the DSM-IV criteria. The procedure has been validated in East African settings [32,33] and both instruments have been used by our team in the Rwandan context previously. Symptoms of trauma can be observed in any culture [34]. The debate about a nosological entity of PTSD in various cultures is not relevant in this context. "PTSD" in this case simply refers to a set of symptoms that obviously can be observed in any culture.

6.1.3.2 ASSESSMENT OF DEPRESSION, ANXIETY, ANTISOCIAL AND AGGRESSIVE BEHAVIOUR IN CHILDREN

With the help of a subscale of the Hopkins Symptom Checklist (HSCL) [32,35], children's anxiety symptoms occurring during the last seven days were assessed. Symptom intensity was rated on a scale from 0 ("not at all") to 3 ("extreme"). Symptoms of depression were acquired with the 10-item short version of the Children's Depression Inventory (CDI-S), an instrument appropriate for children aged 7 to 17 years [36]. Each item is composed in three different questions, which represent the different intensity of a symptom and scores from 0 to 2. For example: (0) "I am sad once in a while"; (1) "I am sad many times" and (2) "I am sad all the times". The summed score of the items ranges from 0 to 20, with a higher score representing greater depressive symptoms. Clinical relevant symptom scores of anxiety and depression were identified according to cut-off recommendations [36,37].

Conduct Disorder (CD) and Oppositional Deviant Disorder (ODD) were assessed with the help of the Sections P and Q of the M.I.N.I. Kid [38]. In order to apply the instrument adequately in the Rwandan context, the cut-off for normal—not normal for every item was discussed in the training with the local interviewers. Additionally, a short version of the aggression scale by Buss and Perry [39] was used to assess aggressive behaviour in the children. It contains 16 items, with subscales for physical and verbal aggression, anger and hostility. Answers range from 0 ("I don't agree") to 4 ("I totally agree"), with a higher score representing higher aggressive behaviour and attitude, with a maximum sum score of 64.

A score of children's psychopathology was generated by adding up the standardized (z-transformed) symptom sum scores for anxiety, depression, aggression, ODD, and CD. The score ranged from -5.7 to 9.8 $(0 \pm SD\ 3.33)$.

6.1.3.3 ASSESSMENT OF FAMILY VIOLENCE IN MOTHERS AND CHILDREN

The Checklist of Family Violence (CFV) [40] was used to assess experiences of family violence in mothers and children. The 36 item checklist defines familial violence as exposure to neglect, physical, emotional or sexual violence as well as witnessing violence between other family members. Additional items at the end of the checklist asked about the identification of the perpetrators of the violence (multiple possible answers), and the interviewee's subjective psychological experience upon experiencing the violence, e.g., "Did you feel helpless?" The participant could answer the questions with "yes" or "no". In this study we asked the child to identify every event where the mother was the perpetrator of the violent act. The questionnaire had previously been used in other cultural contexts with children [41,42]. With the help of this checklist, the mothers' previously experienced family violence during childhood and the children's experienced family violence at home was assessed. For mothers, two items were added to assess intimate partner violence and conjugal rape.

6.1.4 STATISTICAL ANALYSIS

For calculations of Pearson correlations and t-test the following symptom and event sum scores were used: maternal traumatic event types, children's psychopathology, children's experienced maternal violence. Group differences were calculated according to maternal PTSD diagnosis, defined according to DSM-IV criteria. In order to explore how different factors contribute to the psychopathology of the children and children's experienced maternal violence at home, we calculated hierarchical linear regression model. These included potential confounding covariates, such as children's gender, number of siblings, educational level (current school grade) and the family's economical status, all of which did not significantly explain any further variance in children's psychopathology. A priori there was insufficient knowledge to reasonably estimate the effect size, and the usefulness of post-hoc power analyses remains controversial [43]. As Hoenig and Heisey [44] show, all post-hoc power analyses suffer from what is called the "power approach paradox". Given that post-hoc power is a function of the p-value attained, it adds little information. Analyses were performed with SPSS version 21 for Macintosh.

6.2 RESULTS

6.2.1 VIOLENT EXPERIENCES AND PTSD IN MOTHERS

On the CFV nearly all mothers (n = 124, 99%) reported having experienced at least one event of familial violence during their childhood, counting 6.9 different event types on average (range = 0 – 18; SD = 4.71). Most of the mothers (n = 117, 94%) had been exposed to physical violence, 59% (n = 74) to emotional violence, 28% (n = 47) had experienced events of neglect, and 86% (n = 107) had witnessed violent acts committed against a family member. The most frequently mentioned items were being hit with an object (n = 116, 92%), having witnessed a family member being hit with an object (n = 96, 77%), and being slapped on the body, arms or legs (n = 64, 51%). More than every other mother (n = 67, 55%) who was married once in her life reported experiences of physical violence by her husband; 27% (n=33) had been forced into sexual intercourse.

With the help of the adapted event list, the mothers reported an average of 11 different types of traumatic events in their lives (range=4 – 21, SD=4.31) of which 7 (range=1 – 17, SD=4.28) were associated with the genocide in 1994. The most frequently-reported traumatic event types were being forced to flee (n=119, 95%), having witnessed an armed attack (n=109, 87%), and needing to hide (n=86, 69%). The majority (60%) of the traumatic events, which were described as the worst experience, occurred during the genocide in 1994. According to DSM-IV criteria, every fourth mother (n=43, 26%) fulfilled the diagnosis for PTSD, assessed with the PSS-I.

6.2.2 EXPERIENCES OF FAMILY VIOLENCE IN CHILDREN

Questioned with the CFV, nearly all children (n=124, 99%) reported at least one incident of family violence, counting 5.6 different violent events on average (range=0 – 15, SD=3.15). Physical violence was experienced by 99% (n=124), emotional violence by 50% (n=62), neglect by 22% (n=27) and 81% (n=101) witnessed family violence against another family member. The children identified the mother (n=114, 91%), and older siblings (n=62, 50%) as perpetrators of family violence. 39% (n=47) of those children whose mother had ever been married, reported the father as perpetrator of family violence. Most frequently reported items were being hit with an object (n=123, 98%), having witnessed a family member being hit with an object (n=91, 73%), or slapped on the body, arms or legs (n=77, 62%). The majority of the children felt terrified (55%) or helpless (51%) because of family violence.

6.2.3 CHILDREN'S PSYCHOPATHOLOGY IN ASSOCIATION WITH MATERNAL TRAUMATIC EXPERIENCES

According to our first hypothesis, we examined Pearson correlation coefficient. Our results did not indicate an association between the number of traumatic events experienced by the mother and children's psychopathology ($r=-.01$, $p=.94$). See Figure 2 for a scatter plot. This result does not support our first hypothesis.

6.2.4 CHILDREN'S PSYCHOPATHOLOGY IN ASSOCIATION WITH MATERNAL PTSD

Our second hypothesis represents the core hypothesis of our study. No group differences were identified in children's psychopathology, comparing children of mothers with PTSD diagnosis and mothers without PTSD diagnosis ($t=-1.61$, $p=.11$). See Figure 3 for a box plot. The result does not support our second hypothesis.

6.2.5 CHILDREN'S PSYCHOPATHOLOGY IN ASSOCIATION WITH MATERNAL VIOLENCE AT HOME

According to our third hypothesis, we examined whether children's experienced maternal violence at home is associated with children's psychopathology. This was confirmed by a significant Pearson correlation of $r=.59$ ($p<.001$). Figure 4 shows a scatter plot for this association.

6.2.6 LINEAR REGRESSION MODEL WITH CHILDREN'S PSYCHOPATHOLOGY AS DEPENDENT VARIABLE

In a hierarchical linear regression model we predicted in the first step that the children's experienced maternal violence at home would explain a significant portion of the variance of the children's psychopathology. With the addition of mother's PTSD symptom score in the second step, the explained variance increased from 16% to 18% ($F(2, 121)=14.4$, $p<.001$). Contrary to the amount of children's experienced maternal violence at home ($r=.41$, $p<.001$) mother's PTSD symptom ($r=.18$, $p=.06$) score did not achieve a significant contribution. Other confounding variables did not significantly explain any further variance in children's psychopathology.

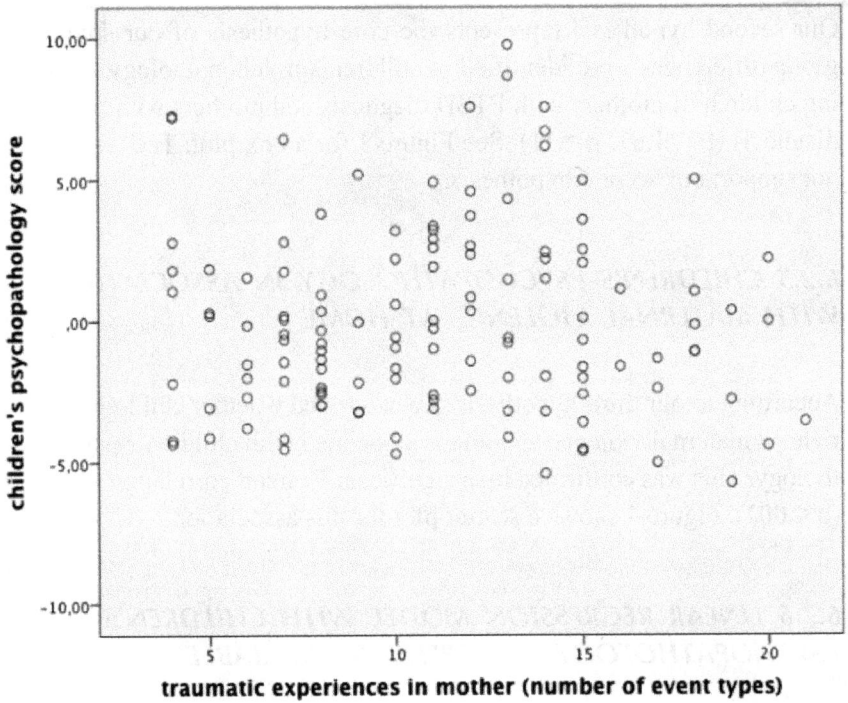

FIGURE 2: Scatter plot and Pearson correlation coefficient for maternal traumatic experiences (number of event types) and children's psychopathology score. r=-.01, p=.94.

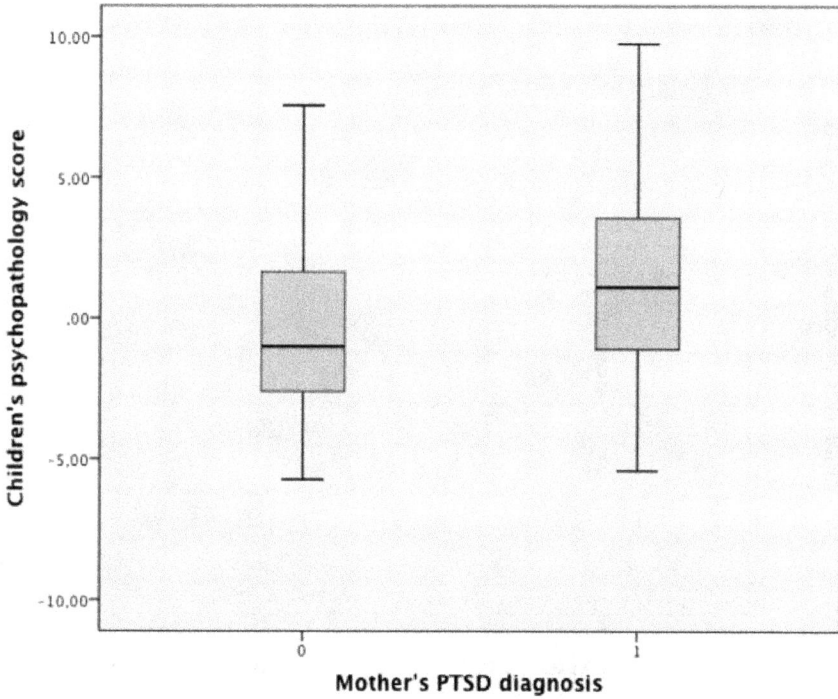

FIGURE 3: Boxplot and t-values of t-Test for independent samples with maternal PTSD diagnosis as group variable and children's psychopathology score as dependent variable. t=- 1.61, p=.11.

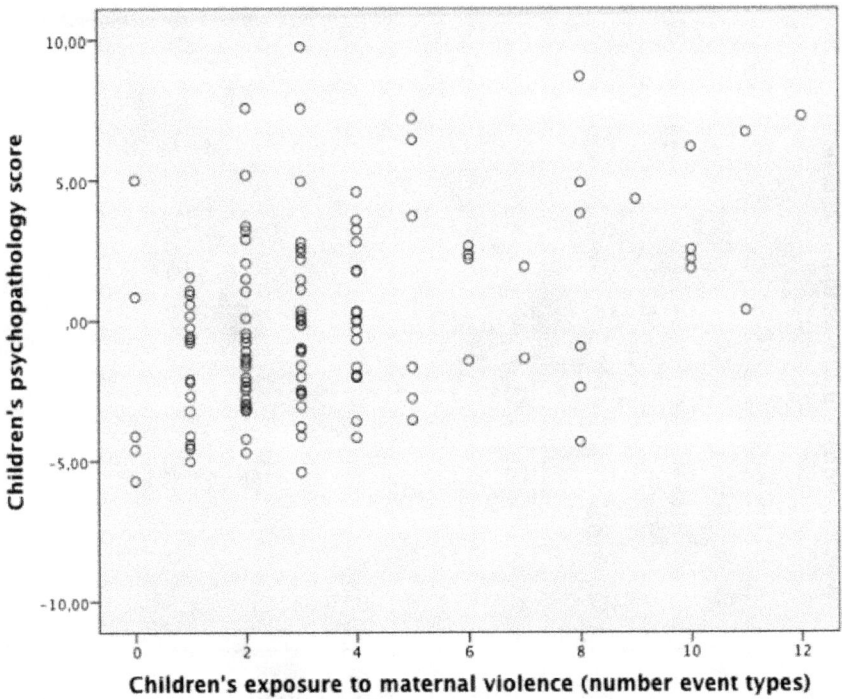

FIGURE 4: Scatter plot and Pearson correlation coefficient for children's exposure to maternal violence (number of event types) and children's psychopathology score. r=.59, p<.001.

For further details, see Table 1. These results support our third hypothesis and confute again our second hypothesis.

TABLE 1: Hierarchical regression model with children's psychopathology score as dependent variable and children's reported family violence conducted by the mother (event sum score) and maternal PTSD symptom score as independent variables

	B	SE B	Beta	Zero-order correlation	p-value
First step					
Constant	-1.84	0.46			< .001
Children's experienced maternal violence at home (sum score of event types)	0.53	0.12	.41	.41	< .001
Second step					
Constant	- 2.44	.55			
Children's experienced maternal violence at home (sum score of event types)	.52	.11	.40	.41	< .001
Mother's PTSD symptom score	.05	.03	.16	.18	.06

Note: Full model's adjusted $R = .18$; $F (2,121) = 14.40, p < .001$.

6.2.7 MATERNAL VIOLENCE AT HOME IN ASSOCIATION WITH MATERNAL PTSD

No group differences were identified in children's experienced maternal violence at home, comparing children of mothers with PTSD diagnosis and mothers without PTSD diagnosis ($t = -.73$, $p = .46$). This result confutes our fourth hypothesis. Figure 5 shows the respective box plot.

6.2.8 MATERNAL VIOLENCE AT HOME IN ASSOCIATION WITH MOTHERS OWN EXPERIENCES OF FAMILY VIOLENCE DURING HER CHILDHOOD

According to our fifth hypothesis, assuming an association between maternal used violence at home and experiences of family violence during her own childhood, we calculated a Pearson correlation coefficient and identified a significant association ($r = .23$, $p < .01$). Figure 6 shows the scatter plot. This result confirms our fifth hypothesis.

6.2.9 LINEAR REGRESSION MODEL WITH MATERNAL VIOLENCE AT HOME AS DEPENDENT VARIABLE

In order to understand how these two factors contribute simultaneously to the occurrence of children's experiences of maternal violence at home, we calculated a hierarchical linear regression model using the maternal violence experienced by the children at home (sum score of event types) as dependent variable. In the first step we predicted that mother's own exposure to family violence in her childhood (sum score of event types) explains a significant portion of the variance of maternal violence at home. With the addition of mother's PTSD symptom score in the second step, 4% of the variance (F $(2, 121) = 3.6$, $p < .05$) could be explained. Other variables, including gender, number of siblings, educational level (current school grade) and family's economical status did not explain any further variance in child psychopathology. For further details, see Table 2. These results contradict our forth hypothesis and support our fifth hypothesis.

6.3 DISCUSSION

Our study did not identify an association between children's psychopathology and maternal traumatic experiences and maternal PTSD. Instead, a significant relationship was found for children's psychopathology and their experienced maternal violence at home. Furthermore, maternal violence against the child was related not only with child's psychopathology but also with mother's own experiences of family violence during their childhood.

The key finding of our study constitutes the missing association of children's psychopathology with maternal PTSD. This result contradicts the common assumption of a direct trans-generational trauma transmission. Obviously, a large-scale catastrophe as the genocide is not necessarily specifically damaging the mental health of the children of survivors. This finding is supported by a number of review articles [45-47] and a comprehensive meta analysis on studies of children of Holocaust survivors, which states that the influence of the parents' traumatic experiences on their children seems to be restricted to studies on clinical participants and cannot be viewed as a common phenomenon [48]. It has also been suggested that the behaviour of Holocaust survivor offspring may not be clinically distinctive but rather a specific personality configuration [47].

The second important finding of our study is that family violence affects the mental health and wellbeing of the children as opposed to maternal PTSD. Our study indicated an association of children's mental health status and their experienced amount of maternal violence at home. Likewise, a number of studies identified psychological consequences of family violence for the children, such as anxiety [49,50], antisocial behaviour [21,51], aggression [52], and depression [51]. The explicit negative psychological consequences of family violence for a child may be explained not only by the experience of a frightening situation in an intimate familial environment but also by the absence of an adequate reaction from the parent and the lack of a trustful relationship. Abusive child-rearing practices do not provide a model for the child to develop adequate emotional regulation mechanisms and interpersonal relatedness, which in turn may lead to antisocial behaviour, such as aggression or Oppositional Deviant Disorder [53,54].

Furthermore, our study shows that children's experienced maternal violence is not associated with maternal PTSD symptom profiles, but with the amount of the mother's own experiences of family violence during her childhood. This sheds a new light on studies that reported that parental PTSD is associated with child rearing practices such as family violence [12-15]. It may not be the PTSD of the mother per se, but the family violence experienced by the mother, that increases the risk for both, the PTSD in the mother and the exposure to family violence in the child. This would support the notion of a Cycle of Violence and fit with results of a series of other studies [52,55-57]. The social learning process was assumed to represent the mechanisms behind this association [58]. Abusive parents represent a role model for abusive behaviour and the moral assurance that such behaviour is appropriate; furthermore, children growing up in an abusive household lack alternative non-violent conflict resolution strategies [59]. As family violence is mostly embedded in other family pathology [60], we assume additional risk factors, such as a violent social environment or lack of family support, which are not assessed in our study but which latently explain the impact of family violence on the children's mental health. Furthermore, it is important to consider that child maltreatment cannot be separated from other disadvantaging factors, such as high everyday life stress or social isolation [60,61].

We conclude that the simple conclusion "a mother with PTSD has children with more symptoms of anxiety, depression and aggressive behaviour" is not valid. At the same time there might be symptoms and mechanisms that are not assessable with the methodology of quantitative measurements. Figure 7 illustrates the different levels that need to be considered when investigating trans-generational trauma transmission.

Some limitations warrant mention. As our data collection was cross-sectional, the cause and effect of relationships cannot be demonstrated. It is therefore possible that family violence was as much a cause as an effect of children's symptoms. Furthermore, data about the father were not assessed, which might have explained additional variance of children's symptoms.

The assessment of children's psychopathology was also limited. Children's anxiety symptoms were measured with the HSCL-25, an instrument designed for adults. Assessment of antisocial behaviour should use different sources of information, such as a parent or a teacher, providing different aspects of a child's functioning [64,65]. As the amount of children's stressful experiences might also represent an important predictor of children's mental wellbeing, children's traumatic experiences should have been assessed. Similarly, school and community violence may play an important role and should be assessed as well.

Still, this study explores the assumption of transgenerational trauma transmission and provides systematic information on two generations, assessed by local B.A. psychologists in a conflict region. All participants are from the same cultural background and allow a comparison of the children of traumatized and non-traumatized mothers. Furthermore, family violence was not just reported by the parents but the children, assuming less bias through social desirability.

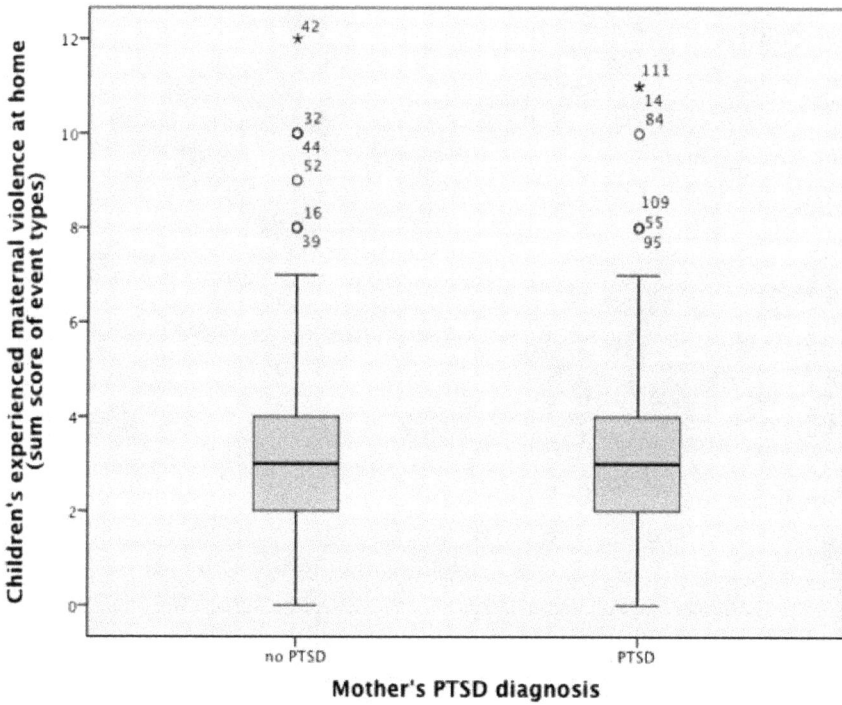

FIGURE 5: Boxplot and t-values of t-Test for independent samples with maternal PTSD diagnosis as group variable and children's experienced maternal violence at home (sum score of event types) as dependent variable. t = - .73, p = .46.

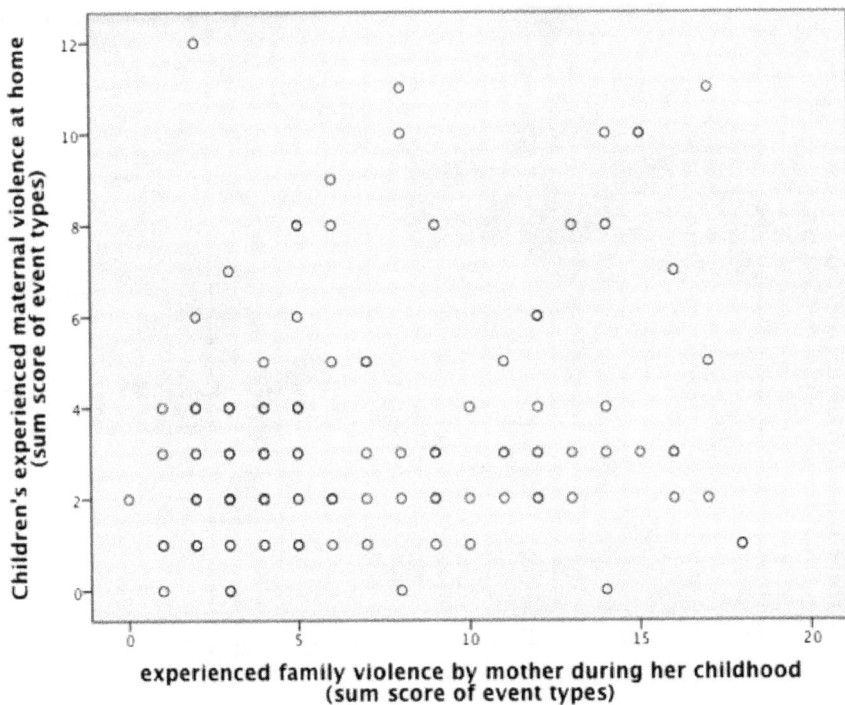

FIGURE 6: Scatter plot and Pearson correlation coefficient for children's experienced maternal violence at home (sum score of event types) and family violence experienced by the mother during her own childhood (sum score of event types). r = .23, p < .01.

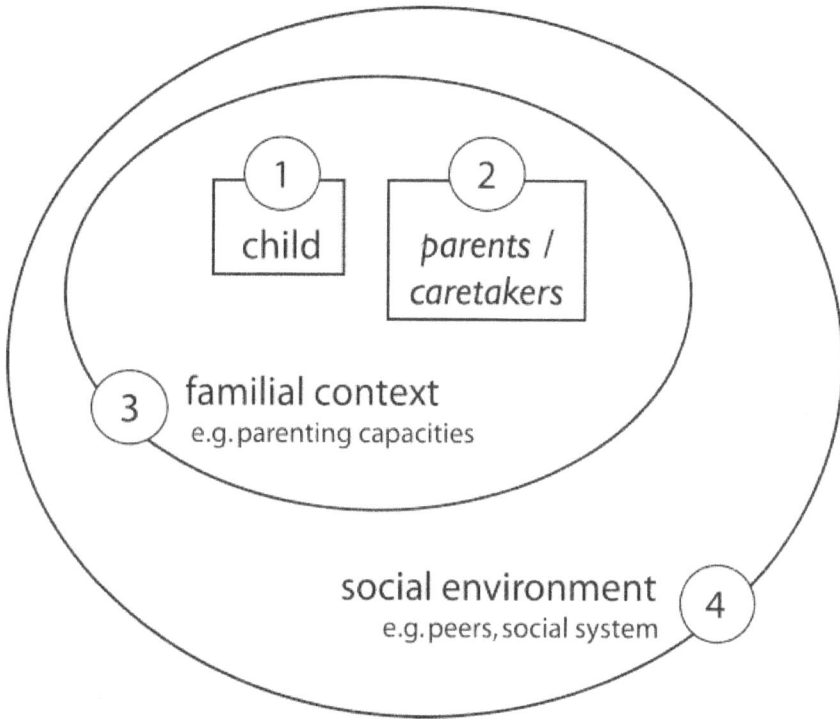

FIGURE 7: Diagram illustrating the complexities of the investigation. The child with all its strength and vulnerabilities should be the central focus of the investigation. Depending on various factors, e.g. genetic predispositions, children may be strengthened or may become more vulnerable by the knowledge of parental traumatic experiences [45]. Second, the mental health status of the child's caretakers – in most cases the biological parents – must be considered. The parent itself may not only show PTSD in consequence of the experience of traumatic events, but develop also other pathological behaviour patterns, symptoms (e.g. complex traumatization, depression), or specific personality configurations. It must be considered that people exposed to traumatic events don't only report negative consequences in their lives. Some show positive changes in their self-perception, in their perception of others and in the objective and meaning of their lives [62,63]. Third, the family context in general must be respected. It implies the impact of siblings or general family functioning, such as patterns of communication, parenting capacity, stress-coping strategies or general worldviews [45,46]. Fourth, the influence of the extra familial support system needs to be taken into account, such as peers, level of integration in the community, which may e.g. concern prejudice of minorities such as refugees or immigrants [45].

The Rwandan women were highly motivated to participate in the study. In our experience, people in resource-poor regions are often highly motivated to make their voice "heard". Usually most people want to contribute to a survey that may document daily living conditions and daily sufferings.

TABLE 2: Hierarchical regression model with children's experienced maternal violence at home (sum score of event types) as dependent variable and mother's experienced family violence during her own childhood (sum score of event types) and maternal PTSD symptom score as independent variables

	B	SE B	Beta	Zero-order correlation	p-value
First step					
Constant	2.61	0.40			< .001
Mother's experienced family violence during childhood (sum score of event types)	0.13	0.05	.23	.23	< .01
Second step					
Constant	2.69	.42			< .001
Mother's experienced family violence during childhood (sum score of event types)	.14	.06	.27	.23	< .05
Mother's PTSD symptom score	- .02	.03	- .07	.07	.51

Note: Full model's adjusted $R = .04$; $F (2,121) = 3.61$, $p < .05$.

6.4 CONCLUSIONS

Our findings do not support the common hypothesis of trans-generational consequences of parental PTSD, as we did not find evidence for an association between maternal PTSD and children's mental health. Instead, experiences of maternal violence represented the most important predictor of children's depression, anxiety, aggression and antisocial behaviour. In contrast with the theory on trans-generational trauma transmission children's experience of maternal violence at home was not associated with maternal PTSD but with mothers own experience of family violence during her own childhood, a result that is in congruence with the hypothesis of the Cycle of Violence. We assume that there might be far more factors affecting child rearing practices and children's mental wellbeing, factors which concern general life and not exclusively PTSD and traumatic past. Our results call for attention for the psychological consequences of family violence in African countries, where family violence is socially accepted as a fundamental child rearing practice. Additionally, our results confirm studies of other countries in the world investigating the Cycle of Violence and therefore support generalization of this hypothesis. The devastating consequences of family violence can be taught to parents, together with alternative child-rearing practices.

REFERENCES

1. Caselli LT, Motta RW: The effect of PTSD and combat level on Vietnam veterans' perceptions of child behavior and marital adjustment. J Clin Psychol 1995, 51(1):4-12.
2. Jordan BK, Marmar CR, Fairbank JA, Schlenger WE, Kulka RA, Hough RL, Weiss DS: Problems in families of male Vietnam veterans with posttraumatic stress disorder. J Consult Clin Psychol 1992, 60(6):916-926.
3. Zalihic A, Zalihic D, Pivic G: Influence of posttraumatic stress disorder of the fathers on other family members. Bosn J Basic Med Sci 2008, 8(1):20-26.
4. Al-Turkait FA, Ohaeri JU: Psychopathological status, behavior problems, and family adjustment of Kuwaiti children whose fathers were involved in the first gulf war. Child Adolesc Psychiatry Ment Health 2008, 2(1):12.
5. Dansby VS, Marinelli RP: Adolescent children of Vietnam combat veteran fathers: a population at risk. J Adolesc 1999, 22:329-340.
6. Daud A, Skoglund E, Rydelius P-A: Children in families of torture victims: transgenerational transmission of parents' traumatic experiences to their children. Int J Soc Welf 2005, 14:23-32.
7. Sack WH, Clarke GN, Seeley J: Posttraumatic stress disorder across two generations of Cambodian refugees. J Am Acad Child Adolesc Psychiatry 1995, 34(9):1160-1166.
8. Davidson AC, Mellor DJ: The adjustment of children of Australian Vietnam veterans: is there evidence for the transgenerational transmission of the effects of war-related trauma? Aust N Z J Psychiatry 2001, 35(3):345-351.

9.   Lauterbach D, Bak C, Reiland S, Mason S, Lute MR, Earls L: Quality of parental relationships among persons with a lifetime history of posttraumatic stress disorder. J Trauma Stress 2007, 20(2):161-172.

10. Ruscio AM, Weathers FW, King DW: Male war-zone veterans' perceived relationship with their children: the importance of emotional numbing. J Trauma Stress 2002, 15(5):351-357.

11. Schechter DS: Intergenerational communication of maternal violent trauma. In September 11: trauma and human bonds. Edited by Coates SW. New York: Analytic Press; 2003:115-142.

12. Banyard VL, Williams LM, Siegel JA: The impact of complex trauma and depression on parenting: an exploration of mediating risk and protective factors. Child Maltreat 2003, 8(4):334-349.

13. Cohen LR, Hien DA, Batchelder S: The impact of cumulative maternal trauma and diagnosis on parenting behavior. Child Maltreat 2008, 13(1):27-38.

14. Kellermann NPF: Perceived parental rearing behavior in children of holocaust survivors. Isr J Psychiatry Relat Sci 2001, 38(1):58-68.

15. Margolin G, Gordis EB: Children's exposure to violence in the family and community. Am Psychol Soc 2004, 13(4):152-155.

16. Taft CT, Kaloupek DG, Schumm JA, Marshall AD, Panuzio J, King DW, Keane TM: Posttraumatic stress disorder symptoms, physiological reactivity, alcohol problems, and aggression among military veterans. J Abnorm Psychol 2007, 116(3):498-507.

17. Harkness LL: Transgenerational transmission of war-related trauma. In International handbook of traumatic stress syndrome. Edited by Wilson JP, Raphael B. New York: Plenum Press; 1993:635-543.

18. Mollica RF, McInnes K, Poole C, Tor S: Dose-effect relationships of trauma to symptoms of depression and post-traumatic stress disorder among Cambodian survivors of mass violence. Br J Psychiatry 1998, 173:482-488.

19. Neuner F, Schauer M, Karunakara U, Klaschik C, Robert C, Elbert T: Psychological trauma and evidence for enhanced vulnerability for posttraumatic stress disorder through previous trauma among West Nile refugees. BMC Psychiatry 2004, 4:34.

20. Grych JH, Jouriles EN, Swank PR, McDonald R, Norwood WD: Patterns of adjustment among children of battered women. J Consult Clin Psychol 2000, 68(1):84-94.

21. Smith C, Thornberry TP: The relationship between childhood maltreatment and adolescent involvement in delinquency. Criminology 1995, 33(4):451-481.

22. Prunier G: Africa's world war. Congo, the Rwandan genocide, and the making of a continental catastrophe. Oxford: Oxford Univ. Press; 2009.

23. Hagengimana A, Hinton D, Bird B, Pollack M, Pitman RK: Somatic panic-attack equivalents in a community sample of Rwandan widows who survived the 1994 genocide. Psychiatry Res 2003, 117(1):1-9.

24. Onyut LP, Neuner F, Schauer E, Ertl V, Odenwald M, Schauer M, Elbert T: The Nakivale Camp mental health project: building local competency for psychological assistance to traumatised refugees. Interv 2004, 2(2):90-107.

25. Pham PN, Weinstein HM, Longman T: Trauma and PTSD symptoms in Rwanda - implications for attitidues toward justice and reconciliation. JAMA 2004, 292(5):602-612.

26. Schaal S, Elbert T: Ten years after the genocide: trauma confrontation and posttraumatic stress in Rwandan adolescents. J Trauma Stress 2006, 19(1):95-105.
27. Bolton P, Neugebauer R, Ndogoni L: Prevalence of depression in rural Rwanda based on symptom and functional criteria. J Nerv Ment Dis 2002, 190(9):631-637.
28. Ancharoff MR, Munroe JF, Fisher LM: The legacy of combat trauma – Clinical implications of intergenerational transmission. In International handbook of multigenerational legacies of trauma. Edited by Danieli Y. New York: Plenum Press; 257-27.
29. Baranowski A, Young M, Johnson-Douglas S, Williams-Keeler L, McCarrey M: PTSD Transmission: a review of secondary traumatization in holocaust survivors families. Can Psychol 1998, 39(4):247-265.
30. Schaal S, Jacob N, Dusingizemungu J-P, Elbert T: Rates and risks for prolonged grief disorder in a sample of orphaned and widowed genocide survivors. BMC Psychiatry 2010, 10(55):9p.
31. Foa EB, Riggs DS, Dancu CV, Rothbaum BO: Reliability and validity of a brief instrument for assessing post-traumatic stress disorder. J Trauma Stress 1993, 6:459-473.
32. Ertl V, Pfeiffer A, Saile R, Schauer E, Elbert T, Neuner F: Validation of a mental health assessment in an African conflict population. Psychol Assess 2010, 22:318-324.
33. Odenwald M, Lingenfelder B, Schauer M, Neuner F, Rockstroh B, Hinkel H, Elbert T: Screening for posttraumatic stress disorder among somali ex-combatants: a validation study. Confl Heal 2007, 1:10.
34. Elbert T, Schauer M: Psychological trauma: burnt into memory. Nature 2002, 419:883.
35. Derogatis LR: Hopkins symptom checklist. In Encyclopedia of psychology. Volume 4. Edited by Kazdin AE. Washington D.C: American Psychological Association; 2000::157-158.
36. Sitarenios G, Kovacs M: Use of the children's depression inventory. In The use of psychological testing for treatment planning and outcome assessment. Edited by Maruish M. Mahwah: Lawrence Erlbaum Association Publishers; 1999:267-298.
37. Mollica RF, Wyshak G, de Marneffe D, Khuon F, Lavelle J: Indochinese versions of the Hopkins symptom checklist-25: a screening instrument for the psychiatric care of refugees. Am J Psychiatry 1987, 144(4):497-500.
38. Sheehan DV, Lecrubier MD, Sheehan KH, Amorim P, Janavs J, Weiller E, Hergueta T, Baker R, Dunbar GC: The Mini-International Neuropsychiatric Interview (M.I.N.I.): the development and validation of a structured diagnostic psychiatric interview for DSM-IV and ICD-10. J Clin Psychiatry 1998, 59(Suppl 20):22-33.
39. Buss AH, Perry M: The aggression questionnaire. J Pers Soc Psychol 1992, 63(3):452-459.
40. Ruf M, Elbert T: Posttraumatische Belastungsstörung im Kindes- und Jugendalter. In Lehrbuch der Verhaltenstherapie – Materialien für die Psychotherapie, Volume 4. Edited by Meinlschmidt G, Schneider S, Margraf J. Berlin, Heidelberg, New York, Tokio: Springer; 2012.
41. Catani C, Jacob N, Schauer E, Kohila M, Neuner F: Family violence, war, and natural disaster: a study of the effect of extreme stress on children's mental health in Sri Lanka. BMC Psychiatry 2008, 8(33):10.

42. Catani C, Schauer E, Elbert T, Missmahl I, Bette J-P, Neuner F: War trauma, child labor, and family violence: life adversitities and PTSD in a sample of school children in Kabul. J Trauma Stress 2009, 22(3):163-171.
43. Thomas L: Retrospective power analysis. Conserv Biol 1997, 11(1):276-280.
44. Hoenig JM, Heisey DM: The abuse of power. Am Stat 2001, 55(1):19-24.
45. Solkoff N: Children of survivors of the Nazi holocaust: a critial review of the literature. Am J Orthopsychiatry 1992, 62(3):342-358.
46. Solomon Z: Transgenerational effects of the holocaust - the Israeli research perspective. In International handbook of multigenerational legacies of trauma. Edited by Danieli Y. New York: Plenum Press; 1998:69-83.
47. Felsen I: Transgenerational transmission of effects of the holocaust – the North American research perspective. In International handbook of multigenerational legacies of trauma. Edited by Danieli Y. New York: Plenum Press; 1998:43-68.
48. Ijzendoorn VMH, Bakermans-Kranenburg MJ, Sagi-Schwartz A: Are children of holocaust survivors less well-adapted? - a meta-analytic investigation of secondary traumatization. J Trauma Stress 2003, 16(5):159-169.
49. Guille L: Men who batter and their children: an integrated review. Aggress Violent Behav 2004, 9(2):129-163.
50. McCloskey LA, Walker M: Posttraumatic stress in children exposed to family violence and single-event trauma. Am Acad Child Adolesc Psychiatry 2000, 39(1):108-115.
51. Zingraff MT, Leiter J, Myers KA, Johnson MC: Child maltreatment and youthful problem behavior. Criminology 1993, 31(2):173-202.
52. Weaver CM, Borkowski JG, Whitman TL: Violence breeds violence: childhood exposure and adolescent conduct problems. J Community Psychol 2008, 36(1):96-112.
53. Cook A, Spinazzola J, Ford J, Lanktree C, Blaustein M, DeRosa R, Cloitre M, Hubbard R, Kagan R, Liautaud J, Mallah K, Olafson E, van der Kolk B: Complex trauma in children and adolescents. Psychiatr Ann 2005, 35(5):390-398.
54. Goldsmith RE, Barlow MR, Freyd JJ: Knowing and not knowing about trauma: inplications for therapy. Psychotherapy: Theor Res Pract Training 2004, 41(4):448-463.
55. Pears KC, Capaldi DM: Intergenerational transmission of abuse: a two-generational prospective study of an at-risk sample. Child Abuse Negl 2001, 25(11):1439-1461.
56. Elbert T, Rockstroh B, Kolassa IT, Schauer M, Neuner F: The influence of organized violence and terror on brain and mind: a co-constructive perspective. In Lifespan development and the brain: the perspective of biocultural co-constructivism. Edited by Baltes PB, Reuter-Lorenz PA, Rösler F. New York: Cambridge University Press; 2006:326-349.
57. Kaufman J, Zigler E: Do abused children become abusive parents? Am J Orthopsychiatry 1987, 57(2):186-192.
58. Straus MA, Gelles RJ, Steinmetz SK: Behind closed doors - violence in the American family. New York: Anchor Press/Doubleday; 1980.
59. Schwartz JP, Hage SM, Bush I, Burns LK: Unhealthy parenting and potential mediators as contributing factors to future intimate violence: a review of literature. Trauma Violence Abuse 2006, 7(3):206-221.

60. Henning K, Leitenberg H, Coffey P, Turner T, Bennett R: Long-term psychological and social impact of witnessing physical conflict between parents. J Interpers Violence 1996, 11(1):35-51.

61. Buchanan A: Intergenerational child maltreatment. In International handbook of multigenerational legacies of trauma. Edited by Danieli Y. New York: Plenum Press; 1998:535-552.

62. Calhoun LG, Tedeschi RG (Eds): Handbook of posttraumatic growth: research and practice. Mahwah, NJ: Erlbaum; 2006.

63. Goldblatt H, Eisikovits Z: Role taking of youths in a family context: adolescents exposed to interparental violence. Am J Orthopsychiatry 2005, 75:644-657.

64. Bird HR: Epidemiology of childhood disorder in a cross-cultural context. J Child Psychol Psychiatry 1996, 37(1):35-49.

65. Granero R, Expeleta L, Domenech JM, de la Osa N: What single reports from children and parents aggregate to attention deficit-hyperactivity disorder and oppositional defiant disorder diagnoses in epidemiological studies. Eur Child Adolesc Psychiatry 2008, 17(6):352-364.

CHAPTER 7

THE INTERGENERATIONAL EFFECTS OF WAR ON THE HEALTH OF CHILDREN

DELAN DEVAKUMAR, MARION BIRCH, DAVID OSRIN, EGBERT SONDORP, AND JONATHAN C.K. WELLS

7.1 BACKGROUND

The adverse effects of war on the health of children have been well documented [1-4], but less well known is how exposure to violence can propagate effects across generations. Conflict causes injury, illness and breakdown in the structures that provide preventive, curative and ameliorative care. It has profound effects on society that form a permissive framework for the effects we describe. The mediators of loss are many, but include population displacement and breakdown of health services and schooling, on a background of economic decline and supply constraint. Figure 1 shows how these indirect effects are related with conflict and have a pervasive influence that reaches down to the next generation.

The Intergenerational Effects of War on the Health of Children. © *Devakumar D, Birch M, Osrin D, Sondorp E, and Wells JCK; licensee BioMed Central Ltd. BMC Medicine, 12,57 (2014), doi:10.1186/1741-7015-12-57. Licensed under Creative Commons Attribution 2.0 Generic License, http://creativecommons.org/licenses/by/2.0/.*

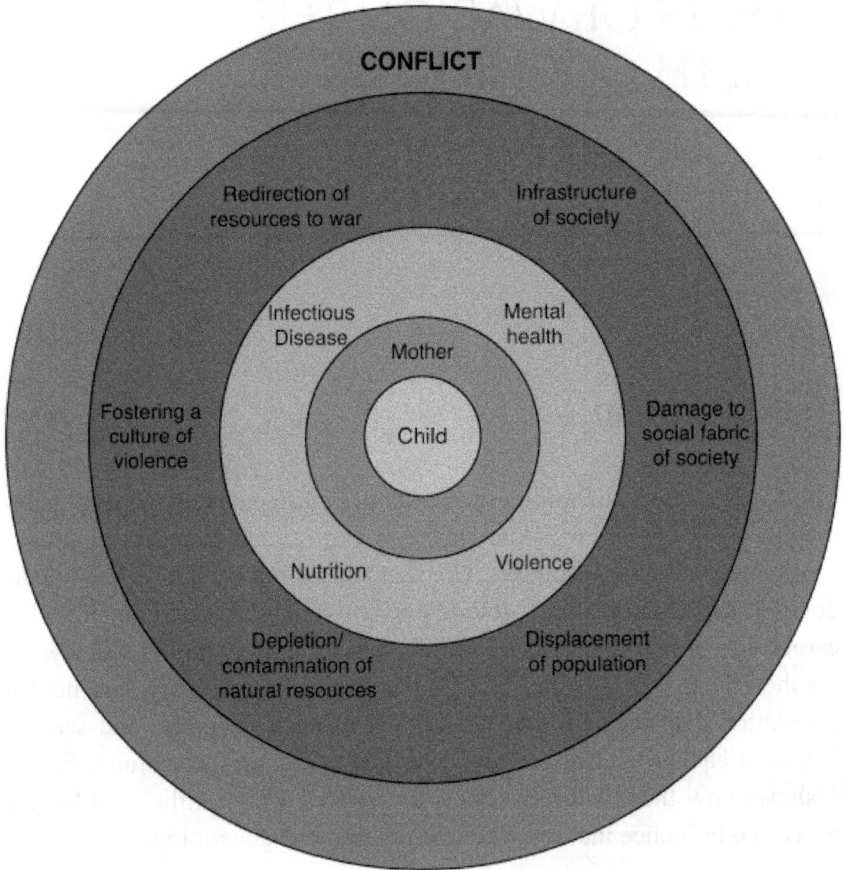

FIGURE 1: Direct effects (orange) and indirect effects- as described by Levy [5] - (brown) of conflict on mother and child.

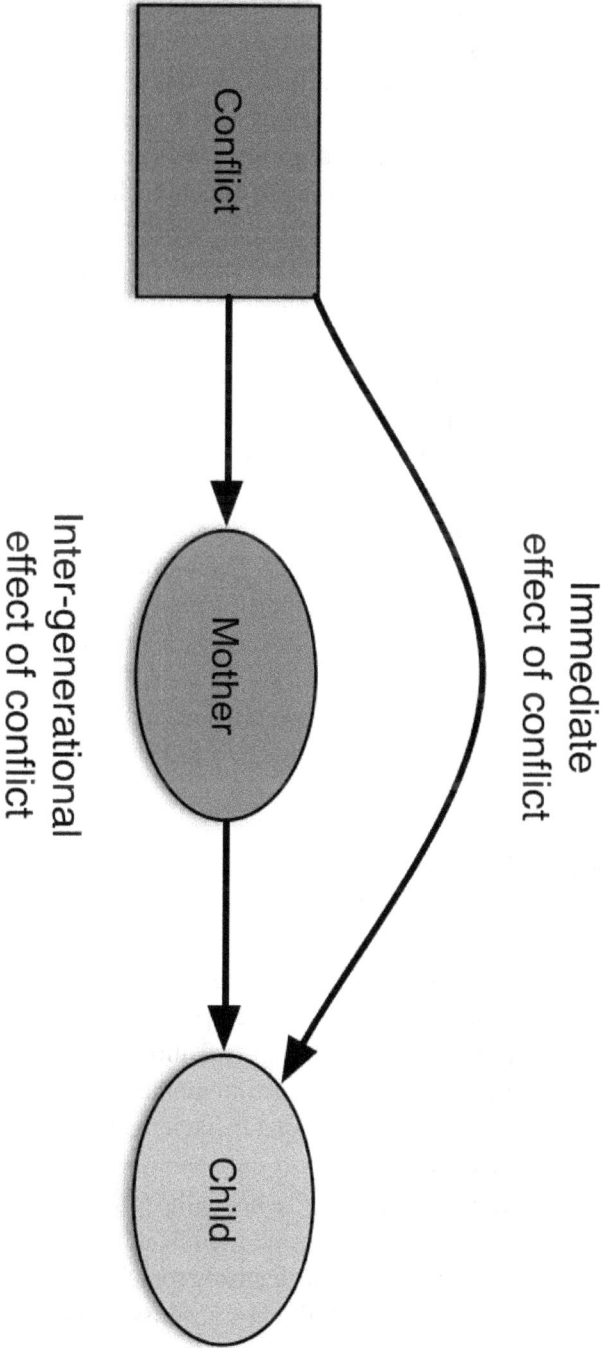

FIGURE 2: Immediate and intergenerational pathways through which conflict affects health.

Conflicts or wars, as defined by the World Health Organizationa, are becoming increasingly complex and involve multiple state and non-state actors [6]. In the last 20 years, conflicts have occurred in 37% of countries. In 2010, there were 30 armed conflicts involving at least one state, 26 non-state conflicts and 18 armed groups involved in one-sided violence [7,8]. It is difficult to know if the nature of conflict has changed, but recent wars provide evidence of the targeting of health facilities to weaken opposition forces and populations. Even schools are coming under attack, either deliberately or as collateral damage [9,10]. The association between conflict and poverty means that conflict-affected populations face major challenges after fighting has ceased. Economic development is affected by war in a number of ways that involve a combination of reduced output and increased expenditure, for example on security, and weakened systems of governance [11]. Most modern wars are short-lived and occur within national boundaries, but some, such as recent conflicts in South Sudan and Afghanistan, continue for decades [6]. Economic breakdown within conflict-afflicted states makes some countries among the poorest in the world, with approximately a third being defined as low-income (gross national income per capita <US$995). The World Bank judges that 80% of the world's 20 poorest countries have experienced major conflicts [12], and it has been estimated that conflict leads to a reduction in annual economic output of 1% to 3% [13,14].

That harms to health may be long-lasting within an individual's lifetime is well established, but there is increasing awareness that adverse effects may continue through intergenerational biological mechanisms. Our life course is sensitive to the environments in which we, our mothers, and grandmothers were conceived and grew up. Many exposures during development are mediated by maternal phenotype and reflect stresses to which mothers were originally exposed. Figure 2 illustrates how the effects of conflict can be mediated through harm to mothers. Recent work has emphasized that maternal physiology and behavior can buffer their offspring against ecological stresses, but this is only partial [15], such that exposure to conflict in one generation may potentially propagate adverse effects to subsequent generations. Epigenetic modifications to DNA expression have emerged as key biological mechanisms contributing to such intergenerational transmission, although direct transmission of epigenetic marks themselves appears rare and the primary impact of maternal phenotype is its influence on de novo marks in the offspring [16,17].

Greater awareness of the potential intergenerational consequences of conflict may lead to their early recognition and improved diagnosis and response. Documentation of the consequences will also add to the overall evidence on the effects of conflict on health, which may weigh more heavily in the balance when violent conflict is an option. A war may end, but its effects do not, and—in an example of intergenerational justice—those who resort to conflict may be held accountable for harms to the health of future generations. For this review, we searched the Medline, Psychinfo and Google Scholar databases using the search strategy described in Additional file 1. Only articles published in English were included, with no date restrictions. After finding an article, we considered the reference list or suggested articles for further evidence. This was supplemented by a general search of the literature on conflict/war and specific searches as questions arose. We summarize the evidence of how four features of conflict—violence, challenges to mental health, infections and malnutrition—may harm more than one generation, responding to emerging ideas about the epigenetic transmission of physiology [18,19]. We also discuss the multiplicative effects of ongoing conflict when hostilities are prolonged.

7.1.1 VIOLENCE

7.1.1.1 MATERNAL EXPOSURE

Violence is ubiquitous in war and pervades all strata of society, although its occurrence is probably underestimated [20-22]. The 20th century saw a secular trend toward a greater proportion of civilians affected, especially women and children [23]. It is estimated that up to 90% of war-related deaths in the last decade were civilian [5]. Conflict creates an ecosystem that persists, but is maladapted to peacetime, and its legacy is frequently an environment that fosters violence. Numbers of small arms remain for years, an example being the 1996 civil war in Guatemala, where rates of gun violence were greater after the war ended [24]. Similarly, increasing armed conflict in land disputes in East Africa is a consequence of prior cold war politics [25], and the 110 million landmines currently thought to remain in 68 countries [26] may lie dormant and harm civilians, both physically and mentally, decades after the original conflict [27,28].

Women are at particular risk of combatant and civilian injury, and of interpersonal violence. Violence against women increases in times of conflict through targeted acts, such as rape and domestic or intimate-partner violence. Sexual violence, including rape, assault, trafficking and prostitution, increases during many conflicts due to the breakdown of traditional safety structures [29]. It may also be used as an intentional strategy of domination, as reported in the former Yugoslavia and Rwanda [20,30]. The magnitude of sexual violence in conflict zones is difficult to quantify and tends to be under-reported [31]. Approximately half of a sample of women interviewed in Liberia had suffered sexual violence [21] and studies in East Timor and Kosovo showed increases to 23% and 15%, respectively, during conflict, compared to 10% and 2% in the post-conflict period [32,33]. A 2006 study from Lebanon suggested that domestic violence increased in areas where there was collective violence [22]. There are other, more complex, links. Substance use is associated with violence against women in non-conflict settings [34-36], although the evidence that it increases during conflict is limited. Clearer is the bidirectional association between violence and alcohol use [37-39].

7.1.1.2 INTERGENERATIONAL ASSOCIATIONS

A clear example of an intergenerational effect is stillbirth after physical violence against a pregnant woman [40,41]. During the siege of Sarajevo, perinatal mortality and morbidity more than doubled, and there was a rise in congenital malformations from 0.4% to 3% [42]. Violence is also associated with an increase in premature birth [43], as was seen during the war in Croatia in the early 1990s [44]. Similar to this in non-conflict settings, a meta-analysis on abuse during pregnancy showed an increased odds ratio for low birth weight of 1.4 (95% confidence interval (CI) 1.1 to 1.8) [45].

Sexual violence has both short- and long-term effects. In the short-term, it is associated with an increase in sexually transmitted diseases, the intergenerational effects of which are discussed later. Maman and colleagues relate HIV infection to violence through three mechanisms: 'forced or coercive sexual intercourse with an infected partner; by limiting women's ability to negotiate safe sexual behaviors; and finally by establishing a pattern of sexual risk taking among individuals assaulted in childhood and adolescence' [46]. Even when services are available, fear of violence may lead to a lower likelihood of accessing treatments to prevent mother-to-child transmission of HIV [47]. In the longer-term, sexual violence may affect parenting capacity. In Rwanda and Darfur, children born after rape have been shown to be at increased risk of neglect, abuse, malnutrition and abandonment [48]. Evidence from hospitals in South Kivu, Democratic Republic of Congo, suggests that when children are born from rape, their mothers are five times more likely to suffer isolation from the community (odds ratio (OR) 4.84; 95% CI 1.41 to 19.53) [49]. Children may also be victims of sexual violence [9], which may change its characteristics in times of conflict: a greater likelihood of gang rape was seen, for example, during conflict in the Democratic Republic of Congo. Sexual violence against children has profound effects on their mental and physical development, with implications for future pregnancies and relationships [50]. Mental illness, affecting a family's ability to function, can persist long after conflict has ended: symptom rates in those who had suffered from mass violence remained elevated for a decade after the Cambodian conflict [51]. More generally, exposure to violence has been associated with long-term effects on children's health, brain structure and neural function [52]. A violent environment may also have long-term effects on the maturational schedule. In Colombia, the secular decline in age at menarche accelerated during periods with high homicide rates, suggesting that psychosocial cues can alter the developmental trajectory [53].

Violence can affect family life, both economically and socially. Among Cambodian families in which one member was injured by a landmine, 61% were pushed into debt [54]. A study from Nicaragua found that women who suffered from abuse had 44% lower earnings [55]. Combat, death and displacement can also lead to the breakdown of family structures. Family members may shift roles, as was noted among women in Nepal who became combatants and replaced those lost during the conflict [56].

It is generally thought that experiencing violence as a child is a risk factor for committing child abuse as an adult [57]. There is some evidence that children who witnessed frightening events (for example, in the Spanish civil war of 1936) are 'more immune to the horrors of violence' [4]. This is especially so for child soldiers, who may experience dehumanizing conditions during a formative period, but there is a danger that maladaptive behaviors are passed on to the next generation. There are few long-term studies in this group. In a 16-year follow-up of child soldiers in Mozambique, men still suffered distress from their traumatic events, but there was no evidence that abusive relationships were passed on to their children [58].

Chemical or radioactive weapons can also damage future generations. While evidence of genetic effects of radiation on the children of survivors of atomic bombs is lacking, follow up studies have found evidence of severe learning difficulties and microcephaly in people exposed in utero. In utero exposure was also associated with decreased school performance and intelligence quotient (IQ) [59,60]. Case–control studies suggest that exposure of men to mustard gas in Iran and mineral contamination (particularly depleted uranium) in Iraq was associated with congenital abnormalities in their children [61,62].

7.1.2 MENTAL HEALTH

7.1.2.1 MATERNAL EXPOSURE

Mental health conditions are common during conflicts, and are augmented by the breakdown of mental health services and community coping strategies, and by increases in stress levels and drug and alcohol use [63]. The most common conditions are depression, anxiety and psychosomatic disorders, but the most widely studied in relation to conflict is post-traumatic stress disorder (PTSD). PTSD is common among combatants, and child soldiers are known to suffer from a much higher than average incidence of psychological disturbances and mental illness [64-67]. PTSD is also found in civilian populations in both women and children [68,69]. De Jong et al. showed that PTSD and anxiety disorder were the most common mental illnesses in all populations, and exposure to violence increased their likelihood in the four conflict zones of Algeria, Cambodia, Ethiopia and Palestine [70]. In Kabul, mothers of children under five were found to have an increase in prevalence of PTSD from 10% to 53% if they experienced at least one armed conflict event [71], and women living in conflict areas in Bosnia and Herzegovina showed a sevenfold increase over a control group in PTSD prevalence [72]. Importantly, mental health disorders also rise in those not directly exposed to violence. Women are generally affected more than men and strong associations exist between the mental health of mothers and their children [63]. For example, in Algeria poor quality of camp housing and the general difficulties of daily living were both associated with increased odds of PTSD (OR 1.8, 95% CI 1.3 to 2.5 and 1.6, 95% CI 1.1 to 2.4, respectively) [73]. Mental illness is also common in children. A systematic review in a long-term conflict in the Middle East showed that children do suffer from a wide range of mental disorders, such as PTSD, depression, anxiety, functional impairment, behavioral problems and Attention Deficit Hyperactivity Disorder [74].

The evidence on drug use in conflict is partial. Drug use increases in groups that have been displaced, especially among combatants and former combatants, for which it may be a way of coping with traumatic situations or memories [75-78]. Economic pressures and increased availability can lead to a rise or change in drug use. For example, the conflict and related drug policy in Afghanistan have been linked to an increase in intravenous opiate use [79,80]. The pattern of illicit drug use depends on the setting: opiates are more common in Pakistan and Afghanistan, while benzodiazepines are common in Bosnia-Herzegovina [81]. A study of khat (a substance that contains a psychoactive compound similar to amphetamines) in north-west Somalia showed that recent use among ex-combatants was 60%, compared with 28% in civilian war survivors and 18% in civilians with no experience of war. Psychotic symptoms were linked with age of onset of khat use and binge consumption. Rates of severe disability due to mental disorders (primarily psychosis) in males over the age of 12 increased in relation to their experience of war, with a prevalence of 16% in ex-combatants, 8% in civilian war survivors and only 3% in those with no experience of war [82].

7.1.2.2 INTERGENERATIONAL ASSOCIATIONS

While evidence is currently limited, parental trauma and psychosocial stress during conflict have been associated with adverse health effects in offspring, through both biological pathways (such as neuroendocrine and immune system modulation) and propagation of stressful social environments [83-85]. Stress may be a mediator through which parents transmit adverse effects to their children, in both conflict and non-conflict settings. In a large population-based cohort study, maternal stress during pregnancy was associated with a number of outcomes in children, including risk of infection and mental disorders [86]. Stress arising from childhood separation from parents during World War II was linked to long-term impairment in offspring social mobility and socio-economic position [87]. A study in people living near Gaza showed a strong association between maternal symptoms of depression, anxiety and PTSD, and PTSD symptoms in children. Avoidance behaviors in children were also associated with the degree of trauma exposure in the mother [88], similar to associations shown in animal studies [89]. Possible mechanisms include epigenetic changes in the hypothalamic-pituitary-adrenal axis (see Box 1) [90,91]. There is also some evidence that paternal PTSD can likewise lead to symptoms in children [92].

Stressful emotions can be passed from one generation to the next, but maternal buffering appears to provide an important damping effect, so that children are less affected than their parents. Children exhibit a form of resilience [93] that is related in turn to their mothers' wellbeing, quality of caregiving and environmental support [94], but traumatic events, such as those occurring in a conflict, may override this buffering. For example, children of Australian veterans of the Vietnam war were found to have a suicide rate three times that of the general community [95] and elevated rates of PTSD and other mental illness have been described in the offspring of Holocaust survivors [96-100]. Mothers, but not fathers, who were themselves offspring of Holocaust survivors had 'higher levels of psychological stress and less positive parenting', while in the grand-offspring generation, children had less positive self-perception and were said by their peers to show 'inferior emotional, instrumental, and social functioning' [101].

TABLE 1: Common reasons for an increase in infectious diseases during conflict

Causes of an increase in infectious disease	Mechanisms of action	Examples
Increased burden of disease	Migration leads to the migration of infectious diseases infecting new non-immune hosts.	The United Nations High Commissioner for Refugees (UNHCR) estimates that there are 15.3 million refugees and a further 26 million internally displaced persons (IDPs) worldwide [116]. Migration in camps that are overcrowded leads to situations where sanitation is not adequate and outbreaks can occur [117], a consideration going back nearly a century to the start of World War II [118].
	Breakdown of prevention programs leading to an increase in vector-borne diseases, such as malaria and trypanosomiasis.	Afghanistan has seen an increase in malaria after it had successfully controlled this disease in the 1970s and the Democratic Republic of Congo has had a rise in trypanosomiasis in conjunction with the rise in conflict [119]. Refugee camps in Sierra Leone and Guinea have both seen outbreaks of Lassa fever from the infestation of rodents [120,121].
Susceptibility of the population to infectious diseases	Reduced immunity from malnutrition, inadequate coverage of immunizations and the loss of herd immunity and the lack of innate immunity to unseen infective organisms.	Afghan refugees from a malaria-free region who fled to Pakistan in 1981 had a prevalence of malaria more than double that of the local population, and a ten-fold increase in burden over the following decade [122].
Breakdown of the healthcare system	Healthcare may be suspended or diminished [2] and funds diverted from it to armed forces or security actors. This leads to reduced detection and treatment of infectious diseases and potentially to increased rates of antibiotic resistance. This is combined with difficulties in accessing the services that do function due to fear of movement or breakdown of the transport networks.	The restriction of transport networks by the Maoist rebels in Nepal in 2005 held up the supply of vaccines, vitamin A, and deworming drugs to nearly 3.6 million Nepalese children [123].

TABLE 1: *Cont.*

Causes of an increase in infectious disease	Mechanisms of action	Examples
		Even normally functioning immunization programs can be affected by security concerns, the polio eradication program in Afghanistan being an example [124]. During the conflict in Bosnia and Herzegovina in the early 1990s, immunization rates fell from approximately 95% pre-conflict to around 30% [125]. Health facilities may themselves come under deliberate attack [8][124,126]. In the Nicaraguan conflict of the mid-1980s, approximately a quarter of the health facilities were partially or completely destroyed [54].
	Movement of healthcare workers	Healthcare workers often have the socioeconomic wherewithal to migrate during conflicts. A report from the International Committee of the Red Cross quotes an Iraqi Ministry of Health estimate that 18,000 of the country's 34,000 doctors left [127]. Liberia is thought to have seen a decrease from 237 to 20 doctors during recent conflict [128].

There is also evidence of intergenerational mental health effects in non-conflict settings, and these are likely to be exacerbated by conflict. A meta-analysis by Surkan et al. showed that maternal depression or depressive symptoms were associated with an OR of 1.5 (95% CI 1.2 to 1.8) for children being underweight and 1.4 (95% CI 1.2 to 1.7) for stunting. The reasons for this include poorer antenatal care, increased risk-taking behaviors and impaired maternal caring [102], with reduced or early cessation of breastfeeding as one possible mediator [103,104]. Maternal mental illness has also been linked to children's cognitive abilities [105]. In India, maternal common mental disorder was associated negatively with mental development in infants at six months of age [106] and, in Barbados, with cognitive outcomes [107]. The latter association persisted when assessed via a school entrance exam at 11 to 12 years of age [108].

There are several mechanisms whereby drug use may exert adverse intergenerational effects. Drug use by pregnant women can have transplacental effects or cause maternal ill-health or altered behavior. The manifestations may be acute - neonatal abstinence syndrome from opiate withdrawal, for example [109]—or lead to longer-term behavioral and cognitive changes [110]. Both drugs and alcohol are closely associated with mental illness in the user, which, in turn, can have detrimental effects on parenting ability and employment. The use of khat has been linked to mental illness, as well as affecting the reproductive system and being teratogenic [111]. However, the magnitude of the intergenerational effect of drug use associated with conflict remains to be established.

7.1.3 INFECTIOUS DISEASES AND HEALTH SYSTEMS

7.1.3.1 MATERNAL EXPOSURE

Mortality in women and children during conflicts is predominantly the result of conditions related indirectly to violence: infectious disease, malnutrition and complications of pregnancy [8]. With the exception of a few examples for which limitation of movement has appeared to prevent transmission [112], higher rates of infectious diseases, such as shigellosis and cholera, are common in conflict zones [113,114]. As described in Table 1, the major drivers are movement of people, infrastructural deterioration, and breakdown in prevention and treatment [115]. Migration of people, for example, both increases infectious disease burden and exposes unimmunized populations to new pathogens.

Sexual violence against women has been mentioned, and sexually transmitted infection rates may rise in conflict settings, as seen with syphilis and gonorrhea in the Second World War [129]. Increased infections are especially common in refugee or IDP populations [130], and in situations characterized by alcohol use and riskier sexual practices [75]. They have also been linked with psychiatric conditions and psychosocial factors. In war-affected Eastern Uganda, major depressive disorder and sexual torture were associated with high-risk sexual activities, which were themselves associated with HIV transmission [131]. It is thought that the conflict in Mozambique led to higher rates of syphilis in pregnant women, some of whom experienced sexual abuse and repeated rape while being held by the insurgents [132]. HIV rates may also be augmented by untreated sexually transmitted infections, lack of condoms, increased incidence of sex work and lack of health education [80,119]. An estimated 70% of Rwanda's rape survivors were infected with HIV [133].

7.1.3.2 INTERGENERATIONAL ASSOCIATIONS

Infectious diseases can affect subsequent generations through direct effects on pregnant women or through the effects of long-term morbidity on their future health, reproductive capacity and finances. The Spanish influenza outbreak, which resulted in up to 40 million deaths, is considered to have originated in and been exacerbated by the conditions of the First World War [134,135], and research on prenatal exposure suggests both long-term health costs, such as increased rates of cardiovascular disease and potentially increased disability, and economic penalties [136,137]. More specifically, infection in utero may lead to abortion or congenital malformations, and many infections can trigger premature birth. A fall in immunization rates may be accompanied by reductions in herd immunity: outbreaks of rubella, which can lead to severe congenital abnormalities, occurred during the conflict in Bosnia and Herzegovina [138]. Congenital infections lead to impaired cognitive development, respiratory and gastro-intestinal disease, and may leave children vulnerable to infections during their lifetime [139].

Infections such as HIV and syphilis can be transmitted vertically from mother to child, causing acute infections, fetal or infant death or chronic childhood conditions. A review of neurodevelopmental outcomes showed that vertical transmission of HIV was associated with poorer neurodevelopmental outcomes in children from resource-poor countries [140]. Likewise, repeated malarial infections and continuing parasitemia are associated with reduced cognitive ability in children in the short- and long-term, with effects on their future economic capacity [141-143].

Lack of human resources adversely affects any future health system. Conflict-driven collapse of the education system, for example, reduces the pool of people who could become health workers. The best-known example is the breakdown of the education system under Cambodia's Khmer Rouge regime, in which teachers were systematically imprisoned or executed. This not only affected the education of children at the time, but also led to a longer-term loss of knowledge and skills from society.

As common users of healthcare services, pregnant women are especially vulnerable to healthcare service disruptions, leading to the exacerbation of illness. An example of this would be the disruption to the supply of drugs and other medical equipment, as described in northern Sri Lanka during the recent civil war. Obstetric complications, such as pre-eclampsia, were common, potentially contributing to the higher rate of low birthweight that was found [144]. In Palestine, military checkpoints delaying access to maternity facilities were associated with an increase in home births from 8% in 1999 to 33% in 2002 [145], while in Nepal's recent civil war, disruption of a hospital's electricity supply led to Caesarean sections being performed by torchlight [123]. More generally, maternal mortality rises during conflict. About half the countries suffering from conflict have maternal mortality ratios >200 per 100,000 live births [8]. The maternal mortality ratio during the conflict in Bosnia and Herzegovina was approximately 75% higher than in the periods immediately before and after [146]. A catastrophic event in its own right, maternal mortality also has damaging effects on the remaining family members, particularly children. Evidence from a non-conflict area of Bangladesh shows very high mortality among younger children—up to 70% for a surviving neonate within two years of the maternal death—approximately 10 times higher than if neither parent had died. Higher mortality persists in children five- to ten-years old, for whom the probability increases five-fold [147]. Similar evidence from Haiti shows increased odds of mortality after a maternal death of 55% for children younger than 12-years-old [148].

7.1.4 NUTRITION

7.1.4.1 MATERNAL EXPOSURE

Malnutrition is common in conflicts and is predominantly manifest in children [149]. During a recent famine in the Horn of Africa, rates of global and severe acute malnutrition reached levels of 50% and 35%, respectively [150]. Food security falls during conflict for reasons ranging from reduced crop production to breaks in the supply chain and trade restrictions [9,151]. Food resources may be destroyed deliberately as a means of harm or population control: in 1980, 140,000 hectares were destroyed by Ethiopian government forces to prevent their use by rebel groups [152]. The diversion of resources away from healthcare and food supply to military expenditure in war can adversely affect population health. Despite an increase in overall gross development product per capita, the early Nazi regime saw an increase in mortality and a decline in child height [153]. International sanctions, a favored government response to civil conflict, may generate similar effects. Neonatal mortality, for example, increased substantially in Iraq during the 1990s [154].

There is some evidence that breastfeeding rates can decline in war times and the adverse effects of this can be greater. In the war in Croatia in the early 1990s, breast-feeding duration was found to be shorter in affected areas [155]. In Guinea Bissau in the late 1990s, infants who were weaned earlier during war periods had higher mortality rates than breastfed infants compared to the pre-war years where this difference was not present [156]. In addition to not having breast milk, we would postulate that disruption to formula milk supplies and unclean water would compound the adverse effects. It was shown that children who were never breastfed were more likely to be malnourished [157].

War may contribute to either acute malnutrition and increased mortality or chronic malnutrition leading to stunting and subtle prolonged deficits associated with lower school attainment and reduced adult income [158]. Nutritional deficiencies may be in macronutrients, providing the basic energy and substrate for growth, or in micronutrients, including vitamins and minerals that promote cellular function. Micronutrient deficiency diseases are common in conflicts: scurvy in Afghanistan from vitamin C deficiency [159], pellagra in Angola from niacin deficiency [160].

7.1.4.2 INTERGENERATIONAL ASSOCIATIONS

Malnourished mothers pass on the stress to their children, whose poor nutritional status may affect subsequent generations. In the Dutch Hunger Winter of 1944 to 1945 during the German occupation, maternal undernutrition was associated with increased risk of low birth weight [161]. Although not directly attributed to malnutrition, a higher proportion of babies were born with moderate low birth weight in Croatia during the war period (1991 to 1995) [162]. Low birth weight is the strongest risk factor for mortality in early infancy [163] and is associated with reduced educational attainment and physical work capacity [158]. Subtler effects include maternal micronutrient deficiencies, such as iron deficiency anemia [164], and conditions that directly affect the fetus, such as neural tube defects associated with folate deficiency [165]. Prenatal malnutrition, leading to low birth weight, results in lower subsequent height and lean mass [166]. Short maternal stature is associated with an increased risk of gestational diabetes, macrosomia, and birth injury and shorter gestation [167-169]. Among Hmong refugees from the Second Indochina war, children displaced during infancy were shorter as adults, whereas children born during the war were found to have greater adiposity, particularly central adiposity [170]. Such growth penalties may take generations to resolve. Maternal short stature is a risk factor for obstructed labor, Caesarean section and low birth weight [171-173], potentially generating a long-term intergenerational cycle [15]. Contrasting with sperm production in men, women's ova are formed primarily early in life, and damage to the reproductive system in young girls, from infections, trauma or harmful substances, for example, can have long-term effects on their reproductive capacity and their children [174,175].

Peri-conceptional, fetal and infant malnutrition can affect the risk of non-communicable disease. People exposed to maternal malnutrition in utero during the Dutch Hunger Winter showed increased risk of obesity, hypertension, cardiovascular disease and type 2 diabetes [176-178]. The longer-term effects depended on when in gestation the lack of nutrition occurred and the period for which there was a deficit, and there is some evidence for a difference in the long-term effects between male and female offspring [179,180]. Although the evidence is conflicting, it may be that the detrimental effects of the Dutch famine extended into the following generation, with the offspring of women born in the famine found to have a lower birth weight [161,181]. Similar associations between early-life famine exposure and subsequent elevated chronic disease risk were reported following the Biafran conflict of 1968 to 1970 [182], and the Chinese famine of 1959 to 1961 [183-186]. In the latter, early-life exposure was also associated with increased risk of schizophrenia [187,188]. In non-conflict settings it is common for chronic disease in adults to affect their offspring, both biologically and economically via loss of earnings. An example of this would be the propensity to obesity and the development of gestational diabetes leading to preterm birth and macrosomia.

Deliberate military efforts may not only impair the capacity for food production but also increase exposure to toxins. For example, bombing and Agent Orange were used in Vietnam to 'deny the enemy sources of food and means of cover' [189]. Approximately 11 to 12 million gallons of Agent Orange were sprayed over nearly 10% of South Vietnam between 1961 and 1971. While research on intergenerational effects continues, the WHO describes dioxin, the active element of Agent Orange, as 'highly toxic' and able to cause 'reproductive and developmental problems' [190,191].

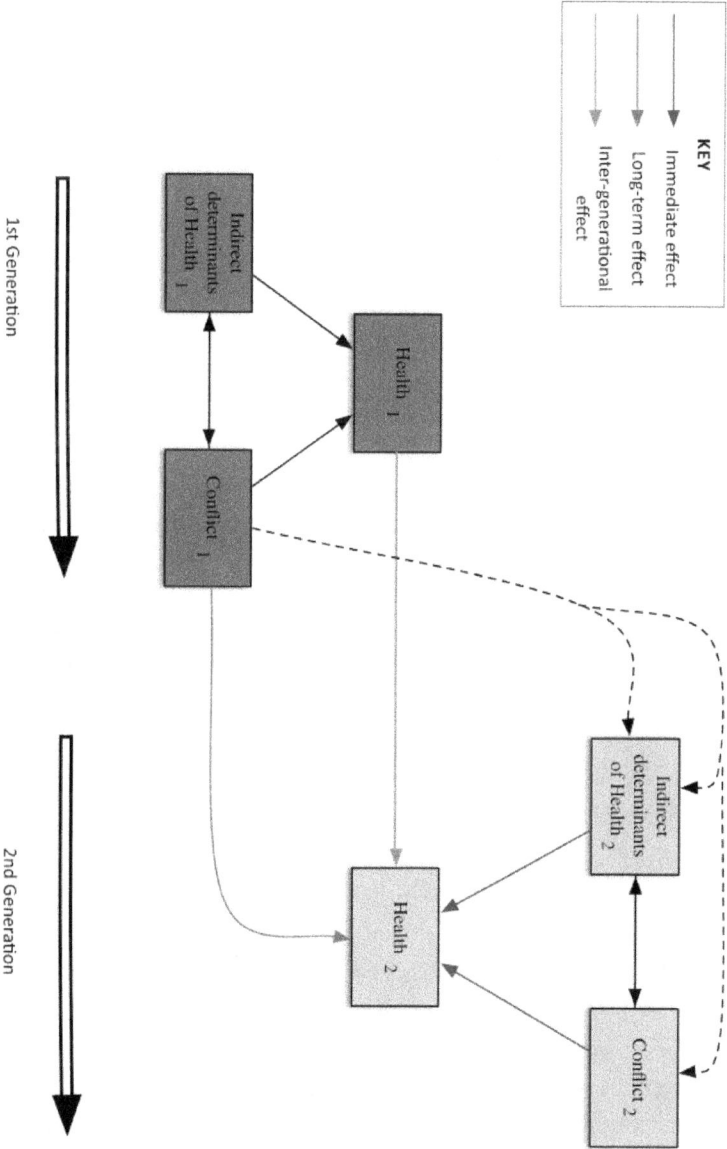

FIGURE 3: Schematic diagram showing how both current and past events affect the health of children across multiple generations.

7.1.5 MULTIPLICATIVE EFFECTS

The intergenerational harms of short conflicts are mitigated by post-conflict recovery of economies, societies and health and schooling systems. In long-lasting conflicts, however, they are exacerbated by on-going fighting to produce a composite effect whereby the immediate effects of conflict combine with long-term and intergenerational effects, as illustrated schematically in Figure 3.

It is difficult to provide definitive evidence for this as prior susceptibility is hard to quantify, but we propose two illustrative scenarios. In the first, an increase in preterm births, perhaps associated with an increase in congenital infections, makes children more susceptible to subsequent infection. This susceptibility is exacerbated by the increased wartime burden of disease. Infection exacerbates wartime under-nutrition, which combines with reduction in the food supply in a downward spiral that reduces a child's capacity to cope with physical insults. These multiple deficits occur within a health system that already cannot cope. In the second scenario, children growing up in a long-lasting conflict region suffer from the intergenerational effects of mental ill-health, as well as an ongoing conflict stress burden. For example, a child inherits an impaired cortisol response through parental stressful experiences, and this makes it harder to cope with the subsequent stressful events the child faces herself.

7.2 DISCUSSION

We have given examples of how conflict can have long-lasting intergenerational effects, working through parental exposure to violence, mental health stressors, infection and nutrition (summarized in Table 2). Much has been written about the health effects of war but the literature on its enduring effects is sparse. With our growing understanding of the developmental origins of health and disease, it is becoming evident that the extreme conditions that conflict imposes can have effects that last for generations, making a 'brief' conflict a misnomer. Many interrelated pathways have been identified between parental exposure and subsequent generations, but further evidence is required to estimate the magnitude of their effects. Given the range of conflict scenarios, there is likely to be a great deal of heterogeneity.

TABLE 2: Summary of maternal and intergenerational effects

Key areas	Maternal exposure—possible consequences	Intergenerational associations—increased risk of
Violence	Domestic violence	Congenital malformations
	Mental illness/physical trauma	Low birth weight
	Rape	Perinatal morbidity and mortality
	Trafficking and prostitution	Premature birth
		Altered physical and mental development
		Neglect and abuse
Mental health	PTSD	Impaired growth
	Depression	Poor educational attainment
	Anxiety	Neuroendocrine and immune system modulation
	Psychosomatic disorders	Infection
	Drug and alcohol abuse	Mental illness
		Higher suicide rates
		Social functioning impairment
Infectious diseases and health systems	Increased transmission of infectious diseases	Fetal or infant mortality
	Malnutrition	Disability
	Obstetric complications	Cardiovascular disease
	Increase in maternal mortality	Congenital malformations
		Impaired cognitive development
Nutrition	Malnutrition including micronutrient deficiencies	Neonatal mortality
	Obstetric complications	Low birth weight
	Maternal mortality	Malnutrition/under-nutrition
		Impaired growth and development
		Educational under-attainment
		Congenital abnormalities
		Non-communicable diseases
		Future reproductive capacity

Our categorization of potential exposures and effects is illustrative and artificial in the sense that their interactions are complex. Physiological and pathological effects of stressors—trauma, infection, malnutrition—are linked in a complex system with institutional factors, such as education and health system challenges, and social factors, such as cultures of alcohol use and violence. Prior conflict creates a population with a reduced capacity to cope with adversity, and ongoing or subsequent conflict may compound this and exacerbate the adverse health effects. The prevention of conflict and its effects on health are crucially important public health concerns [11], but the intergenerational picture has received little attention so far. In many cases, the causal link between conflict and intergenerational outcomes is lacking, and the paucity of research reflects at least partly the challenges of working in current or recent conflict zones. Where evidence from conflict situations is limited, we have hypothesized on the basis of available evidence or discussed evidence from non-conflict situations.

7.2.1 INTERGENERATIONAL JUSTICE

Similar to the growing calls for consideration of future generations in climate change debates, we call for policy makers to consider them with respect to conflict. The notion of intergenerational justice emphasizes a temporal dimension, giving future generations rights that those currently alive should maintain. The extent to which existing legislative powers can be used to uphold these rights is uncertain, but legal bodies could potentially extend their scope to the violation of the rights of future beings. Statutes such as the UN Convention on the Rights of the Child (Articles 38 and 39) already exist to protect the rights of children in war [192]. The arguments we lay out are aligned with gender-based social justice since in many parts of the world women receive fewer resources in general and particularly in terms of access to healthcare [193]. The idea of intergenerational justice can also be aligned with a present day rights-based approach to help protect not only the current population but also future generations. In this sense, we do not see a clash between the two.

It is not within the scope of this paper to adequately review the interventions that may be of benefit in preventing the future adverse effects of war, but we have tried to summarize the main categories in Box 2. Many of these are the same as those required for the current population, but the imperative to protect certain groups, such as pregnant women, is reinforced. Past conflicts may have led to positive changes, such as the removal of oppressive regimes, as well as negative impacts. However, our discussion highlights the importance of minimizing the likelihood of conflict when seeking such positive changes. Interventions to break the cycle of transmission should be examined at the point at which governing bodies and non-state actors are considering going to war, and in its aftermath, as well as during conflict. In examining the health of a population, previous insults need to be considered in order to understand fully the situation and to initiate solutions. Importantly, policy makers should bear in mind that a population may take multiple generations for the adverse health effects of conflict to be negated as a region attempts to return to its premorbid state or moves on to a new post-conflict one and it is possible that a return to the previous state may never happen if conflict changes the status quo within a given area. Conflict-related public health interventions need to be sustained for a number of years and adapted over time to cope with changing needs.

7.3 SUMMARY

In this article, we summarize how the effects of war can propagate across generations. We hope this review will stimulate debate and research on the long-term and intergenerational health effects of conflict and their mechanisms and contribute to the discussion of the costs of war. The evidence we have included strengthens the position that violent conflict should be avoided and indicates that intergenerational effects should be included routinely in the anticipated and estimated consequences of war.

BOX 1: BIOLOGICAL EFFECTS OF PTSD

Increased stress levels in mothers can act in a similar fashion to undernutrition, potentially mediated by changes in the hypothalamic-pituitary-adrenal (HPA) axis [194]. Occurrence of PTSD is thought to be influenced by epigenetic changes, with possibly both genome-wide and specific changes in genes such as DLGP2 [195]. Exposure to massive stress during pregnancy has been associated with epigenetic programming of the HPA axis in utero, leading to an increased susceptibility to mental illness in the child [90]. The mechanism by which this is believed to occur is that traumatic events lead to epigenetic changes to the glucocorticoid GR gene that subsequently alter offspring cortisol response to future events. Radtke et al. showed lasting effects of the methylation of glucocorticoid receptor genes associated with intimate partner violence against the mother around the time of pregnancy [91]. These findings from research on humans are supported by animal studies. For example, expression of the glucocorticoid receptor gene in the rodent hippocampus is modulated by the level of care received by the mother [196,197]. Further to this, the administration of drugs that alter DNA methylation can reverse altered behavior, as shown by the use of the demethylating substance trichostatin and methylating substance methionine [198,199].

BOX 2: USING THE EVIDENCE OF INTERGENERATIONAL CONSEQUENCES OF CONFLICT: SOME POSSIBLE STRATEGIES

PREVENT THE ONSET OF WAR AND VIOLENT CONFLICT

When conflict starts, all options to reach an alternative peaceful solution have rarely been exhausted [200]. There may be strong political or economic motivations behind the decision to go to war or resort to violent conflict. These may include the need to do so for 'humanitarian' reasons, although recent military action initiated on this basis has caused such a degree of mortality, morbidity and destruction that the humanitarian reason has been rather discredited. However, there is potentially a case to be made for going to war to prevent death, injury and destruction.

Viewed objectively, there will be a range of reasons for going to war or taking violent action and a range of reasons for not doing so; evidence of the health consequences of taking violent action will fall within the latter. The greater this evidence is, the harder it will be to justify war. Intergenerational consequences for health are an under-researched result of war that could tip the balance against it, help put a brake on the push to war and ensure that other peaceful options are pursued as a priority.

FACTOR IN A LONGER-TERM PERSPECTIVE IF CONTEMPLATING GOING TO WAR

The link between the likely longer-term health consequences of going to war and the conflict itself can be hard to establish definitively. The more time passes, the more possible confounders have to be taken into account, making direct causal links difficult to prove. However, combining disciplines and research to illustrate these links in the area of child health can be compelling, as there is a general consensus that children should be protected during war and that future generations are innocent. This makes a growing body of evidence that supports the link between conflict and future health problems for children a strong advocacy tool for conflict prevention.

ENSURE A LONG-TERM COMPONENT TO INTERVENTIONS BOTH DURING AND AFTER CONFLICT, TAKING LONG TERM CONSEQUENCES INTO ACCOUNT

The type of interventions used to meet health needs caused by conflict, and the resources that are dedicated to them, should be decided on the basis of need. Much work has been done on how those needs can be accurately assessed [201] and minimum standards of response assured [202]. If need can be shown to be more long-lasting and serious than previously thought, particularly in relation to mother and child health, it could influence needs assessments, minimum standards and intervention planning. This would also help make the case for sufficient and appropriate resource allocation.

ENSURE EXTRA CARE IS PROVIDED FOR VULNERABLE GROUPS, PARTICULARLY PREGNANT WOMEN

Evidence of the intergenerational health consequences of violent conflict will reinforce the degree of vulnerability of pregnant women to health shocks. Pregnant and lactating women are already recognized as a priority group for humanitarian health programs [203], but there is still much to be done before programs are fully integrated, effective and adequately resourced. A better understanding of the consequences of not having optimal and well-resourced programs will be a strong advocacy tool to use with donors and others.

UPHOLDING INTERNATIONAL CONVENTIONS TO SAFEGUARD CHILDREN THROUGH INTERGENERATIONAL JUSTICE

International law that relates to the rights of children is almost universally recognized and key parts of it are considered to be customary law [204]. Better established links between violent conflict and the health and wellbeing of children not yet born could contribute to holding those who initiate war or violent conflict to account for the consequences of their actions. This, in turn, would be a further restraining factor on initiating violent conflict.

REFERENCES

1. Southall D, Carballo M: Can children be protected from the effect of war? BMJ 1996, 313:1493.
2. Goldson E: The effect of war on children. Child Abuse Negl 1996, 20:809-819.
3. Jensen PS, Shaw JO: Children as victims of war: current knowledge and future research needs. J Am Acad Child Adolesc Psychiatry 1993, 32:697-708.
4. Pearn J: Children and war. J Paediatr Child Health 2003, 39:166-172.
5. Levy BS: Health and peace. Croat Med J 2002, 43:114-116.
6. World Health Organization: World Report on Violence and Health. 2002. Available at: http://www.who.int/violence_injury_prevention/violence/world_report/en/

7. Stockholm International Peace Research Institute: SIPRI Yearbook 2012. Oxford: Oxford University Press; 2012.

8. Southall D: Armed conflict women and girls who are pregnant, infants and children; a neglected public health challenge. What can health professionals do? Early Hum Dev 2011, 87:735-742.

9. Watchlist on Children and Armed Conflict: Caught in the Middle: Mounting Violations Against Children in Nepal's Armed Conflict. 2005. Available at: http://watchlist.org/reports/pdf/nepal.report.20050120.pdf

10. O'Malley B: Education Under Attack. UNESCO; 2007. Available at: http://unesdoc. unesco.org/images/0018/001863/186303e.pdf

11. Krug EG, Mercy JA, Dahlberg LL, Zwi AB: The world report on violence and health. Lancet 2002, 360:1083-1088.

12. Bustreo F, Genovese E, Omobono E, Axelsson H, Bannon I: Improving Child Health in Post-Conflict Countries Can the World Bank Contribute? Washington, DC: The World Bank; 2005.

13. Collier P: On the economic consequences of civil war. Oxford Econ Pap 1999, 51:168-183.

14. Chen S, Loayza NV, Reynal-Querol M: The aftermath of civil war. Post-Conflict Transitions Working Paper Number 4. Washington, DC: World Bank; 2007.

15. Wells JC: Maternal capital and the metabolic ghetto: an evolutionary perspective on the transgenerational basis of health inequalities. Am J Hum Biol 2010, 22:1-17.

16. Youngson NA, Whitelaw E: Transgenerational epigenetic effects. Annu Rev Genomics Hum Genet 2008, 9:233-257.

17. Hackett JA, Sengupta R, Zylicz JJ, Murakami K, Lee C, Down TA, Surani MA: Germline DNA demethylation dynamics and imprint erasure through 5-hydroxymethylcytosine. Science 2013, 339:448-452.

18. Barker DJ, Osmond C: Infant mortality, childhood nutrition, and ischaemic heart disease in England and Wales. Lancet 1986, 327:1077-1081.

19. Barker DJ, Osmond C, Winter PD, Margetts B, Simmonds SJ: Weight in infancy and death from ischaemic heart disease. Lancet 1989, 334:577-580.

20. Watts C, Zimmerman C: Violence against women: global scope and magnitude. Lancet 2002, 359:1232-1237.

21. Swiss S, Jennings PJ, Aryee GV, Brown GH, Jappah-Samukai RM, Kamara MS, Schaack RDH, Turay-Kanneh RS: Violence against women during the Liberian civil conflict. JAMA 1998, 279:625-629.

22. Usta J, Farver JA, Zein L: Women, war, and violence: surviving the experience. J Womens Health (Larchmt) 2008, 17:793-804.

23. Rieder M, Choonara I: Armed conflict and child health. Arch Dis Child 2012, 97:59-62.

24. International Action Network on Small Arms: Gun Violence: The Global Crisis. 2008. Available at: http://www.iansa.org/system/files/GlobalCrisis07.pdf

25. Albuja S, Anwar A, Birkeland NM, Caterina M, Charron G, Dolores R, Fajans-Turner A, Ginnetti J, Glatz A, Grayson C, Halff K, Jennings E, Jimenez C, Khalil K, Kok F, Leikvang C, Mancini Beck K, McCallin B, Montemurro M, Perez L, Pierre N, Rothing J, Rushing EJ, Shahinian J, Sheekh NM, Schrepfer N, Spence A, Spurrell C, Tengnäs K, Walick N, et al.: Global Overview 2011. People Internally Displaced by Conflict and Violence. Edited by Birkeland NM, Jennings E, Rushing EJ. Ge-

neva: Norwegian Refugee Council Internal Displacement Monitoring Centre; 2012. Available at: http://www.internal-displacement.org/assets/publications/2012/2012-global-overview-2011-global-en.pdf

26. Machel G: The impact of war on children. UK: C. Hurst & Co; 2001.

27. Bilukha OO, Brennan M, Anderson M: The lasting legacy of war: epidemiology of injuries from landmines and unexploded ordnance in Afghanistan, 2002–2006. Prehosp Disaster Med 2008, 23:493-499.

28. Cardozo BL, Blanton C, Zalewski T, Tor S, McDonald L, Lavelle J, Brooks R, Anderson M, Mollica R: Mental health survey among landmine survivors in Siem Reap province, Cambodia. Med Confl Surviv 2012, 28:161-181.

29. Lindsey-Curtet C, Holst-Roness FT, Anderson L: Addressing the Needs of Women Affected by Armed Conflict. Geneva: International Committee of the Red Cross (ICRC; 2004. Available at: http://www.icrc.org/eng/assets/files/other/icrc_002_0840_women_guidance.pdf

30. Wood EJ: Variation in sexual violence during war. Polit Soc 2006, 34:307-342.

31. Marsh M, Purdin S, Navani S: Addressing sexual violence in humanitarian emergencies. Glob Public. Health 2006, 1:133-146.

32. Hynes M, Robertson K, Ward J, Crouse C: A determination of the prevalence of gender-based violence among conflict-affected populations in East Timor. Disasters 2004, 28:294-321.

33. Women's Wellness Center and the Reproductive Health Response in Crises Consortium: RHRC. 2006. [Prevalence of Gender-Based Violence: Preliminary Findings from a Field Assessment in Nine Villages in the Peja Region, Kosovo]

34. Martin SL, English KT, Clark KA, Cilenti D, Kupper LL: Violence and substance use among North Carolina pregnant women. Am J Pub Health 1996, 86:991-998.

35. Flynn HA, Walton MA, Chermack ST, Cunningham RM, Marcus SM: Brief detection and co-occurrence of violence, depression and alcohol risk in prenatal care settings. Arch Womens Ment Health 2007, 10:155-161.

36. O'Connor MJ, Tomlinson M, LeRoux IM, Stewart J, Greco E, Rotheram-Borus MJ: Predictors of alcohol use prior to pregnancy recognition among township women in Cape Town, South Africa. Soc Sci Med 2011, 72:83-90.

37. World Health Organization: Interpersonal Violence and Alcohol. http://www.who.int/violence_injury_prevention/violence/world_report/factsheets/pb_violencealcohol.pdf

38. Kilpatrick DG, Acierno R, Resnick HS, Saunders BE, Best CL: A 2-year longitudinal analysis of the relationships between violent assault and substance use in women. J Consult Clin Psychol 1997, 65:834-847.

39. Eaton L, Kalichman S, Sikkema K, Skinner D, Watt M, Pieterse D, Pitpitan E: Pregnancy, alcohol intake, and intimate partner violence among men and women attending drinking establishments in a Cape Town, South Africa Township. J Commun Health 2011, 37:208-216.

40. Jejeebhoy SJ: Associations between wife-beating and fetal and infant death: impressions from a survey in rural India. Stud Fam Plann 1998, 29:300-308.

41. Campbell JC: Health consequences of intimate partner violence. Lancet 2002, 359:1331-1336.

42. Simic S, Idrizbegovic S, Jaganjac N, Boloban H, Puvacic J, Gallic A, Dekovic S: Nutritional effects of the siege on new-born babies in Sarajevo. Eur J Clin Nutr 1995, 49:S33-S36.
43. Gazmararian JA, Petersen R, Spitz AM, Goodwin MM, Saltzman LE, Marks JS: Violence and reproductive health: current knowledge and future research directions. Matern Child Health J 2000, 4:79-84.
44. Kuvacic I, Skrablin S, Hodzic D, Milkovic G: Possible influence of expatriation on perinatal outcome. Acta Obstet Gynecol Scand 1996, 75:367-371.
45. Murphy CC, Schei B, Myhr TL, Du Mont J: Abuse: a risk factor for low birth weight? A systematic review and meta-analysis. CMAJ 2001, 164:1567-1572.
46. Maman S, Campbell J, Sweat MD, Gielen AC: The intersections of HIV and violence: directions for future research and interventions. Soc Sci Med 2000, 50:459-478.
47. Heise L, Ellsberg M, Gottemoeller M: Ending violence against women. In Population Reports. Baltimore: Johns Hopkins University, School of Public Health, Population Information Program; 1999:13-18. [Series L, No. 11]
48. Nowrojee B: Shattered Lives: Sexual Violence during the Rwandan Genocide and its Aftermath. New York: Human Rights Watch; 1996.
49. Kelly JT, Betancourt TS, Mukwege D, Lipton R, Vanrooyen MJ: Experiences of female survivors of sexual violence in eastern Democratic Republic of the Congo: a mixed-methods study. Confl Health 2011, 5:25.
50. Nelson BD, Collins L, VanRooyen MJ, Joyce N, Mukwege D, Bartels S: Impact of sexual violence on children in the Eastern Democratic Republic of Congo. Med Confl Surviv 2011, 27:211-225.
51. Mollica RF, McInnes K, Poole C, Tor S: Dose-effect relationships of trauma to symptoms of depression and post-traumatic stress disorder among Cambodian survivors of mass violence. Br J Psychiatry 1998, 173:482-488.
52. Glaser D: Child abuse and neglect and the brain–a review. J Child Psychol Psychiatry 2000, 41:97-116.
53. Villamor E, Chavarro JE, Caro LE: Growing up under generalized violence: an ecological study of homicide rates and secular trends in age at menarche in Colombia, 1940s-1980s. Econ Hum Biol 2009, 7:238-245.
54. Machel G: Impact of Armed Conflict on Children. UNICEF; 1996. Available at: http://www.unicef.org/graca/a51-306_en.pdf
55. Morrison AR, Orlando MB, Biehl ML: Social and economic costs of domestic violence: Chile and Nicaragua. In Too Close to Home: Domestic Violence in the Americas. Edited by Morrison ARaB ML. Washington, D.C: Inter-American Development Bank; 1997:51-80.
56. Sharma M, Prasain D, Hutt M: Gender dimensions of the people's war: some reflections on the experiences of rural women. In Himalayan People's War: Nepal's Maoist rebellion. London: Hurst & Co; 2004:152-165.
57. Cahill L, Sherman P: Child abuse and domestic violence. Pediatr Rev 2006, 27:339-345.
58. Boothby N, Crawford J, Halperin J: Mozambique child soldier life outcome study: lessons learned in rehabilitation and reintegration efforts. Glob Public Health 2006, 1:87-107.
59. Otake M, Schull WJ: Radiation-related small head sizes among prenatally exposed A-bomb survivors. Int J Radiat Biol 1993, 63:255-270.

60. Otake M, Schull WJ: Radiation-related brain damage and growth retardation among the prenatally exposed atomic bomb survivors. Int J Radiat Biol 1998, 74:159-171.
61. Abolghasemi H, Radfar MH, Rambod M, Salehi P, Ghofrani H, Soroush MR, Falahaty F, Tavakolifar Y, Sadaghianifar A, Khademolhosseini SM, Kavehmanesh Z, Joffres M, Burkle FM Jr, Mills EJ: Childhood physical abnormalities following paternal exposure to sulfur mustard gas in Iran: a case–control study. Confl Health 2010, 4:13.
62. Alaani S, Tafash M, Busby C, Hamdan M, Blaurock-Busch E: Uranium and other contaminants in hair from the parents of children with congenital anomalies in Fallujah, Iraq. Confl Health 2011, 5:15.
63. Murthy RS, Lakshminarayana R: Mental health consequences of war: a brief review of research findings. World Psychiatry 2006, 5:25-30.
64. Somasundaram D: Child soldiers: understanding the context. BMJ 2002, 324:1268-1271.
65. Derluyn I, Broekaert E, Schuyten G, De Temmerman E: Post-traumatic stress in former Ugandan child soldiers. Lancet 2004, 363:861-863.
66. Betancourt TS, Borisova II, Williams TP, Brennan RT, Whitfield TH, de la Soudiere M, Williamson J, Gilman SE: Sierra Leone's former child soldiers: a follow-up study of psychosocial adjustment and community reintegration. Child Dev 2010, 81:1077-1095.
67. Moscardino U, Scrimin S, Cadei F, Altoe G: Mental health among former child soldiers and never-abducted children in northern Uganda. Scientific World Journal 2012, 2012:367545.
68. Levy BS, Sidel VW: Health effects of combat: a life-course perspective. Annu Rev Public Health 2009, 30:123-136.
69. Thapa SB, Hauff E: Psychological distress among displaced persons during an armed conflict in Nepal. Soc Psychiatry Psychiatr Epidemiol 2005, 40:672-679.
70. de Jong JT, Komproe IH, Van Ommeren M: Common mental disorders in postconflict settings. Lancet 2003, 361:2128-2130.
71. Seino K, Takano T, Mashal T, Hemat S, Nakamura K: Prevalence of and factors influencing posttraumatic stress disorder among mothers of children under five in Kabul, Afghanistan, after decades of armed conflicts. Health Qual Life Out 2008, 6:29.
72. Klaric M, Klaric B, Stevanovic A, Grkovic J, Jonovska S: Psychological consequences of war trauma and postwar social stressors in women in Bosnia and Herzegovina. Croat Med J 2007, 48:167-176.
73. de Jong JT, Komproe IH, Van Ommeren M, El Masri M, Araya M, Khaled N, van de Put W, Somasundaram D: Lifetime events and posttraumatic stress disorder in 4 postconflict settings. JAMA 2001, 286:555-562.
74. Dimitry L: A systematic review on the mental health of children and adolescents in areas of armed conflict in the Middle East. Child Care Health Dev 2012, 38:153-161.
75. Ezard N, Oppenheimer E, Burton A, Schilperoord M, Macdonald D, Adelekan M, Sakarati A, van Ommeren M: Six rapid assessments of alcohol and other substance use in populations displaced by conflict. Confl Health 2011, 5:1.
76. Bhui K, Warfa N: Drug consumption in conflict zones in Somalia. PLoS Med 2007, 4:e354.
77. Kan PR: Drugs and Contemporary Warfare. Herndon, VA: Potomac Books; 2009.

78. Martz E (Ed): Trauma and Rehabilitation after War and Conflict. Springer; 2010.

79. Strathdee SA, Zafar T, Brahmbhatt H, Ul Hassan S: Higher level of needle sharing among injection drug users in Lahore, Pakistan, in the aftermath of the US-Afghan war. In International Conference on AIDS. Barcelona; 2002.

80. Hankins CA, Friedman SR, Zafar T, Strathdee SA: Transmission and prevention of HIV and sexually transmitted infections in war settings: implications for current and future armed conflicts. AIDS 2002, 16:2245-2252.

81. Bjelosevic E, Hadzikapetanovic H, Loga S, Hodzic M, Skelic D, Savarimooto B: Relation between benzodiazepine abuse and trauma. Med Arh 2003, 57:33-36.

82. Odenwald M, Neuner F, Schauer M, Elbert T, Catani C, Lingenfelder B, Hinkel H, Hafner H, Rockstroh B: Khat use as risk factor for psychotic disorders: a cross-sectional and case–control study in Somalia. BMC Med 2005, 3:5.

83. Federenko IS, Wadhwa PD: Women's mental health during pregnancy influences fetal and infant developmental and health outcomes. CNS Spectr 2004, 9:198-206.

84. Satyanarayana VA, Lukose A, Srinivasan K: Maternal mental health in pregnancy and child behavior. Indian J Psychiatry 2011, 53:351-361.

85. Wachs TD, Black MM, Engle PL: Maternal depression: a global threat to children's health, development, and behavior and to human rights. Child Dev Perspect 2009, 3:51-59.

86. Tegethoff M, Greene N, Olsen J, Schaffner E, Meinlschmidt G: Stress during pregnancy and offspring pediatric disease: a National Cohort Study. Environ Health Perspect 2011, 119:1647-1652.

87. Pesonen AK, Raikkonen K, Kajantie E, Heinonen K, Osmond C, Barker DJ, Forsen T, Eriksson JG: Inter-generational social mobility following early life stress. Ann Med 2011, 43:320-328.

88. Feldman R, Vengrober A: Posttraumatic stress disorder in infants and young children exposed to war-related trauma. J Am Acad Child Adolesc Psychiatr 2011, 50:645-658.

89. Siegmund A, Dahlhoff M, Habersetzer U, Mederer A, Wolf E, Holsboer F, Wotjak CT: Maternal inexperience as a risk factor of innate fear and PTSD-like symptoms in mice. J Psychiatr Res 2009, 43:1156-1165.

90. Seckl JR, Meaney MJ: Glucocorticoid "Programming" and PTSD Risk. Ann N Y Acad Sci 2006, 1071:351-378.

91. Radtke KM, Ruf M, Gunter HM, Dohrmann K, Schauer M, Meyer A, Elbert T: Transgenerational impact of intimate partner violence on methylation in the promoter of the glucocorticoid receptor. Transl Psychiatry 2011, 1:e21.

92. Dekel R, Goldblatt H: Is there intergenerational transmission of trauma? The case of combat veterans' children. Am J Orthopsychiatry 2008, 78:281-289.

93. Betancourt TS, Khan KT: The mental health of children affected by armed conflict: protective processes and pathways to resilience. Int Rev Psychiatry 2008, 20:317-328.

94. Chu AT, Lieberman AF: Clinical implications of traumatic stress from birth to age five. Annu Rev Clin Psychol 2010, 6:469-494.

95. Australian Institute of Health and Welfare: Morbidity of Vietnam Veterans. Suicide in Vietnam Veterans' Children, Supplementary Report 1. 1st edition. Canberra: Australian Institute of Health and Welfare; 2000.

96. Kellerman NP: Psychopathology in children of Holocaust survivors: a review of the research literature. Isr J Psychiatry Relat Sci 2001, 38:36-46.

97. Yehuda R, Bell A, Bierer LM, Schmeidler J: Maternal, not paternal, PTSD is related to increased risk for PTSD in offspring of Holocaust survivors. J Psychiatr Res 2008, 42:1104-1111.
98. Scharf M, Mayseless O: Disorganizing experiences in second- and third-generation holocaust survivors. Qual Health Res 2011, 21:1539-1553.
99. Gangi S, Talamo A, Ferracuti S: The long-term effects of extreme war-related trauma on the second generation of Holocaust survivors. Violence Vict 2009, 24:687-700.
100. Summerfield D: The psychological legacy of war and atrocity: the question of long-term and transgenerational effects and the need for a broad view. J Nerv Ment Dis 1996, 184:375-377.
101. Scharf M: Long-term effects of trauma: psychosocial functioning of the second and third generation of Holocaust survivors. Dev Psychopathol 2007, 19:603-622.
102. Patel V, Rahman A, Jacob KS, Hughes M: Effect of maternal mental health on infant growth in low income countries: new evidence from South Asia. BMJ 2004, 328:820-823.
103. Galler JR, Harrison RH, Biggs MA, Ramsey F, Forde V: Maternal moods predict breastfeeding in Barbados. J Dev Behav Pediatr 1999, 20:80-87.
104. Falceto OG, Giugliani ER, Fernandes CL: Influence of parental mental health on early termination of breast-feeding: a case–control study. J Am Board Fam Pract 2004, 17:173-183.
105. Murray L, Cooper P: Effects of postnatal depression on infant development. Arch Dis Child 1997, 77:99-101.
106. Patel V, DeSouza N, Rodrigues M: Postnatal depression and infant growth and development in low income countries: a cohort study from Goa, India. Arch Dis Child 2003, 88:34-37.
107. Galler JR, Harrison RH, Ramsey F, Forde V, Butler SC: Maternal depressive symptoms affect infant cognitive development in Barbados. J Child Psychol Psychiatry 2000, 41:747-757.
108. Galler JR, Ramsey FC, Harrison RH, Taylor J, Cumberbatch G, Forde V: Postpartum maternal moods and infant size predict performance on a national high school entrance examination. J Child Psychol Psychiatry 2004, 45:1064-1075.
109. Osborn DA, Jeffery HE, Cole MJ: Opiate treatment for opiate withdrawal in newborn infants. Cochrane Database Syst Rev 2010., (10) CD002059
110. Shankaran S, Lester BM, Das A, Bauer CR, Bada HS, Lagasse L, Higgins R: Impact of maternal substance use during pregnancy on childhood outcome. Semin Fetal Neonatal Med 2007, 12:143-150.
111. Mwenda JM, Arimi MM, Kyama MC, Langat DK: Effects of khat (Catha edulis) consumption on reproductive functions: a review. East Afr Med J 2003, 80:318-323.
112. Strand RT, Fernandes Dias L, Bergstrom S, Andersson S: Unexpected low prevalence of HIV among fertile women in Luanda, Angola. Does war prevent the spread of HIV? Int J STD AIDS 2007, 18:467-471.
113. Guerin PJ, Brasher C, Baron E, Mic D, Grimont F, Ryan M, Aavitsland P, Legros D: Shigella dysenteriae serotype 1 in west Africa: intervention strategy for an outbreak in Sierra Leone. Lancet 2003, 362:705-706.
114. Griffith DC, Kelly-Hope LA, Miller MA: Review of reported cholera outbreaks worldwide, 1995–2005. Am J Trop Med Hyg 2006, 75:973-977.

115. Gayer M, Legros D, Formenty P, Connolly MA: Conflict and emerging infectious diseases. Emer Infect Dis 2007, 13:1625-1631.
116. United Nations High Commissioner for Refugees [http://www.unhcr.org/]
117. Shears P, Berry AM, Murphy R, Nabil MA: Epidemiological assessment of the health and nutrition of Ethiopian refugees in emergency camps in Sudan, 1985. Med J (Clin Res Ed) 1987, 295:314-318.
118. Brewer IW: The control of communicable diseases in camps. Am J Pub Health 1918, 8:121-124.
119. Connolly MA, Heymann DL: Deadly comrades: war and infectious diseases. Lancet 2002, 360:s23-s24.
120. Fair J, Jentes E, Inapogui A, Kourouma K, Goba A, Bah A, Tounkara M, Coulibaly M, Garry RF, Bausch DG: Lassa virus-infected rodents in refugee camps in Guinea: a looming threat to public health in a politically unstable region. Vector Borne Zoonotic Dis 2007, 7:167-171.
121. Bonner PC, Schmidt WP, Belmain SR, Oshin B, Baglole D, Borchert M: Poor housing quality increases risk of rodent infestation and Lassa fever in refugee camps of Sierra Leone. Am J Trop Med Hyg 2007, 77:169-175.
122. Rowland M, Rab MA, Freeman T, Durrani N, Rehman N: Afghan refugees and the temporal and spatial distribution of malaria in Pakistan. Soc Sci Med 2002, 55:2061-2072.
123. Singh S, Bohler E, Dahal K, Mills E: The state of child health and human rights in Nepal. PLoS Med 2006, 3:e203.
124. Health care in danger http://www.icrc.org/eng/what-we-do/safeguarding-health-care/index.jsp
125. Mann J, Drucker E, Tarantola D: Bosnia: the war against public health. Med Global Survival 1994, 1:130-144.
126. Nathanson V: Delivering healthcare in situations of conflict or violence. BMJ 2011, 343:d4671.
127. ICRC: Iraq: Civilians without Protection: the Ever-Worsening Humanitarian Crisis. 2007. Available at: http://www.icrc.org/eng/assets/files/other/iraq-report-icrc.pdf
128. Msuya C, Sondorp E: Interagency Health Evaluation Liberia. 2005. Available at: http://www.alnap.org/resource/3392.aspx
129. De Schryver A, Meheus A: Epidemiology of sexually transmitted diseases: the global picture. Bull World Health Organ 1990, 68:639-654.
130. Ward J, Vann B: Gender-based violence in refugee settings. Lancet 2002, 360:s13-s14.
131. Kinyanda E, Weiss HA, Mungherera M, Onyango-Mangen P, Ngabirano E, Kajungu R, Kagugube J, Muhwezi W, Muron J, Patel V: Psychiatric disorders and psychosocial correlates of high HIV risk sexual behaviour in war-affected Eastern Uganda. AIDS Care 2012, 24:1323-1332.
132. Cossa HA, Gloyd S, Vaz RG, Folgosa E, Simbine E, Diniz M, Kreiss JK: Syphilis and HIV infection among displaced pregnant women in rural Mozambique. Int J STD AIDS 1994, 5:117-123.
133. Civilians in war zones; women and children worst Economist 2009. Available at: http://www.economist.com/node/13145799

134. Oxford JS, Sefton A, Jackson R, Innes W, Daniels RS, Johnson NP: World War I may have allowed the emergence of "Spanish" influenza. Lancet Infect Dis 2002, 2:111-114.
135. Erkoreka A: Origins of the Spanish Influenza pandemic (1918–1920) and its relation to the First World War. J Mol Genet Med 2009, 3:190-194.
136. Mazumder B, Almond D, Park K, Crimmins EM, Finch CE: Lingering prenatal effects of the 1918 influenza pandemic on cardiovascular disease. J Dev Orig Health Dis 2010, 1:26-34.
137. Almond D: Is the 1918 influenza pandemic over? Long-term effects of in utero influenza exposure in the post-1940 U.S. population. J Polit Econ 2006 1918, 114:672-712.
138. Novo A, Huebschen JM, Muller CP, Tesanovic M, Bojanic J: Ongoing rubella outbreak in Bosnia and Herzegovina, March-July 2009--preliminary report. Euro Surveill 2009., 14 pii: 19343
139. Saigal S, Doyle LW: An overview of mortality and sequelae of preterm birth from infancy to adulthood. Lancet 2008, 371:261-269.
140. Le Doare K, Bland R, Newell ML: Neurodevelopment in children born to HIV-infected mothers by infection and treatment status. Pediatrics 2012, 130:e1326-e1344.
141. Fernando D, Wickremasinghe R, Mendis KN, Wickremasinghe AR: Cognitive performance at school entry of children living in malaria-endemic areas of Sri Lanka. Trans R Soc Trop Med Hyg 2003, 97:161-165.
142. Clarke SE, Jukes MC, Njagi JK, Khasakhala L, Cundill B, Otido J, Crudder C, Estambale BB, Brooker S: Effect of intermittent preventive treatment of malaria on health and education in schoolchildren: a cluster-randomised, double-blind, placebo-controlled trial. Lancet 2008, 372:127-138.
143. Kihara M, Carter JA, Newton CR: The effect of Plasmodium falciparum on cognition: a systematic review. Trop Med Int Health 2006, 11:386-397.
144. Simetka O, Reilley B, Joseph M, Collie M, Leidinger J: Obstetrics during civil war: six months on a maternity ward in Mallavi, northern Sri Lanka. Med Confl Surviv 2002, 18:258-270.
145. Childbirth at checkpoints in the occupied Palestinian territory Abstract available at: http://download.thelancet.com/flatcontentassets/pdfs/palestine/palestine2011-4.pdf
146. Hudic I, Radoncic F, Fatusic Z: Incidence and causes of maternal death during 20-year period (1986–2005) in Tuzla Canton, Bosnia and Herzegovina. J Matern Fetal Neonatal Med 2011, 24:1286-1288.
147. Strong MA: The health of adults in the developing world: the view from Bangladesh. Health Transit Rev 1992, 2:215-224.
148. Anderson FW, Morton SU, Naik S, Gebrian B: Maternal mortality and the consequences on infant and child survival in rural Haiti. Matern Child Health J 2007, 11:395-401.
149. Complex Emergency Database [http://www.cedat.be/]
150. World Health Organization: Public Health Risk Assessment and Interventions. The Horn of Africa: Drought and Famine Crisis. Geneva; 2011.
151. Egal F: Nutrition in conflict situations. Br J Nutr 2006, 96:S17-19.
152. Hendrie B: Relief aid behind the lines: the cross-border operation in Tigray. In War and Hunger Rethinking International Responses to Complex Emergencies. Edited by Macrae J, Zwi A, Duffield M, Slim M. London: Zed Books; 1994:125-139.

153. Baten J, Wagner A: Autarchy, market disintegration, and health: the mortality and nutritional crisis in Nazi Germany, 1933–1937. Econ Hum Biol 2002, 1:1-28.
154. Ali MM, Shah IH: Sanctions and childhood mortality in Iraq. Lancet 2000, 355:1851-1857.
155. Zakanj Z, Armano G, Grguric J, Herceg-Cavrak V: Influence of 1991–1995 war on breast-feeding in Croatia: questionnaire study. Croat Med J 2000, 41:186-190.
156. Jakobsen M, Sodemann M, Nylen G, Bale C, Nielsen J, Lisse I, Aaby P: Breastfeeding status as a predictor of mortality among refugee children in an emergency situation in Guinea-Bissau. Trop Med Int Health 2003, 8:992-996.
157. Andersson N, Paredes-Solis S, Legorreta-Soberanis J, Cockcroft A, Sherr L: Breastfeeding in a complex emergency: four linked cross-sectional studies during the Bosnian conflict. Public Health Rep 2010, 13:2097-2104.
158. Victora CG, Adair L, Fall C, Hallal PC, Martorell R, Richter L, Sachdev HS: Maternal and child undernutrition: consequences for adult health and human capital. Lancet 2008, 371:340-357.
159. Cheung E, Mutahar R, Assefa F, Ververs MT, Nasiri SM, Borrel A, Salama P: An epidemic of scurvy in Afghanistan: assessment and response. Food Nutr Bull 2003, 24:247-255.
160. Seal AJ, Creeke PI, Dibari F, Cheung E, Kyroussis E, Semedo P, van den Briel T: Low and deficient niacin status and pellagra are endemic in postwar Angola. Am J Clin Nutr 2007, 85:218-224.
161. Lumey LH: Decreased birthweights in infants after maternal in utero exposure to the Dutch famine of 1944–1945. Paediatr Perinat Epidemiol 1992, 6:240-253.
162. Brialic I, Rodin U, Vrdoljak J, Plavec D, Capkun V: Secular birth weight changes in liveborn infants before, during, and after 1991–1995 homeland war in Croatia. Croat Med J 2006, 47:452-458.
163. Hogue CJ, Buehler JW, Strauss LT, Smith JC: Overview of the national infant mortality surveillance (NIMS) project–design, methods, results. Public Health Rep 1987, 102:126-138.
164. Pena-Rosas JP, Viteri FE: Effects and safety of preventive oral iron or iron+folic acid supplementation for women during pregnancy. Cochrane Database Syst Rev 2009., 4 CD004736
165. De-Regil LM, Fernandez-Gaxiola AC, Dowswell T, Pena-Rosas JP: Effects and safety of periconceptional folate supplementation for preventing birth defects. Cochrane Database Syst Rev 2010., 10 CD007950
166. Wells JC, Chomtho S, Fewtrell MS: Programming of body composition by early growth and nutrition. Proc Nutr Soc 2007, 66:423-434.
167. Gudmundsson S, Henningsson AC, Lindqvist P: Correlation of birth injury with maternal height and birthweight. BJOG 2005, 112:764-767.
168. Moses RG, Mackay MT: Gestational diabetes: is there a relationship between leg length and glucose tolerance? Diab Care 2004, 27:1033-1035.
169. Myklestad K, Vatten LJ, Magnussen EB, Salvesen KA, Romundstad PR: Do parental heights influence pregnancy length? A population-based prospective study, HUNT 2. BMC Pregnancy Childbirth 2013, 13:33.
170. Clarkin PF: Adiposity and height of adult Hmong refugees: relationship with war-related early malnutrition and later migration. Am J Hum Biol 2008, 20:174-184.

171. Fishman SM, Caulfield L, de Onis M: Childhood and maternal underweight. In Comparative Quantification of Health Risks: Global and Regional Burden of Disease Attributable to Selected Major Risk Factors. Edited by Ezzati M, Lopez AD, Rodgers A, Murray CLJ. Geneva: World Health Organization; 2004:39-161.
172. Maternal anthropometry and pregnancy outcomes. A WHO collaborative study. Bull World Health Organ 1995, 73:1-98.
173. Horta BL, Gigante DP, Osmond C, Barros FC, Victora CG: Intergenerational effect of weight gain in childhood on offspring birthweight. Int J Epidemiol 2009, 38:724-732.
174. Greenfeld C, Flaws JA: Renewed debate over postnatal oogenesis in the mammalian ovary. BioEssays 2004, 26:829-832.
175. Bukovsky A, Caudle MR, Svetlikova M, Wimalasena J, Ayala ME, Dominguez R: Oogenesis in adult mammals, including humans: a review. Endocrine 2005, 26:301-316.
176. Ravelli G-P, Stein ZA, Susser MW: Obesity in young men after famine exposure in utero and early infancy. N Engl J Med 1976, 295:349-353.
177. Roseboom TJ, van der Meulen JH, Ravelli AC, Osmond C, Barker DJ, Bleker OP: Effects of prenatal exposure to the Dutch famine on adult disease in later life: an overview. Mol Cell Endocrinol 2001, 185:93-98.
178. Stein AD, Zybert PA, van der Pal-de Bruin K, Lumey LH: Exposure to famine during gestation, size at birth, and blood pressure at age 59 Y: evidence from the Dutch famine. Eur J Epidemiol 2006, 21:759-765.
179. Ravelli AC, van Der Meulen JH, Osmond C, Barker DJ, Bleker OP: Obesity at the age of 50 y in men and women exposed to famine prenatally. Am J Clin Nutr 1999, 70:811-816.
180. Stein AD, Kahn HS, Rundle A, Zybert PA, van der Pal-de Bruin K, Lumey LH: Anthropometric measures in middle age after exposure to famine during gestation: evidence from the Dutch famine. Am J Clin Nutr 2007, 85:869-876.
181. Stein AD, Lumey LH: The relationship between maternal and offspring birth weights after maternal prenatal famine exposure: the Dutch famine birth cohort study. Hum Biol 2000, 72:641-654.
182. Hult M, Tornhammar P, Ueda P, Chima C, Edstedt Bonamy AK, Ozumba B, Norman M: Hypertension, diabetes and overweight: looming legacies of the Biafran famine. PloS One 2010, 5:e13582.
183. Zheng X, Wang Y, Ren W, Luo R, Zhang S, Zhang JH, Zeng Q: Risk of metabolic syndrome in adults exposed to the great Chinese famine during the fetal life and early childhood. Eur J Clin Nutr 2012, 66:231-236.
184. Yang Z, Zhao W, Zhang X, Mu R, Zhai Y, Kong L, Chen C: Impact of famine during pregnancy and infancy on health in adulthood. Obes Rev 2008, 9:95-99.
185. Li Y, Jaddoe VW, Qi L, He Y, Wang D, Lai J, Zhang J, Fu P, Yang X, Hu FB: Exposure to the Chinese famine in early life and the risk of metabolic syndrome in adulthood. Diab Care 2011, 34:1014-1018.
186. Huang C, Li Z, Wang M, Martorell R: Early life exposure to the 1959–1961 Chinese famine has long-term health consequences. J Nutr 2010, 140:1874-1878.
187. St Clair D, Xu M, Wang P, Yu Y, Fang Y, Zhang F, Zheng X, Gu N, Feng G, Sham P, He L: Rates of adult schizophrenia following prenatal exposure to the Chinese famine of 1959–1961. JAMA 2005, 294:557-562.

188. Xu MQ, Sun WS, Liu BX, Feng GY, Yu L, Yang L, He G, Sham P, Susser E, St Clair D, He L: Prenatal malnutrition and adult schizophrenia: further evidence from the 1959–1961 Chinese famine. Schizophr Bull 2009, 35:568-576.

189. Westing AH: Warfare in a fragile world: military impacts on the human environment. London: Taylor and Francis; 1980.

190. World Health Organization: Dioxins and their effects on human health. Fact Sheet No 225, May 2010. Available at: http://www.who.int/mediacentre/factsheets/fs225/en/

191. Martin M: Vietnamese victims of Agent Orange and US–Vietnam relations. Congressional Research Service 7–5700 CRS Report for Congress May 28 2009 (re level of Agent Orange used); 2009.

192. United Nations Convention on the Rights of the Child Available at: [http://www.unicef.org/crc]

193. Osmani S, Sen A: The hidden penalties of gender inequality: fetal origins of ill-health. Econ Hum Biol 2003, 1:105-121.

194. Holsboer F: The corticosteroid receptor hypothesis of depression. Neuropsychopharmacol 2000, 23:477-501.

195. Schmidt U, Holsboer F, Rein T: Epigenetic aspects of posttraumatic stress disorder. Dis Markers 2011, 30:77-87.

196. Francis D, Diorio J, Liu D, Meaney MJ: Nongenomic transmission across generations of maternal behavior and stress responses in the rat. Science 1999, 286:1155-1158.

197. Liu D, Diorio J, Tannenbaum B, Caldji C, Francis D, Freedman A, Sharma S, Pearson D, Plotsky PM, Meaney MJ: Maternal care, hippocampal glucocorticoid receptors, and hypothalamic-pituitary-adrenal responses to stress. Science 1997, 277:1659-1662.

198. Weaver IC, Champagne FA, Brown SE, Dymov S, Sharma S, Meaney MJ, Szyf M: Reversal of maternal programming of stress responses in adult offspring through methyl supplementation: altering epigenetic marking later in life. J Neurosci 2005, 25:11045-11054.

199. Weaver IC, Meaney MJ, Szyf M: Maternal care effects on the hippocampal transcriptome and anxiety-mediated behaviors in the offspring that are reversible in adulthood. Proc Natl Acad Sci U S A 2006, 103:3480-3485.

200. Gardner H, Kobtzeff O {Eds): The Ashgate Research Companion to War: Origins and Prevention. Ashgate: Farnham; 2012.

201. ICRC/IFRC: Guidelines for Assessment in Emergencies. Geneva, Switzerland: ICRC and the IFRCRC; 2008. Available at: http://psychosocial.actalliance.org/default.aspx?di=66841

202. The Sphere Project: The Sphere Handbook: Humanitarian Charter and Minimum Standards in Humanitarian Response. 2011.

203. World Health Organization: Integrating Sexual and Reproductive Health into Health Emergency and Disaster Risk Management. Geneva; 2012.

204. Office of the Special Representative of the Secretary-General for Children and Armed Conflict: The Six Grave Violations Against Children During Armed Conflict: The Legal Foundation Working Paper 1. New York; 2009.

PART III

THE DEVELOPMENTAL IMPACT ON MENTAL AND PHYSICAL HEALTH

CHAPTER 8

CHILDHOOD ADVERSITY, RECENT LIFE STRESSORS, AND SUICIDAL BEHAVIOR IN CHINESE COLLEGE STUDENTS

ZHIQI YOU, MINGXI CHENG, SEN YANG, ZONGKUI ZHOU, AND PING QIN

8.1 INTRODUCTION

Suicidal behavior in young people has become a significant public health problem and has been the focus of many studies world-wide. Consequently it is urgent to study the associated risk factors for a better understanding of this problem and to establish assessment and prevention systems. In China, suicide among young people has become a particularly serious challenge for public health. There were up to 2,000,000 Chinese attempting suicide every year, with yearly suicide casualties of 287, 000 in the period of 1995–1999 [1]. Although it is the leading cause of death for young people in China, suicide in this population has not been much investigated and relevant evidence of significant correlates is meager compared with that of western countries.

Suicidality, including suicidal ideation and suicide attempt, may be influenced by many factors, ranging from genetics [2], family functions [3], social-economic status [4], personality [5] and psychiatric comorbidity [6]. The experience of adverse events during childhood has long been known to be a significant risk factor for suicidal behaviors among young adults. A large body of research, either with clinical samples [7], community samples [8], or specific groups such as drug abusers [9] and males with hyperactivity-inattention symptoms [10], has revealed that a higher number of adverse experiences in childhood were linked with higher risks for suicidal ideation or suicide attempt. Similar results were also found in one study focusing on college students [11]. At the same time, recent negative life events confer another striking risk factor for suicidal behaviors among young people. Consistent evidence has shown that recent negative life events are associated with an increased risk for onset of suicidal ideation and suicide attempt [12], and that the number or the severity of recent life events could predict the severity of suicidality and its repetition [13].

Though childhood adversity and recent negative events are individually known as prominent risk factors for suicidal behavior, few studies have explored the combinative role of these two exposures on suicidality. According to the stressor-diathesis model of suicidal behaviors proposed by Dr van Heeringen [14], suicidal behavior should be not only influenced by the independent effects of diathesis and stress, but also further formed by their interaction. Moreover, certain diatheses (usually associated with early childhood experience and genetics) could increase the likelihood of people encountering stressful events later in life [14]. It is therefore very likely that childhood adversities and recent life stressors have a multiplicative impact on suicidality.

Available studies on childhood adversities and suicidal behavior have delved into the influence of sexual abuse and neglect, leaving the influence of many common adversities in one's early life unascertained [15]. To our awareness, in research on negative events prior to suicidal behaviors, no study has simultaneously considered types of childhood adversity and recent negative events as well as their joint effects on suicidality.

To amend the missing knowledge in the area, this study aims: a) to examine the independent association of childhood adversities and recent life stressors with suicidality in a large sample of Chinese college students;

b) to explore the interactive effect of the two exposures; and c) to probe the specific impacts of different types of childhood adversities and recent school life stressors on suicidal behaviors in this population.

8.2 METHODS

8.2.1 ETHICAL APPROVAL

The study was approved by the Ethical Committee for Scientific Research at Central China Normal University. A signed consent form was collected from each student.

8.2.2 PARTICIPANTS OF STUDY

Of eight universities in Wuhan, a city in central China, six agreed to join in the survey. All were attached directly to the ministries of P. R. China. Stratified cluster sampling was used first to identify 10% of students at each university and then to randomly select participants from classes. Of a total 7022 students selected into the study, 6096 students participated in the survey (response rate: 86.8%). 5989 respondents completed all question items designed for the present study and therefore were considered as study population in the data analyses. The sample comprised 3156 (52.8%) male and 2768 (46.2%) female students. There were 56 respondents who did not report their gender. The age range of the sample was from 14 to 26 years old (M = 19.94; SD = 1.38).

8.2.3 INSTRUMENT FOR ASSESSMENT

8.2.3.1 CHILDHOOD ADVERSITIES (CA)

In this section, participants were asked to report the worst adverse experience in the first 10 years of their life. The Childhood Adversity questionnaire listed 6 adversities that children might experience: divorce of parents, poor parental relationship, loss of a parent, family financial problems, sexual abuse, and severe physical illness, together with the option of "None of the above". Participants were asked to review each item in this part and to report if they had ever undergone any of these adversities, and if yes, then to specify which adverse experience had the worst impact on them. The score range of CA was 0–1. Students reporting "None of the above" were assigned a score with "0" and classified as "without childhood adversity", while those reporting they had experienced one or more adversities were assigned a score of "1" and classified as cases "with childhood adversity".

8.2.3.2 SCHOOL LIFE STRESSORS (SLS)

To assess recent negative life events in college students, the SLS questionnaire was created to measure frustrations in different domains that college students might encounter. Based upon results from the pilot investigation for this study, nine stressors were considered: 1) poor school performance, 2) rupture of romantic relationships, 3) difficulty of adapting college life, 4) financial problems, 5) employment stress, 6) conflicts with classmates, 7) failure in making close friends and 8) other frustrations. The participants were asked which frustrations they had encountered during the past one year period. Students who reported at least one of the listed stressors were assigned a score of "1" and regarded as "with school life stressor', while those reporting "None of the above" were assigned a score of "0" and classified as "without school life stressor".

8.2.3.3 SUICIDALITY

Participants' suicidal ideation and suicide attempts were assessed by a questionnaire comprising 5 questions: 1) Did you ever seriously consider killing yourself in the past year; 2) Have you ever seriously considered killing yourself in your life; 3) Did you ever try or attempt to kill your-self within the past one year; 4) Have you ever tried or attempted to kill yourself in your life; and 5) Have you ever had a nonfatal suicide action. Participants answered the first 4 questions by marking 0 (never), 1 (some-times) or 2 (very often). For the last question respondents had to answer only "Yes" or "No". Participants were asked to respond to all items. Stu-dents who answered "never" for both items about suicidal ideation (items 1 and 2) were classified as "Without suicidal ideations", while the others were classified as "With suicidal ideations". Similarly, students who chose "no" or "never" as the answer to all three questions about suicide attempts (items 3–5) were classified as "Without suicidal attempts"; otherwise, they were regarded as "With suicidal attempts."

8.2.3.4 DEMOGRAPHIC INFORMATION

Personal demographic information was also collected during the survey. Respondents reported personal details including age, gender, specialty of study, and region of permanent family residence (urban or rural).

8.2.4 PROCEDURE

An independent website was designed for this project with all relevant ques-tionnaires and the site was accessible only through a unique password as-signed to each selected student. The students were asked to complete the survey online. Before the survey, they were given a brief introduction to the study and were ensured of the confidentiality of personal data. Students who agreed to participate signed a consent form. The on-line survey started with an overall introduction about the research purposes, and then moved to spe-cific instructions for each questionnaire. Several pilot studies were carried out to examine whether the questionnaires were suitable and understandable, and also to test the functionality of the website. There was no report of techni-cal problems during the final online survey collecting data from the students.

8.2.5 DATA ANALYSES

Data were first generated into a spreadsheet file and then analyzed with SPSS17.0. Firstly, a t-test was used to detect if there was any difference in the number of school life stressors according to the presence of childhood adversity. Secondly, three logistic regression models were conducted to assess the effects of gender, region, childhood adversity and school life stressors on risks for suicidal ideation and for suicide attempts. Model 1 estimated the individual effect of each of these variables; Model 2 estimated the separate effects of CA and the SLS with the adjustment for gender and region; while in Model 3 the effects of gender, region, SLS and CA on suicidality were considered simultaneously in one analytic model. Lastly, separate regression analyses were conducted to examine specific CA and SLS events as risk factors for suicidal ideation and suicide attempt.

TABLE 1: Prevalence of suicidal ideation and suicide attempts in the study population.

Variables under study		Number	Suicidal ideation		Suicide attempts	
		N	%	(n)	%	(n)
Gender	Male	3165	12.02	(412)	1.33	(42)
	Female	2768	20.38	(564)	2.60	(72)
Region	Urban	3942	16.39	(646)	2.23	(88)
	Rural	2044	16.39	(335)	1.32	(27)
School life stressor	No	953	6.40	(61)	0.84	(8)
	Yes	5036	18.29	(921)	2.13	(107)
Childhood adversity	No	3698	13.63	(504)	1.33	(49)
	Yes	2291	20.86	(478)	2.88	(66)
Total		5989	16.40	(982)	1.92	(115)

Note. In the study population, 56 students did not report gender information and 3 students did not report the region of permanent family residence.

8.3 RESULTS

Among the 5989 college students, 982 (16.40%) presented a positive answer to suicidal ideation some time during their life course, while 115

(1.92%) reported the presence of a suicide attempt. The prevalence of both suicidal ideation and suicide attempt was significantly higher in female students than in male students. Table 1 shows the prevalence of suicidal behaviors by variables of interest in the present study. Examination of the relationship between childhood adversities and school life stressors showed that in the group of students "with childhood adversities", the mean number of school life stressors was 2.51±1.47, whereas the corresponding number was 1.86±1.34 for the group "without childhood adversities". The t-test result indicated that compared to those without any adversity in childhood, individuals who had one or more adverse childhood experience experienced more recent negative events in school (t = 30.28, p<0.001).

Table 2 shows the effect of study variables on risk for suicidal ideation, derived from three logistic regression models. Results from model 1 revealed that gender, recent school life stressors and childhood adversities all had a significant association with suicidal ideation, while region of family residence did not. Compared with model 1, the OR values associated with SLS and CA in Model 2 were slightly reduced after adjustments for the effects of gender and region. When all variables were simultaneously included in model 3, gender, region, SLS and CA all had a notable influence on suicidal ideation. Moreover, compared with the estimates from model 2, the OR associated with SLS decreased by 3.60% and the OR associated with CA reduced by 15.38%, suggesting that there was an interactive effect of SLS and CA on risk for suicidal ideation.

Table 2 also displayed the results of regression analyses focusing on suicide attempt. Again, the effect sizes associated with the variables under study, as well the pattern of the effects, were very similar to those found in the analyses on suicidal ideation. From model 2 to model 3, there was a 4.35% reduction of the OR value associated with SLS and a 15.89% reduction of the OR associated with CA, suggesting an interactive effect of the two exposures on risk for suicide attempt.

Analyses were then conducted to examine the associations between suicidality and each item in the CA and SLS questionnaires. Associations between each specific childhood adversity and suicidality are shown in Table 3. Family financial problems constituted the most common childhood negative event (21.8%) for the Chinese college students, followed by poor parental relationship (9.5%).

TABLE 2: Effects of gender, region, school life stressors and childhood adversities on risk for suicidal ideation and for suicide attempt.

Variables	Model I				Model II				Model III			
	Wald	p	OR	95% CI	Wald	p	OR	95% CI	Wald	p	OR	95% CI
Suicidal ideation												
Gender (0/1 = male/female)	57.87	0.00	1.71	1.49–1.97					60.19	0.00	1.76	1.53–2.03
Region (0/1 = urban/rural)	0.71	0.94	0.94	0.82–1.08					8.62	0.00	0.80	0.70–0.93
School life stressors (0/1 = no/yes)	180.24	0.00	1.37	1.31–1.44	184.99	0.00	1.39	1.32–1.45	141.72	0.00	1.34	1.28–1.40
Childhood adversities (0/1 = no/yes)	87.64	0.00	1.93	1.68–2.22	100.39	0.00	2.08	1.80–2.40	56.48	0.00	1.76	1.52–2.04
Suicide attempt												
Gender (0/1 = male/female)	12.26	0.00	1.99	1.35–2.92					11.24	0.00	1.94	1.32–2.86
Region (0/1 = urban/rural)	6.64	0.01	0.60	0.41–0.89					11.34	0.00	0.51	0.34–0.75
School life stressors (0/1 = no/yes)	28.84	0.00	1.36	1.22–1.52	31.04	0.00	1.38	1.23–1.54	21.18	0.00	1.32	1.17–1.48
Childhood adversities (0/1 = no/yes)	17.85	0.00	2.24	1.54–3.25	23.54	0.00	2.58	1.76–3.79	14.96	0.00	2.17	1.47–3.22

Notes: Model 1: Analyses without any adjustment. Model 2: only adjusted for gender and region. Model 3: adjusted for all variables listed in the table.

Among the childhood adverse experiences, sexual abuse, divorce of parents, poor parental relationship and loss of a parent were associated with significantly increased risks for suicidal ideation ($p<0.01$ for all) and suicide attempt ($p<0.01$ for all). Though financial problems and severe physical illness in childhood had a significant effect on suicidal ideation ($p<0.01$), they did not have a significant influence on suicidal attempt ($p = 0.20$ and $p = 0.26$, respectively). Among all childhood adversities under study, the three carrying the most risk for suicidal ideation were sexual abuse, poor parental relationship and loss of a parent; for suicide attempts, the top three risk factors were sexual abuse, loss of a parent and divorce of parents. It is worth mentioning that even with the limited number of college students who reported sexual abuse, this form of childhood adversity carried the highest risk for suicidality.

Table 4 shows the relationships between each specific stressor on the SLS and suicidal behaviors in the study population. Poor school performance was the most common stressor in college life, presenting in 56.44% of the study population. Poor school performance, rupture of a romantic relationship, failure to adapt, financial problems, conflicts with classmates, failure to make close friends, and other frustrations, all had a significant effect ($p<0.01$) on suicidal ideation. For suicide attempts, only poor school performance ($p<0.05$), rupture of romantic relationships ($p<0.01$), failure in adaptation ($p<0.01$) and financial problems ($p<0.05$) had a significant influence. Conflicts with classmates, poor school performance and other frustrations carried the highest risk for suicidal ideation, while rupture of romantic relationships, difficulty in adaptation, and financial problems were carried the highest risk for suicidal attempt. Furthermore, there was no significant effect of stress from employment competition on suicidal behavior in the study population.

8.4 DISCUSSION

8.4.1 DEMOGRAPHIC STRUCTURE OF SUICIDALITY IN CHINESE COLLEGE STUDENTS

The present study demonstrates that both suicidal ideation and suicide attempts were significantly more common in female students as compared with their male counterparts. This observation is consistent with the conclusion of a previous study on Chinese college students [16], and also in high concordance with many reports internationally [17]–[19]. As for the effect of region, there was no significant rural-urban difference for suicidal ideation, but the risk of suicide attempt was significantly higher among students coming from urban areas than those from rural China. This finding is somewhat different from the previous view that the suicide rate in rural China is much higher than that in urban places [1], [20]. A possible reason could be that the sample population in the current study is very different from those in previous reports. College students coming from rural areas were now studying and hence living in a city of central China. They were pursuing an education and enjoying a much better living environment than what they had in the rural area. It is therefore understandable that these students are at a relatively lower risk for attempting suicide compared with counterpart students coming from the urban areas.

8.4.2 CHILDHOOD ADVERSITY, SCHOOL LIFE STRESSORS AND SUICIDALITY

This study shows that both adverse experiences in childhood and recent life stressors in school life are strongly associated with risk for suicidal behaviors in young people studying in university. These results are consistent with previous reports focusing on early life adversities [7], [8], and also studies on recent stressful life events in relation to suicidality [12], [13].

This study adds to the literature demonstrating that experience of childhood adversity (CA) could increase the likelihood of exposure to negative life events (SLS) during young adulthood and that there is an interactive effect between SLS and CA on suicidality. Such observations support the stress-diathesis model of suicidal behaviors, proposed by Dr van Heeringen [14]. Apart from the respectively independent effect of school life stressors and childhood adversities on suicidality, the two types of exposure combined to exert an interactive role on suicidality. According to the stress-diathesis model, childhood adversities could act as a diathesis that could predispose individuals to more negative events in their future life; the occurrence of later stressful events could in turn further predispose these people to become more vulnerable to the effects of stressful events; and consequently, risk for suicidal behavior becomes higher and higher through an interactive process. There are a number of published studies providing evidence of the proposed impact pathway. For example, childhood adversity was found to be linked with personality characteristics such as aggression; the aggressiveness made the subjects more maladapted and therefore induced more stressful events [21]. Childhood adversity could increase the tendency to form specific cognitive characteristics, such as negative attribution style [22] and hopelessness [23], which could in turn increase the vulnerability to new stressors.

The observed interaction between childhood adversity and recent school life stressors could also be interpreted from developmental perspectives. One possible explanation lies in the association between attachment and suicidality. Secure attachment has been acknowledged as a strong, if not the most important, protective factor for children's psychosocial development. Especially in the face of troubles or frustrations, secure attachment could be the child's major psychological resource [24]. As well established, early adversities or traumas are detrimental for the formation of secure attachment [25].Therefore, children with severe childhood adversity might show less secure attachment during their upbringing and show greater vulnerability in response to stressful events compared to peer youth raised in families that experienced no obvious adversity. It is also more difficult for them to retain stable and durable relationship with others, including with family members and classmates [26]—factors strongly associated with suicidality among young people [27]. The current results are consistent with the attachment hypothesis, in that interpersonal stress and conflicts with classmates showed high prevalence among students with suicidal behavior.

Moreover, childhood adversity and recent life stressors may share certain characteristics as risk factors for suicidality, the most notable being difficult family relationships. Family circumstances are usually enduring and related both socially and psychologically to the adjustment of individual family members. Children from such families may experience ongoing suffering and are more likely to experience stressors from childhood through adolescence to adulthood. This is supported by early research demonstrating strong associations between a problematic family background, early life adversity and recent stressful life events [28]. It is also evident that children from family backgrounds characterized by low socio-economic status, poor communication or troublesome life are at an increased risk for suicidal behaviors [24].

TABLE 3: Logistic regression results showing risk of suicidal behaviors associated with specific adverse experiences in childhood.

			Suicidal ideation				Suicide attempts			
		cases	Wald	p	OR	95% CI	Wald	p	OR	95% CI
Step 1	Gender		53.25	0.00	1.70	1.48–1.96	1.24	0.27	1.19	0.88–1.60
	Region		2.10	0.15	0.90	0.78–1.04	4.26	0.04	0.72	0.53–0.98
Step 2	Divorce of parents	140	13.92	0.00	2.16	1.44–3.28	18.71	0.00	4.06	2.15–7.66
	Poor parental relationship	566	95.58	0.00	2.83	2.30–3.49	47.37	0.00	3.86	2.63–5.68
	Loss of parent(s)	110	17.92	0.00	2.62	1.68–4.10	16.20	0.00	4.39	2.14–9.02
	Financial problems	1307	28.05	0.00	1.62	1.36–1.94	1.64	0.20	1.32	0.86–2.01
	Sexual abuse	19	9.83	0.00	4.36	1.74–10.98	11.04	0.00	8.45	2.40–29.78
	Severe physical illness	149	19.4	0.00	2.44	1.64–3.62	1.30	0.26	1.71	0.68–4.29

Note: ORs were adjusted for all childhood adversities as well as demographic variables listed in the table.

8.4.3 INFLUENCE OF SPECIFIC LIFE STRESSORS OR NEGATIVE EVENTS

The present study indicates that different types of life stressors or negative events, either in childhood or in school life, had different effects on suicidal behavior in Chinese college students. Compared with other stressful events, poor school performance was the most common stressor that Chinese college students encountered within a one year period. Among all stressors under study, those that were significantly associated with suicidality (both suicidal ideation and suicide attempts) were poor school performance, rupture of romantic relationships, difficulty in adapting school life and financial problems; conflicts with classmates, failure to make close friends and other frustrations were linked with suicidal ideation but not suicide attempts. These findings are mostly in agreement with another study of college students, showing that suicidality was especially associated with interpersonal affairs, such as interpersonal conflicts and ruptured relationships as well as school performance [29].

TABLE 4: Logistic regression results showing risk of suicidal behaviors associated with specific stressors in school life.

		cases	Suicidal ideation				Suicide attempts			
			Wald	p	OR	95% CI	Wald	p	OR	95% CI
Step 1	Gender		56.72	0.00	1.74	1.51–2.01	3.35	0.06	1.32	0.98–1.79
	Region		2.07	0.15	0.90	0.80–1.04	6.15	0.01	0.68	0.50–0.92
Step 2	Poor school performance	3380	28.15	0.00	1.50	1.29–1.74	4.40	0.04	1.41	1.02–1.93
	Rupture of love affairs	1269	9.30	0.00	1.30	1.10–1.53	9.00	0.00	1.65	1.19–2.29
	Difficulty in adapting to college life	1545	21.91	0.00	1.45	1.24–1.69	8.89	0.00	1.62	1.18–2.22
	Financial problems	1229	12.52	0.00	1.36	1.15–1.61	4.54	0.03	1.45	1.03–2.04
	Employment stress	1176	0.10	0.75	0.97	0.81–1.16	0.61	0.43	1.15	0.81–1.64
	Conflicts with classmates	706	21.09	0.00	1.59	1.30–1.93	3.03	0.08	1.42	0.96–2.10
	Failure in making close friends	2011	14.68	0.00	1.34	1.15–1.56	1.75	0.18	1.24	0.90–1.70
	Other frustration	1516	26.40	0.00	1.49	1.28–1.74	0.34	0.56	1.10	0.79–1.53

Note: ORs were adjusted for all school life stressors as well as demographic variables listed in the table.

It is worth noting that employment stress did not confer significant risk for suicidal behavior in the present study. In earlier research the association between unemployment and suicidality has been viewed as ambiguous and conclusions have varied under different research conditions [27]. To our awareness, however, no study has focused on suicidal behavior in relation to stress from possible employment competition, let alone in a sample of Chinese college students. Yet we could not simply conclude from the present data that employment stress has no significant effect on suicidal behaviors in Chinese undergraduates, because the present sample mostly consisted of students who had not yet completed their third year at their universities. Due to their limited experiences in the labor market, it is likely that job competition is not yet an urgent consideration for the subjects of the present study. On the other hand, our data demonstrate that recent stress from financial problems is strongly associated with risk for both suicidal ideation and suicide attempt. This is in line with previous studies of young adults [30], [31], and underlines the importance of financial support for college students and of students' proper management of their economic situation during school life.

Regarding childhood adversities, it is interesting to see that all parent-related stressors during childhood—including divorce of parents, poor parental relationship and loss of a parent– were associated with a significantly increased risk for suicidal behavior. This finding is in line with the literature [17], [31], and makes particular sense when thinking of the stress-diathesis model and attachment theory discussed in the previous section. Although very few students reported the experience of sexual abuse during childhood, this exposure denoted the highest risk for suicidal ideation and attempt. On the other hand, the experience of family financial problems during childhood was the most frequently reported childhood stressor in this population, although compared to other negative childhood experiences it had the lowest influence on suicidality. Of course, family financial problems during childhood do not necessarily mean low economic status, because the problems could be due to a short term crisis. Nevertheless, the results from this study indicate that compared with insufficient resources caused by financial problems, family stressors such as parental divorce or a poor parent-child relationship play a more important role in the development of suicidality.

8.4.4 LIMITATIONS

There are several limitations in the present study. One limitation is that the study is a cross-sectional investigation, which does not allow detection of any causal relationship between exposure to adversity and suicidality. It would be ideal to test the findings from this study using a cohort design, following children from their early life. Another limitation concerns generalizability. The sample was obtained strictly by a stratified cluster sampling method in six of eight universities in a major city in Central China. Although we are confident that our sample represents well the undergraduate college students in the area of Central China, it is uncertain to us if it could represent undergraduates in other places of China such as the more developed coastal or the less developed western regions. It is therefore preferable that more studies should be carried out in larger and more diverse samples to test the present findings and evaluate their generalizability.

8.5 CONCLUSION

Based on a large sample of undergraduate students in China, the present study reports a 16.40% rate of suicidal ideation and a 1.92% rate of suicide attempts. The prevalence differed significantly by gender and region of family residence, with higher rates in females than males and lower rates among students from rural areas compared to urban areas. At the same time, students with suicidal behavior more often reported the experience of negative life stressors in both childhood and recent school life. While childhood adversity and recent school life stressors each denoted significant risk for suicidal behavior, the two types of exposure tended to co-occur and act interactively to increase the risk for suicidal behavior. With noticeable variation of effects associated with specific stressors, family relationship problems during childhood and recent interpersonal conflicts in school are of great importance in predicting risk for suicidality. These findings should be taken into account when planning programs of mental health promotion, suicide prevention and suicide intervention in university settings in China, and perhaps internationally.

REFERENCES

1. Phillips MR, Li X, Zhang Y (2002) Suicide rates in China, 1995–99. Lancet 359: 835–840 doi: 10.1016/S0140-6736(02)07954-0.
2. Pedersen N, Fiske A (2010) Genetic influences on suicide and nonfatal suicidal behavior: Twin study findings. Eur Psychiatry 25: 264–267 doi: 10.1016/j.eurpsy.2009.12.008.
3. Kwok SYCL (2011) Perceived family functioning and suicidal ideation: Hopelessness as mediator or moderator. Nurs Res 60: 422–429 doi: 10.1097/NNR.0b013e31823585d6.
4. Hawton K, Harriss L, Hodder K, Simkin S, Gunnell D (2001) The influence of the economic and social environment on deliberate self-harm and suicide: an ecological and person-based study. Psychol Med 31: 827–836 doi: 10.1017/S0033291701003993.
5. Yen S, Shea MT, Sanislow CA, Skodol AE, Grilo CM, et al. (2009) Personality traits as prospective predictors of suicide attempts. Acta Psychiatr Scand 120: 222–229 doi: 10.1111/j.1600-0447.2009.01366.x.
6. Pompili M, Di Cosimo D, Innamorati M, Lester D, Tatarelli R, et al. (2009) Psychiatric comorbidity in patients with chronic daily headache and migraine: A selective overview including personality traits and suicide risk. J Headache Pain 10: 283–290 doi: 10.1007/s10194-009-0134-2.
7. Skopp NA, Luxton DD, Bush N, Sirotin A (2011) Childhood adversity and suicidal ideation in a clinical military sample: Military unit cohesion and intimate relationships as protective factors. J Soc Clin Psychol 30: 361–377 doi: 10.1521/jscp.2011.30.4.361.
8. Buchmann A, Blomeyer D, Laucht M (2012) Suicidal behaviors among young adults: Risk factors during development from early childhood to adolescence. Prax Kinderpsychol Kinderpsychiatr 61: 32–49.
9. Sundin M, Spak F, Spak L, Sundh V, Waern M (2011) Substance use/abuse and suicidal behavior in young adult women: A population-based study. Subst Use Misuse 46: 1690–1699 doi: 10.3109/10826084.2011.605414.
10. Galéra C, Bouvard M, Encrenaz G, Messiah A, Fombonne E (2008) Hyperactivity-inattention symptoms in childhood and suicidal behaviors in adolescence: The Youth Gazel Cohort. Acta Psychiatr Scand 118: 480–489 doi:10.1111/j.1600-0447.2008.01262.x.
11. Singh S, Manjula M, Philip M (2012) Suicidal risk and childhood adversity: A study of Indian college students. Asian J Psychiatr 5: 154–159 doi: 10.1016/j.ajp.2012.02.024.
12. Cupina D (2009) Life events, gender and suicidal behaviors in the acute community setting. Australas Psychiatry 17: 233–236 doi: 10.1080/10398560802680746.

13. Grover KE, Green KL, Pettit JW, Monteith LL, Garza MJ, et al. (2009) Problem solving moderates the effects of life event stress and chronic stress on suicidal behaviors in adolescence. J Clin Psychol 65: 1281–1290 doi: 10.1002/jclp.20632.

14. Van Heeringen K (2000) A stress-diathesis model of suicidal behavior. Crisis 21: 192a doi: 10.1201/b12215-7.

15. Sfoggia A, Pacheco MA, Grassi-Oliveira R (2008) History of childhood abuse and neglect and suicidal behavior at hospital admission. Crisis 29: 154–158 doi: 10.1027/0227-5910.29.3.154.

16. Tang J, Yu Y, Wu Y, Du Y, Ma Y, et al. (2011) Association between non-suicidal self-injuries and suicide attempts in Chinese adolescents and college students: A cross-section study. PloS One 6: e17977 doi: 10.1371/journal.pone.0017977.

17. Bedi S, Nelson EC, Lynskey MT, McCutcheon VV, Heath AC, et al. (2011) Risk for suicidal thoughts and behavior after childhood sexual abuse in women and men. Suicide Life Threat Behav 41: 406–415 doi: 10.1111/j.1943-278X.2011.00040.x.

18. Hawton K (2000) Sex and suicide gender differences in suicidal behaviour. Br J Psychiatry 177: 484–485 doi: 10.1192/bjp.177.6.484.

19. Mościcki EK (1994) Gender differences in completed and attempted suicides. Ann Epidemiol 4: 152–158 doi: 10.1016/1047-2797(94)90062-0.

20. Zhang J, Jia S, Jiang C, Sun J (2006) Characteristics of Chinese suicide attempters: An emergency room study. Death Stud 30: 259–268 doi: 10.1080/07481180500493443.

21. Sarchiapone M, Jaussent I, Roy A, Carli V, Guillaume S, et al. (2009) Childhood trauma as a correlative factor of suicidal behavior - via aggression traits. Similar results in an Italian and in a French sample. Eur Psychiatry 24: 57–62 doi: 10.1016/j.eurpsy.2008.07.005.

22. Kleiman EM, Miller AB, Riskind JH (2012) Enhancing attributional style as a protective factor in suicide. J Affect Disord 143: 236–240 doi: 10.1016/j.jad.2012.05.014.

23. Spokas M, Wenzel A, Stirman SW, Brown GK, Beck AT (2009) Suicide risk factors and mediators between childhood sexual abuse and suicide ideation among male and female suicide attempters. J Trauma Stress 22: 467–470 doi: 10.1002/jts.20438.

24. Violato C, Arato JE (2004) Childhood attachment and adolescent suicide: A stepwise discriminant analysis in a case-comparison study. Individ Differ Res 2: 162–168.

25. Hill EM, Young JP, Nord JL (1994) Childhood adversity, attachment security, and adult relationships: A preliminary study. Ethol Sociobiol 15: 323–338 doi: 10.1016/0162-3095(94)90006-X.

26. Frederick J, Goddard C (2008) Living on an island: consequences of childhood abuse, attachment disruption and adversity in later life. Child Fam Soc Work 13: 300–310 doi: 10.1111/j.1365-2206.2008.00554.x.

27. Van Orden KA, Witte TK, Cukrowicz KC, Braithwaite SR, Selby EA, et al. (2010) The interpersonal theory of suicide. Psychol Rev 117: 575–600 doi: 10.1037/a0018697.

28. Ackerman BP, Brown ED, Izard CE (2004) The relations between persistent poverty and contextual risk and children's behavior in elementary school. Dev Psychol 40: 367–377 doi: 10.1037/0012-1649.40.3.367.

29. Vázquez JJ, Panadero S, Rincón PP (2010) Stressful life events and suicidal behaviour in countries with different development levels: Nicaragua, El Salvador, Chile and Spain. J Community Appl Soc Psychol 20: 288–298 doi: 10.1002/casp.1036.

30. Wang Y, Sareen J, Afifi TO, Bolton SL, Johnson EA, et al. (2012) Recent stressful life events and suicide attempt. Psychiatr Ann 42: 101–108 doi: 10.3928/00485713-20120217-07.

31. Zhang J, Ma Z (2012) Patterns of life events preceding the suicide in rural young Chinese: A case control study. J Affect Disord 140: 161–167 doi: 10.1016/j.jad.2012.01.010.

CHAPTER 9

CHILDHOOD SEXUAL ABUSE AND THE DEVELOPMENT OF RECURRENT MAJOR DEPRESSION IN CHINESE WOMEN

JING CHEN, YIYUN CAI, ENZHAO CONG, YING LIU, JINGFANG GAO, YOUHUI LI, MING TAO, KERANG ZHANG, XUMEI WANG, CHENGGE GAO, LIJUN YANG, KAN LI, JIANGUO SHI, GANG WANG, LANFEN LIU, JINBEI ZHANG, BO DU, GUOQING JIANG, JIANHUA SHEN, ZHEN ZHANG, WEI LIANG, JING SUN, JIAN HU, TIEBANG LIU, XUEYI WANG, GUODONG MIAO, HUAQING MENG, YI LI, CHUNMEI HU, YI LI, GUOPING HUANG, GONGYING LI, BAOWEI HA, HONG DENG, QIYI MEI, HUI ZHONG, SHUGUI GAO, HONG SANG, YUTANG ZHANG, XIANG FANG, FENGYU YU, DONGLIN YANG, TIEQIAO LIU, YUNCHUN CHEN, XIAOHONG HONG, WENYUAN WU, GUIBING CHEN, MIN CAI, YAN SONG, JIYANG PAN, JICHENG DONG, RUNDE PAN, WEI ZHANG, ZHENMING SHEN, ZHENGRONG LIU, DANHUA GU, XIAOPING WANG, XIAOJUAN LIU, QIWEN ZHANG, YIHAN LI, YIPING CHEN, KENNETH S. KENDLER, SHENXUN SHI, AND JONATHAN FLIN

Childhood Sexual Abuse and the Development of Recurrent Major Depression in Chinese Women. © Chen J et al. PLoS ONE **9**,1 *(2014), doi:10.1371/journal.pone.0087569. Licensed under a Creative Commons Attribution 4.0 International License, http://creativecommons.org/licenses/by/4.0/.*

9.1 INTRODUCTION

Studies carried out in Western populations indicated that childhood sexual abuse (CSA) increases the risk of developing major depression (MD) [1], [2], [3], [4], [5], [6], [7], [8], [9], [10], [11], [12], [13], [14], [15]. Furthermore, these studies also show that depressed patients who reported CSA differ in some clinical features from MD patients without a history of CSA. For example, they had been shown to have more severe depressive symptoms, longer duration of episodes, earlier onset, and higher levels of comorbidity [16], [17], [18], [19].

Some studies carried out in China reported higher levels of depressive symptoms in participants who experienced CSA [20]. However, none of these studies examined the association between CSA exposure and the risk of developing MD. The China, Oxford and VCU Experimental Research on Genetic Epidemiology (CONVERGE) study has been examining risk factors for MD reported in Western populations, using a large cohort of Chinese women with recurrent MD (rMD). We previously reported an analysis of CSA in a preliminary sample from this study consisting of 1,970 cases and 2,597 controls. Our findings were broadly similar to those seen in Western samples and can be summarized as follows: 1) Any form of CSA was significantly associated with rMD; this association strengthened with increasing CSA severity from non-genital, to genital, to intercourse. 2) The association between any form of CSA and rMD remained significant after accounting for parental history of depression, childhood emotional neglect (CEN), childhood physical abuse (CPA) and a measure of perceived parenting (derived from the parental bonding instrument (REF). 3) Among the depressed women, those with CSA had an earlier age of onset, longer depressive episodes and an increased risk for generalized anxiety disorder and dysthymia [21].

We now report analyses of CSA and rMD with our final sample of 5,983 controls and 6,017 cases. Our study had the following major aims. First, could we replicate our findings from our preliminary sample? Second, we examined in more detail the relationship between rMD and the nature of the CSA. In addition to the nature of the abuse, we asked which other features of CSA (including the age and gender of the perpetrator, and the relationship of the perpetrator to the victim) increased the risk of rMD. Third, we examined the association between CSA and individual depressive symptoms to find out whether the nature of the illness differed between those who have and those who did not have a history of CSA.

9.2 METHODS

9.2.1 SAMPLE

The data for the present study were drawn from the China, Oxford and VCU Experimental Research on Genetic Epidemiology (CONVERGE) study of MD. These analyses were based on a total of 6017 cases recruited from 58 provincial mental health centres and psychiatric departments of general medical hospitals in 45 cities and 23 provinces, and 5983 controls who were recruited from patients undergoing minor surgical procedures at general hospitals (37%) or from local community centres (63%). Where controls were obtained from a hospital, this was always from the same hospital as the cases.

All cases and controls were female and had four Han Chinese grandparents. Cases and controls were excluded if they had a pre-existing history of bipolar disorder, any type of psychosis or mental retardation. Cases were between 30 and 60 years old, had two or more episodes of MD, with the first episode occurring between ages 14 and 50, and had not abused drugs or alcohol prior to their first depressive episode. Controls were chosen to match the region of origin of cases, were aged between 40 and 60, had never experienced an episode of MD and were not blood relatives of cases. An older minimal age of controls was used to reduce the chances that they might have a subsequent first onset of MD. The mean (S.D.) age of cases and controls in the dataset was similar: 44.4 (8.9) years for cases and 47.7 (5.6) years for controls.

All subjects were interviewed using a computerized assessment system. All interviewers were medical professionals and were trained by the CONVERGE team for a minimum of 1 week in the use of the interview. The interview includes assessment of demographic factors, psychopathology, psychosocial functioning and personal characteristics. Interviews were tape recorded and a proportion of them were listened to by the trained editors who provided feedback on the quality of the interviews. The study protocol was approved centrally by the Ethical Review Board of Oxford University and the ethics committee in participating hospitals in China.

9.2.2 MEASURES

The diagnoses of lifetime MD was established with the Composite International Diagnostic Interview (CIDI; [22]), which classifies diagnoses according to DSM-IV criteria [23]. The interview was originally translated into Mandarin by a team of psychiatrists in Shanghai Mental Health Centre, with the translation reviewed and modified by members of the CONVERGE team.

Additional information using instruments developed for the Virginia Adult Twin Study of Psychiatric and Substance Use Disorders (VATSP-SUD; [24]), translated and reviewed for accuracy by members of the CONVERGE team, was collected on stressful life events, CSA, family history and parent–child relationships etc. The stressful life events section assessed 16 traumatic lifetime events and the age of their occurrence. The CSA module was a shortened version of the more detailed module used in the VATSP-SUD study, which is in turn based on the instrument developed by Martin et al. [25]. We assessed separately the history of MD in mothers and fathers of our cases and controls using the Family History Research Diagnostic criteria [26], and parent–child relationships were measured with the 16-item Parental Bonding Instrument (PBI) modified by Kendler [27] based on Parker's original 25-item instrument [28]. Three factors were extracted from these 16 items and labeled warmth, protectiveness and authoritarianism. The computerized interview system is described elsewhere [21].

Symptoms reported during the most severe MD episode were classified according to DSM-IV diagnostic "A criteria" such as loss of interest, weight loss/gain, insomnia/hypersomnia, etc.

There is evidence that sensitive subjects such as CSA are more accurately reported with more confidential methods of assessment [29], and therefore participants were asked to fill in a paper questionnaire about CSA [25]. The questions asked whether, before the subject was 16 years old, did any adult or any other older person involve the subject in any unwanted incidents such as (1) inviting or requesting them to do something sexual, (2) kissing or hugging in a sexual way, (3) touching or fondling private parts, (4) showing their sex organs, (5) making them touch the person in a sexual way, or (6) attempting or having sexual intercourse. The possible responses were 'never', 'once' and 'more than once'. We used these responses to define three forms of CSA [5]: (1) non-genital CSA including sexual invitation, sexual kissing, and exposing (2) genital CSA including fondling and sexual touching and (3) attempted or completed intercourse.

We assessed childhood physical abuse (CPA) through the question in our stressful life events section: 'Were you ever physically abused as a child?' We assessed childhood emotional neglect (CEN) through the question in this section: 'Were you ever seriously neglected as a child?' Emotional neglect refers to a lack of emotional support and inadequate attention to a child's emotional needs, including the need for affection. Physical abuse refers to bodily assaults on a child by an older person that pose a risk of, or result in, injury.

Thirty-nine participants (6.4%) in the rMD group and 26 participants (17.2%) in the control group were more than 16 years old when sexual abuse first occurred (Chi square test, p<0.001). These subjects were not incluced as CSA cases.

9.2.3 STATISTICAL ANALYSIS

We examined the association between CSA and rMD using logistic regression in R [30], from which we derived estimates of odds ratios (ORs) and their associated 95% confidence intervals (CIs). We examined the degree to which the association between self-reported CSA and rMD changed with the inclusion of variables that reflect parental family history of depression, CPA, CEN and parent–child relationships according to the PBI. We controlled only for age, social class, occupation and education in the first step of the logistic regression model, and then for family history of MD in the second step. In the third step, we added CPA, CEN and PBI. The above analysis was carried out in samples recruited before June 2010 (Cohort 1, MD n = 1970, controls n = 2597) and after June 2010 (Cohort

2, MD n = 4169, controls n = 3473). Logistic regression was carried out in three steps to analyze the effect of cohort and the interaction between cohort and CSA. To examine the relationship between CSA and MD co-morbidity, we predicted, in case only, the risk of depressive patients with CSA having dysthymia, generalized anxiety disorder (GAD), panic disorder (PD), postnatal depression and phobia with MD, building logistic regression models in three steps.

The impact of the nine DSM-IV criteria depressive symptoms on CSA were assessed by logistic regression. The association between specific features of CSA and rMD was also assessed by logistic regression. Associations between variables were expressed as ORs and 95% CIs. The age at which CSA occurred in rMD and non-MD participants was analyzed by Student's t-test. R [30] was used in data analysis.

TABLE 1: Childhood sexual abuse (CSA) of all participants.

	Any CSA	Non-genital	Genital	Intercourse
Cohort 1				
MD (n = 1920)	189 (9.8%)***	67 (34.5%)***	76 (4.0%)***	46 (2.4%)***
Controls (n = 2588)	70 (2.7%)	31 (1.2%)	29 (1.1%)	10 (0.4%)
Cohort 2				
MD (n = 4041)	392 (9.7%)***	108 (2.7)***	171 (4.2)***	113 (2.8)***
Controls (n = 3439)	68 (2.0%)	42 (1.2)	19 (0.6)	7 (0.2)
Combined				
MD (n = 5295)	560 (10.6%)***	167 (3.2)***	237 (4.5)***	156 (3.0)***
Controls (n = 5820)	125 (2.1%)	66(1.1)	44 (0.7)	15 (0.3)

Values are given as n (%). ***p<0.001.

9.3 RESULTS

9.3.1 PREVALENCE OF CSA

Data on CSA were obtained from 5,295 cases of recurrent MD and 5,820 controls. Table 1 shows the prevalence of specific forms of CSA in cases versus controls in our preliminary and final samples. The rates of the specific forms of CSA were consistently higher in cases versus controls in two cohorts. In the combined sample, any form of CSA was reported by 10.6% of the women with a history of rMD versus 2.1% of controls. Unwanted attempted or completed intercourse before the age of 16 was reported by 3.0% of women with rMD versus 0.3% of controls in full samples.

We analyzed the association between CSA and rMD in cohort 1 and cohort 2 and found no significant differences (p > 0.05) between results from the two cohorts (Table 2). Indeed, the results showed remarkable consistency. The consistency justified combining the entire sample. In the rest of this paper, all results are given for the complete sample.

TABLE 2: Childhood sexual abuse (CSA) and the odds ratios for major depression (MD).

	Cohort 1	Cohort 2	P value of difference	Combined
Any CSA Model 1	3.26 (1.95–5.45)***	4.06 (3.10–5.40)***	0.696	4.06 (3.19–5.24)***
Model 2	2.63 (1.55–4.46)***	3.79 (2.80–4.95)***	0.555	3.62 92.82–4.70)***
Model 3	1.86 (1.06–3.29)*	2.06 (1.45–2.95)***	0.843	2.17 (1.60–2.98)***
Non-genital Model 1	2.47 (1.17–5.23)*	2.01 (1.38–2.99)***	0.522	2.21 (1.58–3.15)***
Model 2	1.91 (0.88–4.16)	1.96 (1.32–2.95)***	0.857	2.01 (1.42–2.90)***
Model 3	1.47 (0.66–3.29)	1.38 (0.84–2.30)	0.980	1.44 (0.93–2.26)
Genital Model 1	2.77 (1.32–5.83)**	5.82 (3.69–9.74)***	0.212	5.24 (3.52–8.15)***
Model 2	2.31 (1.07–4.98)*	5.32 (3.33–8.98)***	0.222	4.77 (3.17–7.48)***
Model 3	1.57 (0.66–3.74)	3.22 (1.80–6.15)***	0.387	3.09 (1.88–5.35)***
Intercourse Model 1	13.35 (1.83–97.42)*	10.39 (5.18–24.73)***	0.906	10.65 (5.56–23.71)***
Model 2	10.87 (1.47–80.38)*	8.73 (4.30–20.94)***	0.899	9.02 (4.67–20.22)***
Model 3	6.99 (0.92–53.22)	2.45 (1.10–6.23)*	0.552	3.07 (1.49–7.18)**

*Values are given as odds ratio (95% confidence interval). Model 1 includes control variables for age and educational background. Model 2 includes in addition parental family history of depression. Model 3 includes in parent-child relationships as assessed by the PIB, childhood physical abuse (CPA) and childhood emotional neglect (CEN). *p<0.05, **p<0.01, ***p<0.001. Cohort 1: MOD n = 1920, Controls n = 2588; Cohort 2: MD n = 4041, Controls n = 3439; Combined MD n = 5295, Controls n = 5820.*

While all attempts were made to match cases and controls, the groups differed in a number of features, previously reported as risk factors for MD. In general, cases had less education, and lower social and occupational status than controls. These, and related features are described in detail in other publications [31], [32], [33], [34]. For the analyses, reported in this paper, we controlled for social, occupational and educational differences where necessary.

9.3.2 THE RELATIONSHIP BETWEEN RMD AND CSA

Any form of CSA was strongly associated with a history of rMD (OR 4.06)(model 1 in Table 2). Looking at specific forms of CSA, the association with rMD strengthened with increasingly severe abuse: non-genital (OR 2.21), genital (OR 5.24) and intercourse (OR 10.65). We considered whether the relationship between CSA and rMD reflected the presence of mental illness in the parents. We therefore repeated the analyses, adding in family history diagnoses of mother and father (model 2 in Table 2). The magnitude of the association between CSA and rMD decreased, but remained significant.

CSA is also correlated with childhood adversity, in particular CPA and CEN, and with the nature of the relationship between parent and child. To explore whether parent–child relationships and childhood adversity explain the association between CSA and rMD, we added into model 3 (from Table 2) the results from the PBI, and the assessments of CPA and CEN. We found that the OR for the effect of CSA on rMD was decreased (Table 2). That is, controlling for the parent–child relationship, CPA and CEN, any form of CSA, genital CSA, and intercourse CSA remained significantly associated with a history of rMD in our sample.

9.3.3 THE RELATIONSHIP BETWEEN THE CSA AND COMORBIDITY OF RMD AND PHENOMENOLOGY OF RMD

We next considered the possibility that the experience of CSA could increase the rate of comorbid disorders in patients with rMD. We examined the association between self-reported CSA and major depression with dysthymia, postnatal depression, generalized anxiety disorder (GAD), panic disorder (PD) and phobia. Controlling only for age and education (table 3, model 1) a lifetime history of GAD, dysthymia, panic disorder, postnatal depression and phobia was associated with CSA (p<0.05). These associations all remained significant with the inclusion of parental MD history (table 3, model 2). Adding PBI, CPA and CEN into the model, the association between CSA and dysthymia and between CSA and phobia remained significant (p<0.05).

TABLE 3: Childhood sexual abuse (CSA) and the odds ratios for co-morbid disorders.

	Any CSA	No CSA	Model 1	Model 2	Model 3
MD and dysthymia (n = 588)	107 (18.2%)	465 (79.1%)	2.22 (1.73–2.83)***	2.13 (1.66–2.72)***	1.60 (1.11–2.27)*
MD and postnatal depression (n = 982)	144 (14.7%)	829 (84.4%)	1.43 (1.14–1.79)**	1.39 (1.11–1.74)**	1.35 (0.99–1.83)
MD and GAD (n = 1516)	178 (11.7%)	1309 (86.3%)	1.28 (1.05–1.55)*	1.24 (1.02–1.51)*	1.06 (0.81–1.39)
MD and PD (n = 400)	56 (14.0%)	336 (84.0%)	1.74 (1.26–2.36)***	1.68 (1.22–2.28)**	1.39 (0.88–2.12)
MD and phobia (n = 2333)	273 (11.7%)	2036 (87.3%)	1.46 (1.22–1.75)***	1.40 (1.16–1.68)***	1.41 (1.09–1.80)**

*MD, major depression; GAD, generalized anxiety disorder; PD, panic disorder. Values are given as n (%) or odds ratio (95% confidence interval). Model 1 includes control variables for age and educational background. Model 2 includes in addition parental family history of depression. Model 3 includes in parent-child relationships as assessed by the PIB, childhood physical abuse (CPA) and childhood emotional neglect (CEN). *p<0.05, **p<0.01, ***p<0.001.*

Within cases (table 4, model 1), we found that depressed patients with CSA had a significantly earlier age of onset of MD. This result was significant when we included parental history of MD (model 2) and when including parental child relation, CPA and CPN in model 3. The number of reported depressive episodes for those with CSA was significantly more than those without CSA in model 1 and model 2. In model 3 the relationship was not significant. The duration of the longest episode of MD for those with CSA was significantly greater than those without CSA and this was seen in all models.

TABLE 4: The relationship between childhood sexual abuse (CSA) and clinical features of major depression (MD).

	Age of onset of MD[a]			Numbers of episodes of MD[b]			Duration of the longest episode of MD[c]		
	Model 1	Model 2	Model 3	Model 1	Model 2	Model 3	Model 1	Model 2	Model 3
Coefficients	−1.89	−1.80	−1.27	0.095	0.086	−0.031	0.301	0.301	0.231
p-value	9.61e-08	3.63e-7	0.005	5.80e-6	4.01e-5	0.291	<2e-16	<2e-16	<2e-16

Model 1 includes control variables for age and educational background. Model 2 includes in addition parental family history of depression. Model 3 includes in parent-child relationships as assessed by the PIB, childhood physical abuse (CPA) and childhood emotional neglect (CEN). [a]The results from a linear regression model with age of onset of MD as response and was "any CSA" as predictor. [b]The results from a Poisson regression model with numbers of episodes of MD as response and was "any CSA" as predictor. [c]The results from a Poisson regression model with duration of the longest episodes of MD as response and was "any CSA" as predictor.

Table 5 summarizes the association between CSA and individual DSM-IV criteria for MD reported at the worst lifetime episode. Any form of CSA was significantly associated with suicidal ideation or attempt (OR 1.50) and feelings of worthlessness or guilt (OR 1.41). Looking at specific forms of CSA, the association with genital (OR 1.66) and intercourse (OR 1.69) was only significant with suicidal ideation or attempt.

9.3.4 FEATURES OF CSA THAT INCREASE RISK OF RMD

The mean age of first reported CSA in rMD patients 10.99 (sd 3.55), and 11.75 (sd 3.49) for the controls. The difference between two groups was significant (t = −2.19, df = 185.802, p = 0.031). All other CSA characteristics including attempted or completed intercourse, age of perpetrator, gender of perpetrator, abuse by a relative, whether forced or threatened, how affected at the time, of individuals with rMD versus controls were assessed by logistic regression (results showed in table 6). Only the attempted or completed intercourse (OR 3.47, 95%CI 1.66–8.22, p<0.01), use of force and threats (OR 1.95, 95%CI 1.05–3.82, p<0.05) and how strongly the victims were affected at the time (OR 1.39, 95%CI 1.20–1.64, p<0.001) were associated with risk for rMD.

TABLE 5: Association of Childhood sexual abuse (CSA) major depression (MD) symptoms.

	Any CSA	Non-genital	Genital	Intercourse
Depressed mood	1.95 (0.56–12.33)	0.57 (0.16–3.65)	2.05e6 (5.12e-11–NA)	2.14e6 (7.22e-15–NA
Loss of interest	1.78 (0.71–5.97)	0.72 (0.26–3.01)	2.97 (0.63–52.92)	1.50e6 (0.0007–4.26e83)
Weight loss/ gain, appetite changes	0.93 (0.70–1.25)	0.85 (0.54–1.40)	1.19 (0.77–1.94)	0.73 (0.46–1.21)
Insomnia/ hypersomnia	1.05 (0.71–1.60)	1.37 (0.68–3.29)	0.73 (0.45–1.25)	1.69 (0.76–4.83)
Psychomotor agitation/ retardation	1.15 (0.86–1.58)	1.17 (0.71–2.03)	1.02 (0.68–1.60)	1.44 (0.82–2.77)
Fatigue/loss of energy	0.93 (0.67–1.32)	1.47 (0.78–3.16)	0.82 (0.52–1.34)	0.77 (0.45–1.43)
Feelings of worthlessness/ guilt	1.41 (1.02–2.02)*	1.09 (0.66–1.92)	1.68 (1.01–3.00)	1.58 (0.87–3.24)
Concentrate/ indecisiveness	1.31 (0.72–2.63)	0.62 (0.30–1.51)	2.04 (0.75–8.42)	3.90 (0.86–69.00)
Suicidal ideation/attempt	1.50 (1.20–1.89)***	1.21 (0.85–1.77)	1.66 (1.19–2.35)**	1.69 (1.12–2.63)*

*Values are given as odds ratio (95% confidence interval). *p<0.05, **p<0.01, ***p<0.001*

9.4 DISCUSSION

Our study produced four major findings. First, we were able to replicate the findings from analysis of the first 2,000 cases of the CONVERGE study. We found in Han Chinese women that CSA is robustly associated with an increased risk of developing rMD. This increases our confidence in the validity of this important finding. Second, CSA affected the clinical features of rMD. In women with rMD, those with a history of CSA had an earlier age of onset, longer depressive episodes and an increased risk to suffer from dysthymia and phobia. Third, we found that any form of CSA was associated with suicidal ideation or attempt and feelings of worthlessness or guilt. Genital and intercourse forms of CSA were associated with suicidal ideation or attempt. Fourth, the use of force or threats, the magnitude of the upset experienced by the subject at the time of abuse, and younger age at CSA were significantly associated with rMD.

TABLE 6: Characteristics of sexual abuse in major depression (MD) patients and controls who reported childhood sexual abuse (CSA).

	MD N = 560	Controls N = 125	OR (95% CI)/t
Age at time of abuse	10.99 (3.55)	11.75 (3.49)	t = –2.19, df = 185.802, p = 0.031
Intercourse vs. others	156/404	15/110	3.47 (1.66–8.22)**
Age of perpetrator			0.96 (0.77–1.19)
Under 15 years	13	70	
15–18 years	22	104	
19–24 years	27	110	
25–49 years	53	234	
Older than 50 years	10	42	
Male/female or both	39/521	9/116	1.30 (0.47–4.62)
Relative or not	187/373	32/93	1.57 (0.87–2.98)
Forced or note	187/373	24/101	1.95 (1.05–3.82)*
How affected			1.39 (1.20–1.64)***
1	188	65	
2	83	23	
3	68	16	
4	43	7	
5	50	5	
6	33	4	
7	95	5	

*Values are given as n (%) and odds ratio (95% confidence interval). *p<0.05, **p<0.01, ***p<0.001*

In our full sample, any form of CSA was reported by 10.6% of the women with a history of rMD versus 2.1% of controls. This frequency of CSA is lower than in other Chinese studies, in which at least one type of CSA has been reported in 16.7% to 22.1% of female students [35], [36], [37]. However, our study differs in that we studied an older group of women (the mean age of our sample is 46 years). The marked economic and cultural changes occurring in China may be one of the reasons for the different rates.

The association of CSA with the risk of MD has been extensively documented in Western populations [5], [12], [38], [39], [40], [41], [42], as has the dose–response relationship between CSA and risk for developing MD [38], [39], and the finding that CSA involving intercourse has the largest odds ratio [12], . Our findings indicate that these observations about the relationship between MD and CSA also hold true in China. Our findings are likely to be robust because of the large sample we have surveyed: the largest sample previously studied included 3982 subjects [38].

On average, parents with psychiatric illness provide poorer environments for their children, potentially not attending to their daughters' well-being and so increasing the risk of abuse. This means CSA could be an indirect or a direct manifestation of parental depressive disorder. In our sample, any form of CSA was significantly associated with a parental history of depression (OR 3.51, 95% CI 2.90–4.23, p<0.001). When we controlled for parental MD history, the association between CSA and rMD decreased mildly.

Some researchers have reported that poor parental care, high control, overprotection, and alienation in the relationship between parent and child increases the risk of developing MD [43], [44], [45], [46], [47], [48], [49], [50], [51], [52]. In our sample, any form of CSA was significantly associated with perceived parenting. Others studies obtained significant associations between CPA, CEA and MD [43], [53], [54], [55], [56]. Some reported that CPA and CEN in part explain the effect of CSA on MD [12], [39], [40]. There was some evidence that CEN is more strongly related to the presence of MD in adulthood than either CPA or CSA [57]. One study showed that childhood adversities were highly interrelated [58]. In our sample, CEN (OR 6.58, 95% CI 5.39–8.00, p<0.001) and CPA (OR 7.88, 95% CI 6.04–10.19, p<0.001) were strongly related. When we controlled for the effect of parent–child relationship, CPA and CEN, we found that the strength of the relationship between the risk of rMD and any CSA remained significant, but the OR decreased substantially, especially for intercourse (from 10.39 to 2.45) in cohort 2. This suggested that part of the impact of CSA on risk for rMD is a relatively non-specific index of disruption and poor treatment in the home of origin. However a substantial part of the effect appears to be specific to CSA itself.

Our results showed that increasing severity of abuse is associated with an increased risk of rMD. CSA had a systematic 'dose–response' relationship with risk for rMD: the greater the severity of CSA, the stronger is the observed association with rMD. Controlling for potential confounders (specifically parental history of MD, parent–child relationship and other childhood adversities) attenuated the CSA–MD association but the association between rMD and 'any CSA', genital, and intercourse still remained significant. This suggests that CSA in part causes rMD. When controlled for the family history of depression, parent-child relationship, CPA, and CEN, the ORs decreased. It should be noted that exposure to multiple forms of abuse, including physical and emotional neglect, also increases the risk of rMD. Thus, although the evidence seems to be consistent with a causal model, we cannot exclude more complex relationships between CSA and rMD.

We also considered whether the effect of CSA on rMD might result in characteristic symptomatology. The greater prevalence of co-morbid dysthymia and phobia, together with an earlier age of onset and longer episodes, indicates that this may be true. Some studies found that MD patients, with a history of CSA, had more severe depressive symptoms, longer duration of index depressive episode, earlier onset, and higher comorbidity [16], [17], [18], [19]. Our findings were consistent with these studies.

Significant CSA-associated risk for suicidal thoughts and behavior has been reported in non-clinical, twins, population-representative adolescent cohorts, students, patients in primary care, and other clinical populations [38], [41], [42], [43], [44], [45], [46], [47], [48], [49], [50], [51]. Fewer studies have examined CSA as a risk factor for suicidal thoughts and attempt in MD patients. Sarchiapone et al. (2007) reported that childhood trauma was significantly associated with making a suicide attempt in unipolar depression patients [52]. Our research found that CSA, especially "genital" and "intercourse", increased the risk of having suicidal ideation or attempt in female Chinese rMD patients.

Some studies demonstrated a positive association between shame, poor or impaired self-esteem and childhood abuse [53], [54], [55], [56]. In our study, we found a significant relationship between CSA and feelings of worthlessness or guilt. Our result is consistent with these studies.

Many aspect of CSA may have a role in the pathogenesis of MD. Few studies have so far examined the relationship between characteristics of CSA and MD. One study identified a number of CSA features that increased the risk of MD: these were the age of abuse occurrence, the presence of attempted or completed intercourse, more than one perpetrator, gender of perpetrator, abuse by a relative, forced or threatened abuse, how strongly the victims were affected at that time [59]. Another study found that greater numbers of CEA and CSA perpetrators were associated with a greater number of depressive episodes in adulthood [60]. Age of onset has been significantly linked to depression by some investigators; an early age of onset predicted depression [61], [62], [63]. Abuse perpetrated by a father figure has also been significantly related to the presence of depression in adult survivors [57]. Mennen and Meadow (1995) found that force used by a non-father figure was significantly related to increased rates of depression in sexually abused girls [64]. In our study, we also found that earlier age onset of CSA was associated with rMD. Greater effect at that time and the use of force by perpetrator predicted rMD. These findings are consistent with previous findings.

Our study has several potential limitations. First, as in most epidemiological studies, CSA in our sample was assessed retrospectively. Recall may be inaccurate and/or biased [49], [65]. Estimates for the rates of CSA in our control sample (2.64% for any CSA and only 0.30% for unwanted intercourse) are lower than estimates obtained from other, non-Chinese samples (24.7–30.4% for any CSA and 5.6–8.4% for intercourse) [5], [38], [66]. These low rates may reflect either under-reporting in Chinese populations or truly lower rates of CSA in China versus most Western populations.

Subjects reported CSA in a self-report questionnaire, so the low rates of CSA in our sample were not the result of hesitance to admit to CSA during a face-to-face interview. If cultural factors influenced subjects to underreport CSA, the general expectation is that this bias would impact equally on our cases and controls. However, we cannot rule out the possibility that our cases (because of depressed mood or greater contact with health professionals) were more willing to report CSA than were our controls. In our sample, more participants in the control group (17.2%) than in the rMD group (6.4%) were older than 16 at first abuse. Although, analysis excluding or these participants yielded same results, we cannot exclude the possibility that our observed association between CSA and rMD could arise from biased reporting rather than a true causal association.

Second, our assessments of CEN and CPA were obtained from a single item. Despite covering important potential traumas, our coverage was far from exhaustive. It is possible that our aspects of the home environment predisposed to both CSA and rMD, thereby biasing upwards our estimates of their association.

Third, our assessment of socio-economic status was based on the highest educational attainment of study participants. Various markers of familial dysfunction are associated with MD in adult. We did not assess additional family characteristics, such as personality and cognitive abilities, which might confound the relationship between CSA and MD.

Fourth, our findings may not apply to other groups. Our cases were obtained from subjects attending psychiatric clinics in general hospitals, and this population may differ from the population undergoing minor surgery in general hospitals or attending community centers. In our study, 63% of of control were recruited from community centers. We observed no differences in demographic features between controls obtained in community centres and in hospitals but it is possible that some unacknowledged differences within the control groups contribute to our findings.

Fifth, our sample had recurrent MD. The impact of CSA on individuals with a single episode of MD who do not present for treatment may be different; we do not know whether our results generalize to other groups of MD patients.

In summary, we have found that CSA is strongly associated with rMD in Chinese women. The association shows a strong dose–response relationship and is mildly attenuated when controls are added for parental depression and other childhood environmental adversities. These results suggest, but do not prove, that the CSA–MD association in China is causal, as has been suggested in US and Australian samples [5], [38]. We also found that CSA was associated with suicide ideation or attempt and some subtype of MD in female patients; early age of onset, being forced and greater affected at the time of CSA was more likely to have rMD.

It is important for healthcare practitioners to know that CSA could increase the risk of developing MD. When dealing with a patient with CSA, clinicians should assess the relevance of such a history and address it therapeutically, as this may be helpful for the patient.

REFERENCES

1. Jumper SA (1995) A meta-analysis of the relationship of child sexual abuse to adult psychological adjustment. Child Abuse Negl 19: 715–728. doi: 10.1016/0145-2134(95)00029-8

2. Neumann DA, Houskamp BM, Pollock VE, Briere J (1996) The long-term sequelae of childhood sexual abuse in women: a meta-analytic review. Child Maltreatment 1: 6–16. doi: 10.1177/1077559596001001002

3. Rind B, Tromovitch P (1997) A meta-analytic review of findings from national samples on psychological correlates of child sexual abuse. J Sex Res 34: 237–255. doi: 10.1080/00224499709551891

4. Fergusson DM, Mullen PE, editors (1999) Childhood Sexual Abuse : An Evidence-Based Perspective. Thousand Oaks, CA.: Sage Publications.

5. Kendler KS, Bulik CM, Silberg J, Hettema JM, Myers J, et al. (2000) Childhood sexual abuse and adult psychiatric and substance use disorders in women: an epidemiological and cotwin control analysis. Arch Gen Psychiatry 57: 953–959. doi: 10.1001/archpsyc.57.10.953

6. Paolucci EO, Genuis ML, Violato C (2001) A meta-analysis of the published research on the effects of child sexual abuse. J Psychol 135: 17–36. doi: 10.1080/00223980109603677

7. Kaplow JB, Widom CS (2007) Age of onset of child maltreatment predicts long-term mental health outcomes. J Abnorm Psychol 116: 176–187. doi: 10.1037/0021-843x.116.1.176

8. Young MS, Harford KL, Kinder B, Savell JK (2007) The relationship between childhood sexual abuse and adult mental health among undergraduates : victim gender doesn't matter. J Interpers Violence 22: 1315–1331. doi: 10.1177/0886260507304552

9. Bonomi AE, Cannon EA, Anderson ML, Rivara FP, Thompson RS (2008) Association between self-reported health and physical and/or sexual abuse experienced before age 18. Child Abuse Negl 32: 693–701. doi: 10.1016/j.chiabu.2007.10.004

10. Carey PD, Walker JL, Rossouw W, Seedat S, Stein DJ (2008) Risk indicators and psychopathology in traumatised children and adolescents with a history of sexual abuse. Eur Child Adolesc Psychiatry 17: 93–98. doi: 10.1007/s00787-007-0641-0

11. Draper B, Pfaff JJ, Pirkis J, Snowdon J, Lautenschlager NT, et al. (2008) Long-term effects of childhood abuse on the quality of life and health of older people: results from the Depression and Early Prevention of Suicide in General Practice Project. J Am Geriatr Soc 56: 262–271. doi: 10.1111/j.1532-5415.2007.01537.x

12. Fergusson DM, Boden JM, Horwood LJ (2008) Exposure to childhood sexual and physical abuse and adjustment in early adulthood. Child Abuse Negl 32: 607–619. doi: 10.1016/j.chiabu.2006.12.018

13. Rohde P, Ichikawa L, Simon GE, Ludman EJ, Linde JA, et al. (2008) Associations of child sexual and physical abuse with obesity and depression in middle-aged women. Child Abuse Negl 32: 878–887. doi: 10.1016/j.chiabu.2007.11.004

14. Powers A, Ressler KJ, Bradley RG (2009) The protective role of friendship on the effects of childhood abuse and depression. Depress Anxiety 26: 46–53. doi: 10.1002/da.20534

15. Chen LP, Murad MH, Paras ML, Colbenson KM, Sattler AL, et al. (2010) Sexual abuse and lifetime diagnosis of psychiatric disorders: systematic review and meta-analysis. Mayo Clin Proc 85: 618–629. doi: 10.4065/mcp.2009.0583

16. Gladstone G, Parker G, Wilhelm K, Mitchell P, Austin MP (1999) Characteristics of depressed patients who report childhood sexual abuse. Am J Psychiatry 156: 431–437.

17. Zlotnick C, Mattia J, Zimmerman M (2001) Clinical features of survivors of sexual abuse with major depression. Child Abuse Negl 25: 357–367. doi: 10.1016/s0145-2134(00)00251-9

18. Gamble SA, Talbot NL, Duberstein PR, Conner KR, Franus N, et al. (2006) Childhood sexual abuse and depressive symptom severity: the role of neuroticism. J Nerv Ment Dis 194: 382–385. doi: 10.1097/01.nmd.0000218058.96252.ac

19. Widom CS, DuMont K, Czaja SJ (2007) A prospective investigation of major depressive disorder and comorbidity in abused and neglected children grown up. Arch Gen Psychiatry 64: 49–56. doi: 10.1001/archpsyc.64.1.49

20. Chen JP, Han P, Dunne MP (2004) Child sexual abuse: a study among 892 female students of a medical school. Zhonghua Er Ke Za Zhi 42: 39–43.

21. Cong E, Li Y, Shao C, Chen J, Wu W, er al (2012) Childhood sexual abuse and the risk for recurrent major depression in Chinese women. Psychol Med 42: 409–417. doi: 10.1017/s0033291711001462

22. WHO (1997) Composite International Diagnostic Interview (CIDI), Version 2.1. Geneva: World Health Organization.

23. APA (1994) Diagnostic and Statistical Manual of Mental Disorders. Washington, DC: American Psychiatric Association.

24. Kendler KS, Prescott CA (2006) Environment, and Psychopathology : Understanding the Causes of Psychiatric and Substance Use Disorders. New York: Guildford Press.

25. Martin J, Anderson J, Romans S, Mullen P, O'Shea M (1993) Childhood sexual abuse and adult psychiatric and substance use disorders in women: an epidemiological and cotwin control analysis. Child Abuse Negl 17: 383–392.

26. Endicott J, Andreasen N, Spitzer RL (1992) Family History-Research Diagnostic Criteria. Biometrics Research. New York: New York State Psychiatric Institute.

27. Kendler KS (1996) Parenting: a genetic-epidemiologic perspective. Am J Psychiatry 153: 11–20.

28. Parker G, Tupling H, Brown LB (1979) A Parental Bonding Instrument. Br J Psychiatry 52: 1–10. doi: 10.1111/j.2044-8341.1979.tb02487.x

29. Laumann EO, Gagnon JH, Michael RT, Michaels S (1994) The Social Organization of Sexuality. Chicago, IL.: University of Chicago Press.

30. R Development Core Team (2010) R: A language and environment for statistical computing. R Foundation for Statistical Computing. Vienna, Austria.

31. Tao M, Li Y, Xie D, Wang Z, Qiu J, et al. (2011) Examining the relationship between lifetime stressful life events and the onset of major depression in Chinese women. J Affect Disord 135: 95–99. doi: 10.1016/j.jad.2011.06.054

32. Li Y, Shi S, Yang F, Gao J, Tao M, et al. (2011) Patterns of co-morbidity with anxiety disorders in Chinese women with recurrent major depression. Psychol Med: 1–9.

33. Gao J, Li Y, Cai Y, Chen J, Shen Y, et al. (2011) Perceived parenting and risk for major depression in Chinese women. Psychol Med: 1–10.

34. Gan Z, Li Y, Xie D, Shao C, Yang F, et al. (2011) The impact of educational status on the clinical features of major depressive disorder among Chinese women. J Affect Disord 136: 988–992. doi: 10.1016/j.jad.2011.06.046

35. Sun YP, Zhang B, Dong ZJ, Yi MJ, Sun DF, et al. (2008) Psychiatric state of college students with a history of childhood sexual abuse. World J Pediatr 4: 289–294. doi: 10.1007/s12519-008-0052-4

36. Chen J, Dunne MP, Han P (2006) Child sexual abuse in Henan province, China: associations with sadness, suicidality, and risk behaviors among adolescent girls. J Adolesc Health 38: 544–549. doi: 10.1016/j.jadohealth.2005.04.001

37. Chen J, Dunne MP, Han P (2004) Child sexual abuse in China: a study of adolescents in four provinces. Child Abuse Negl 28: 1171–1186. doi: 10.1016/j.chiabu.2004.07.003

38. Nelson EC, Heath AC, Madden PA, Cooper ML, Dinwiddie SH, et al. (2002) Association between self-reported childhood sexual abuse and adverse psychosocial outcomes: results from a twin study. Arch Gen Psychiatry 59: 139–145. doi: 10.1001/archpsyc.59.2.139

39. Spinhoven P, Elzinga BM, Hovens JG, Roelofs K, Zitman FG, et al. (2010) The specificity of childhood adversities and negative life events across the life span to anxiety and depressive disorders. J Affect Disord 126: 103–112. doi: 10.1016/j.jad.2010.02.132

40. Cohen P, Brown J, Smaile E (2001) Child abuse and neglect and the development of mental disorders in the general population. Dev Psychopathol 13: 981–999.

41. Silverman AB, Reinherz HZ, Giaconia RM (1996) The long-term sequelae of child and adolescent abuse: a longitudinal community study. Child Abuse Negl 20: 709–723. doi: 10.1016/0145-2134(96)00059-2

42. Martin G, Bergen HA, Richardson AS, Roeger L, Allison S (2004) Sexual abuse and suicidality: gender differences in a large community sample of adolescents. Child Abuse Negl 28: 491–503. doi: 10.1016/j.chiabu.2003.08.006

43. McCauley J, Kern DE, Kolodner K, Dill L, Schroeder AF, et al. (1997) Clinical characteristics of women with a history of childhood abuse: unhealed wounds. JAMA 277: 1362–1368. doi: 10.1001/jama.277.17.1362

44. Brodsky BS, Oquendo M, Ellis SP, Haas GL, Malone KM, et al. (2001) The relationship of childhood abuse to impulsivity and suicidal behavior in adults with major depression. Am J Psychiatry 158: 1871–1877. doi: 10.1176/appi.ajp.158.11.1871

45. Ullman SE, Najdowski CJ (2009) Correlates of serious suicidal ideation and attempts in female adult sexual assault survivors. Suicide Life Threat Behav 39: 47–57. doi: 10.1521/suli.2009.39.1.47

46. Peters DK, Range LM (1995) Childhood sexual abuse and current suicidality in college women and men. Child Abuse Negl 19: 335–341. doi: 10.1016/s0145-2134(94)00133-2

47. Bedi S, Nelson EC, Lynskey MT, McCutcheon VV, Heath AC, et al. (2011) Risk for suicidal thoughts and behavior after childhood sexual abuse in women and men. Suicide Life Threat Behav 41: 406–415. doi: 10.1111/j.1943-278x.2011.00040.x

48. Davidson JR, Hughes DC, George LK, Blazer DG (1996) The association of sexual assault and attempted suicide within the community. Arch Gen Psychiatry 53: 550–555. doi: 10.1001/archpsyc.1996.01830060096013

49. Fergusson DM, Horwood LJ, Woodward LJ (2000) The stability of child abuse reports: a longitudinal study of the reporting behaviour of young adults. Psychol Med 30: 529–544. doi: 10.1017/s0033291799002111

50. Basile KC, Black MC, Simon TR, Arias I, Brener ND, et al. (2006) The association between self-reported lifetime history of forced sexual intercourse and recent health-risk behaviors: findings from the 2003 National Youth Risk Behavior Survey. J Adolesc Health 39: 752.e751–757. doi: 10.1016/j.jadohealth.2006.06.001

51. Molnar BE, Berkman LF, Buka S (2001) L (2001) Psychopathology, childhood sexual abuse and other childhood adversities: relative links to subsequent suicidal behaviour in the US. Psychol Med 31: 965–977. doi: 10.1017/s0033291701004329

52. Sarchiapone M, Carli V, Cuomo C, Roy A (2007) Childhood trauma and suicide attempts in patients with unipolar depression. Depress Anxiety 24: 268–272. doi: 10.1002/da.20243

53. Cavaiola AA, Schiff M (1989) Self-esteem in abused chemically dependent adolescents. Child Abuse Negl 13: 327–334. doi: 10.1016/0145-2134(89)90072-0

54. Tong L, Oates K, McDowell M (1987) Personality development following sexual abuse. Child Abuse Negl 11: 371–383. doi: 10.1016/0145-2134(87)90011-1

55. Andrews B (1997) Bodily shame in relation to abuse in childhood and bulimia: a preliminary investigation. Br J Clin Psychol 36 (Pt 1): 41–49. doi: 10.1111/j.2044-8260.1997.tb01229.x

56. Andrews B (1995) Bodily shame as a mediator between abusive experiences and depression. J Abnorm Psychol 104: 277–285. doi: 10.1037//0021-843x.104.2.277

57. Roesler TA, McKenzie N (1994) Effects of childhood trauma on psychological functioning in adults sexually abused as children. J Nerv Ment Dis 182: 145–150. doi: 10.1097/00005053-199403000-00003

58. Kessler RC, McLaughlin KA, Green JG, Gruber MJ, Sampson NA, et al. (2010) Childhood adversities and adult psychopathology in the WHO World Mental Health Surveys. Br J Psychiatry 197: 378–385. doi: 10.1192/bjp.bp.110.080499

59. Bulik CM, Prescott CA, Kendler KS (2001) Features of childhood sexual abuse and the development of psychiatric and substance use disorders. Br J Psychiatry 179: 444–449. doi: 10.1192/bjp.179.5.444

60. Liu RT, Jager-Hyman S, Wagner CA, Alloy LB, Gibb BE (2012) Number of child-hood abuse perpetrators and the occurrence of depressive episodes in adulthood. Child Abuse Negl 36: 323–332. doi: 10.1016/j.chiabu.2011.11.007

61. Wozencraft T, Wagner W, Pellegrin A (1991) Depression and suicidal ideation in sexually abused children. Child Abuse Negl 15: 505–511. doi: 10.1016/0145-2134(91)90034-b

62. Rodriguez N, Ryan SW, Rowan AB, Foy DW (1996) Posttraumatic stress disorder in a clinical sample of adult survivors of childhood sexual abuse. Child Abuse Negl 20: 943–952. doi: 10.1016/0145-2134(96)00083-x

63. Epstein JN, Saunders BE, Kilpatrick DG (1997) Predicting PTSD in women with a history of childhood rape. J Trauma Stress 10: 573–588. doi: 10.1002/jts.2490100405

64. Mennen FE, Meadow D (1995) The relationship of abuse characteristics to symptoms in sexually abused girls. J Interpers Violence 10: 259–274. doi: 10.1177/088626095010003002

65. Kendler KS, Aggen SH (2013) Clarifying the causal relationship in women between childhood sexual abuse and lifetime major depression. Psychol Med 13: 1–9. doi: 10.1017/s0033291713001797

66. Dube SR, Anda RF, Whitfield CL, Brown DW, Felitti VJ, et al. (2005) Long-term consequences of childhood sexual abuse by gender of victim. Am J Prev Med 28: 430–438. doi: 10.1016/j.amepre.2005.01.015

CHAPTER 10

DIFFERENCES IN THE ASSOCIATION BETWEEN CHILDHOOD TRAUMA AND BMI IN BLACK AND WHITE SOUTH AFRICAN WOMEN

J. H. GOEDECKE, J. FORBES, AND D. J. STEIN

10.1 INTRODUCTION

The prevalence of obesity (body mass index [BMI] $>30kg/m^2$) in women in South Africa is high, with black women being more commonly affected than white women (31.8% vs. 22.7%). [1] Although many studies have examined traditional risk factors for obesity in South African women, including genetics, diet, physical activity [2], very few studies have examined childhood psychosocial circumstances and their effect on obesity risk.

Childhood psychological trauma has been associated with poor mental health, as well as poor physical health. [3] For example, Batten et al [4] indicated that reported history of childhood abuse or neglect was associated with an increased risk of lifetime depressive disorders in both men and women. Further, in women only, reported history of childhood abuse or neglectwas also associated with a 9- fold increase in cardiovascular disorders. Obesity, a major risk factor for cardiovascular diseases, has also

Differences in the Association Between Childhood Trauma and BMI in Black and White South African Women. Goedecke JH, Forbes J, and Stein DJ. African Journal of Psychiatry 16 (2013), doi: http://dx.doi.org/10.4314/ajpsy.v16i3.27. The African Journal of Psychiatry is an Open Access Publication which allows re-use.

been associated with childhood abuse. [5–10] In a retrospective cohort study including 13,177 participants aged 19–92 years, Williamson et al. [5] found that the fraction of adult obesity cases that were attributable to childhood abuse were 8% for a BMI $\geq$30 kg/m^2 and 17% for BMI $\geq$40 kg/ m^2. Further, the risk of obesity increased with the number and severity of each type of abuse, i.e. neglect, sexual, emotional and physical abuse. [5]

Many factors/moderators may impact the relationship between childhood abuse and obesity risk, including age, gender, socioeconomic status, as well as ethnicity. [7] Notably, Medei and Matthews [7], in their systematic review incorporating studies from mainly high-income countries, reported that the relationship between childhood abuse and obesity is more consistent in females than males, and that more black women reported histories of physical abuse than other races. Further, they reported that lower socioeconomic status is associated with increased risk of both childhood abuse and obesity.

The prevalence of child neglect and trauma is high in South Africa. In a nationally representative sample of South Africans (South African Stress and Health Study), Williams et al. [11] found that the prevalence of childhood abuse was as high as 11.6%, with the black population most affected. To our knowledge, no research has been undertaken examining the effects of childhood trauma on obesity risk in South Africa. South Africa provides a unique laboratory to explore the pathogenesis of different phenotypes, by examining whether different population groups, which have been exposed to quite different environments, show variance in such phenotypes. Accordingly, the aim of the study was to examine ethnic differences in the association between childhood trauma and obesity in black and white South African women matched for body fatness.

10.2 METHODS

10.2.1 SUBJECTS

The study included 44 urbanized premenopausal South African women, comprising eight normal-weight (BMI <25 kg/m^2) black, 12 normal-weight white and 9 obese (BMI >30 kg/m^2) black and 15 obese white

South African women. The terms black and white are not meant to reify racial categories, but rather to reflect ongoing disparities that reflect different histories.Subjects were recruited by advertisement in local newspapers and from local church groups, community centers and universities. Inclusion criteria were: (i) age 18–45 years, (ii) no known diseases or taking medication for any metabolic disorders, and (iii) not currently pregnant, lactating or postmenopausal.

10.2.2 ETHICS

The study was approved by the Research Ethics Committee of the Faculty of Health Sciences of the University of Cape Town. Prior to participating in the study, participants gave written informed consent.

10.2.3 MEASUREMENTS

Socioeconomic status (SES) was assessed on the basis of asset index, housing density, education and employment, as previously described. [12] Asset index was based on 14 items reflecting individual and household wealth. Education was categorized by grades passed. Housing density was defined as the number of persons per room living in the household. Subjects were categorized as unemployed, students, informally employed or formally employed. Based on a rank sum of these scores, a SES score was devised which showed good internal reliability (Standardized Cronbach's $\alpha=0.829$).

Weight, height, and waist (level of umbilicus) circumferences were taken. Body fatness was measured using dual-energy-X-ray absorptiometry (DXA, Discovery-W, Software version 4.40, Hologic Inc., Bedford, MA). Body composition of subjects that exceeded the scanning region was calculated using the arm-replaced method. [13]

Self-reported exposure to childhood trauma was measured using the short form of the Childhood Trauma Questionnaire (CTQ). [14] The 28-item version of CTQ comprises the following subscales: physical and emotional neglect, and physical, emotional and sexual abuse. Each subscale score ranges from 5 to 25, with higher scores indicative of greater abuse. A total abuse score (ranging from 25 to 125) was calculated by summing the values obtained on the five subscales.

TABLE 1: Characteristics of the participants according to ethnicity and BMI

	Normal-weight black (n=8)	Normal-weight white (n=12)	Obese black (n=9)	Obese white (n=15)
Demographics				
Age (yrs)	24±1	25±3B	27±1	31±2B
Tertiary education (%)	22.2C	100C	0D	78.6D
Unemployment (%)	77.8C	0C	62.5D	13.3D
Housing density (people/room)	2.2±0.6C	0.4±0.1C	2.0±0.3D	0.4±0.2D
Asset Index (%)	39.7±9.0C	82.1±5.04C	27.7±4.8D	86.2±2.7D
Total SES score	11.9±1.7C	22.3±0.8C	10.6±1.2D	23.0±0.5D
Body composition				
Height (cm)	157±3C	169±2C	157±3D	167±2D
Weight (kg)	56.9±2.4A	64.9±1.3B	95.1±3.4A	106.6±6.6B
BMI (kg/m^2)	22.9±0.6A	22.7±0.4B	38.6±0.9A	37.8±1.7B
Body fat (%)	31.9±2.2A	30.5±2.0B	47.2±1.0A	45.2±1.0B
Childhood trauma questionnaire (CTQ) scores adjusted for age and SES				
Total CTQ score *	38.8±7.9	43.1±6.3	33.2±9.0	45.9±6.0
Physical neglect	8.6±1.6	7.7±1.2	8.4±1.8	7.1±1.2
Emotional neglect *	7.0±2.1	10.9±1.7	8.7±2.4	11.5±1.6
Physical abuse	9.0±1.9	7.7±1.5	6.2±2.1	7.2±1.4
Emotional abuse *	5.6±2.1	11.0±1.7	4.2±2.4	11.7±1.6
Sexual abuse	8.6±1.9C	5.9±1.5C	5.7±2.1	8.4±1.4

*Values are mean ± standard error. Demographic and body composition variables adjusted for age. Childhood trauma questionnaire (CTQ) scores adjusted for age and total socioeconomic status (SES) score. aP<0.05 and AP<0.01 for normal-weight black vs. obese black; bP<0.05 and BP<0.01 for normal-weight white vs. obese white; cP<0.05 and CP<0.01 for normal-weight black vs. normal-weight white; dP<0.05 and DP<0.01 for obese black vs. obese white. * represents a significant effect of SES score.*

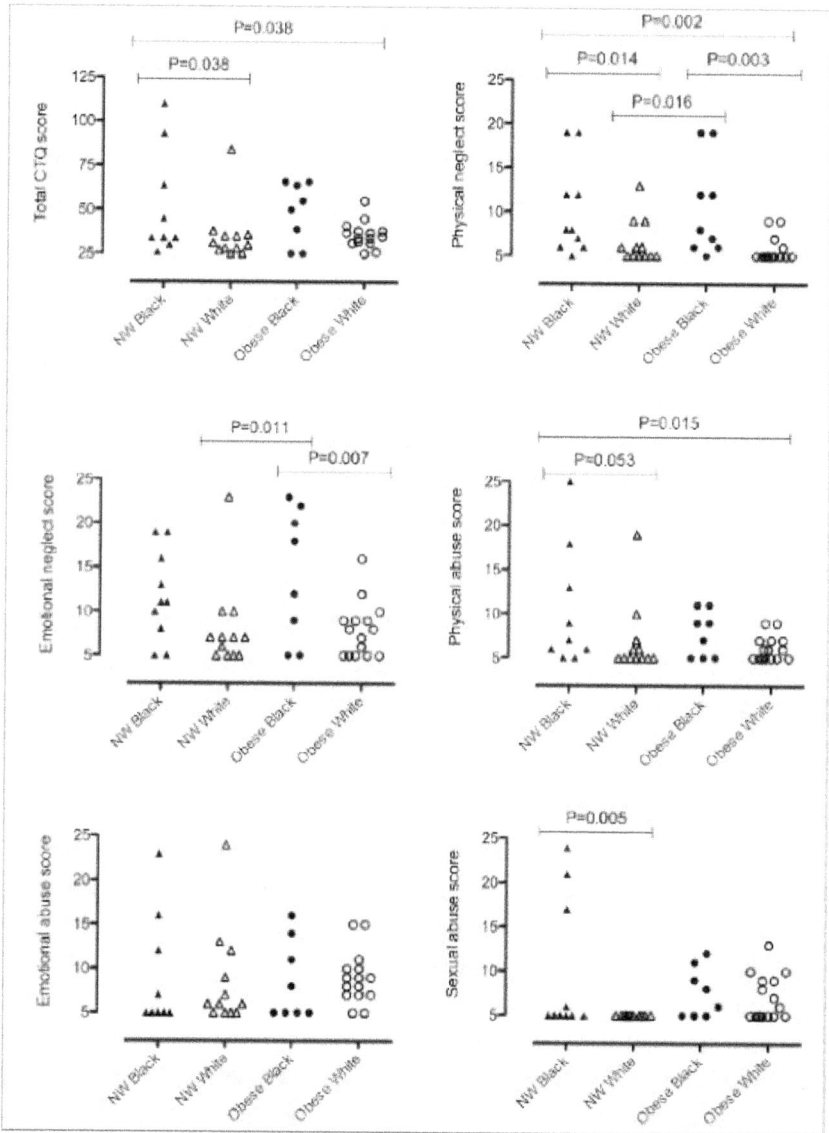

FIGURE 1: Comparison of self-reported exposure to childhood trauma between normal-weight (NW) and obese, black and white women, measured using the Childhood Trauma Questionnaire (CTQ) and its sub-scales [14]

10.2.4 DATA ANALYSIS

The data was analyzed using STATISTICA Version 10 (Statsoft Inc., Tulsa, OK). Demographics and body composition of the normal-weight and obese, black and white women are presented as mean ± standard error and were compared using a two-way analysis of variance (ANOVA) with Fisher LSD post-hoc analysis, adjusting for age. CTQ data of the normal-weight and obese, black and white women are presented as raw values (Figure 1), as well as adjusted (for age and SES) mean ± standard error (Table 1). Differences in CTQ scores between ethnic and BMI groups were compared using a two-way ANOVA with Fisher LSD post-hoc analysis, with and without covarying for age and SES.

10.3 RESULTS

The characteristics of the participants are presented in Table 1. Obese white women were older than their normalweight counterparts, and consequently all subsequent analyses were adjusted for age. Irrespective of BMI group, black women had a significantly lower total SES score, based on lower levels of education, higher unemployment, a lower asset index and a higher housing density.

Black women were shorter than white women, but both the normal-weight and obese black and white women were well matched for BMI and body fat %. By design, obese women were heavier and had higher BMI and body fat % than normal-weight women.

The raw (unadjusted) scores for the CTQ and the CTQ subscales are presented in Figure 1. The total CTQ score, as well as all the scores for the subscales, apart from emotional abuse, were higher in black than white women (P<0.05 for ethnicity), but did not differ by BMI group (P>0.05 for BMI group). Specifically, total CTQ and physical abuse scores were higher in normal-weight black than normal-weight and obese white women, whereas emotional neglect was higher in obese black than normalweight and obese white women. Physical neglect was higher in all black than white women, and physical abuse was higher in normal-weight black than normal-weight white women. However, apart from the sexual abuse score, the differences in these scores were no longer significant after adjusting for ethnic differences in age and SES (Table I). For sexual abuse, there was a significant interaction between ethnicity and BMI group (P=0.04), with scores in normal weight women being higher in black than white women, but scores in obese women not differing by ethnicity.

10.4 DISCUSSION

The main finding of this study was that ethnicity altered the association between childhood sexual abuse and BMI status such that in normal-weight women, sexual abuse was higher in black than white women, whereas in obese women, sexual abuse score did not differ by ethnicity. In contrast, no associations between the other subscales of childhood trauma, including physical and emotional neglect/abuse and BMI status were found. Rather, we found that childhood trauma was higher in black than white women (Figure 1), but this difference was largely driven by differences in socioeconomic status rather than ethnicity per se (Table 1).

Many studies have shown an association between childhood abuse and obesity [5-10], but few have examined specific subtypes of abuse or examined the interaction with ethnicity. In support of our findings, Midei et al. [8] in a sample of 311 black and white women in the USA, assessed childhood abuse using the CTQ, and showed that obesity was related to physical and sexual abuse, as opposed to neglect and emotional abuse. However, the interaction with ethnicity was not reported.

In our study we showed that ethnicity altered the relationship between childhood sexual abuse and BMI status, which may possibly be explained by ethnic differences in body image and perceptions regarding body size. We have recently shown that white women associate beauty, respect and happiness with a smaller body size than their black counterparts. [15] Studies in largely white populations have suggested that eating is regulated as a 'protective function'. [9] These studies imply that white women who are sexually abused may become obese, in order to be viewed as less attractive and therefore are protected against future sexual advances/abuses. [9] In contrast to white women, black women in South Africa regard a larger BMI as attractive, showing greater wealth, dignity and respect, while being lean is regarded as being less beautiful, and associated with having HIV. [16,17] Extending the theorythat eating is regulated as a 'protective function' [9], our data suggest that being lean may protect black women against sexual advances/abusers. We therefore hypothesize that after early adversity there is emotional dysregulation, resulting in altered eating responses (e.g. altered eating patterns after exposure to stressors). In particular environments (e.g. those which emphasize that a low BMI is attractive), this may express itself as relative weight gain, while in other environments (e.g. those which emphasize that a high BMI is attractive), this may express itself as relative weight loss.It must be noted that there is a shift in black middle socio-economic classes that weight loss and a smaller body size is considered attractive, and that this sample is largely drawn from a disadvantaged community. This still leaves the question of whether the results are mediated by ethnicity or whether the effects of ethnicity are mediated by socioeconomic status.

Irrespective of body size, childhood trauma scores were higher in black than white women, supporting previous studies from South Africa [11] and the USA. [8] However, when adjusting for ethnic differences in socioeconomic status, we found that these differences were no longer significant. An association between interpersonal violence and socioeconomic status has been previously established [7] and possibly explains the higher childhood trauma in black women who were of a significantly lower socioeconomic status than the white women.

The strength of the study is the use of DXA as a precise measure of body fatness, compared to BMI estimates used in other studies [7], and the use of the CTQ, which has been shown to have good test-retest reliability, measurement invariance across diverse populations and good criterion-related validity against clinical interview and therapist ratings. [14,18,19] Limitations of the study include the small sample size and theretrospective design, from which we cannot infer causality. The present study also relied on a self-report measure of abuse, which may result in either over- or under reporting. A study that includes a measure of collateral history to support the experience of trauma/abuse would have more predictive power. A more representative sample including larger numbers, as well as older adults and men would provide more information on these relationships. Further, information on resilience and recovery would be informative, as

well as inclusion of additional measures to addressthe mechanisms underlying the relationship, are importantfor future research.

10.5 CONCLUSION

In this small study we showed that ethnicity alters the association between
childhood sexual abuse and BMI status. In our setting, ethnic population
is partly a proxy for differences in views about body weight and beauty.
If replicated in more extensive studies, this finding may provide a very
useful model for exploring the pathogenesis of obesity in general, and the
way in which early adversity interacts with societal views of weight gain
in particular.

REFERENCES

1. Puoane T, Steyn K, Bradshaw D, et al. Obesity in South Africa: The South African
    Demographic and Health Survey. Obesity Research 2002;10:1038-48.
2. Goedecke JHJ, C.; Lambert, E.V. Obesity in South Africa: 1995- 2005. South Afri-
    can Medical Research Council Cape Town, 2006.
3. Wegman HL, Stetler C. A meta-analytic review of the effects of childhood abuse on
    medical outcomes in adulthood. Psychosom Med 2009;71:805-12.
4. Batten SV, Aslan M, Maciejewski PK, Mazure CM. Childhood maltreatment as
    a risk factor for adult cardiovascular disease and depression. J Clin Psychiatry
    2004;65:249-54.
5. Williamson DF, Thompson TJ, Anda RF, Dietz WH, Felitti V. Body weight and obe-
    sity in adults and self-reported abuse in childhood. Int J Obes Relat Metab Disord
    2002;26:1075-82.
6. Bentley T, Widom CS. A 30-year follow-up of the effects of child abuse and neglect
    on obesity in adulthood. Obesity (Silver Spring) 2009;17:1900-5.
7. Midei AJ, Matthews KA. Interpersonal violence in childhood as a risk factor for
    obesity: a systematic review of the literature and proposed pathways. Obes Rev
    2011;12:e159-72.
8. Midei AJ, Matthews KA, Bromberger JT. Childhood abuse is associated with adi-
    posity in midlife women: possible pathways through trait anger and reproductive
    hormones. Psychosom Med 2010;72:215-23.
9. Gustafson TB, Sarwer DB. Childhood sexual abuse and obesity. Obes Rev
    2004;5:129-35.

10. Rohde P, Ichikawa L, Simon GE, et al. Associations of child sexual and physical abuse with obesity and depression in middle-aged women. Child Abuse Negl 2008;32:878-87.
11. Williams SL, Williams DR, Stein DJ, Seedat S, Jackson PB, Moomal H. Multiple traumatic events and psychological distress: the South Africa stress and health study. J Trauma Stress 2007;20:845-55.
12. Goedecke JH, Levitt NS, Lambert EV, et al. Differential Effects of Abdominal Adipose Tissue Distribution on Insulin Sensitivity in Black and White South African Women. Obesity.(Silver.Spring) 2009;17:1506-12.
13. Micklesfield LK, Reid S, Bewerunge L, Rush EC, Goedecke JH. A proposed method to measure body composition in obese individuals using dual-energy X-ray absorptiometry. International Journal of Body Composition Research 2007;5:147-51.
14. Bernstein DP, Stein JA, Newcomb MD, et al. Development and validation of a brief screening version of the Childhood Trauma Questionnaire. Child Abuse Negl 2003;27:169-90.
15. McHiza ZJ, Goedecke JH, Lambert EV. Intra-familial and ethnic effects on attitudinal and perceptual body image: a cohort of South African mother-daughter dyads. BMC Public Health 2011;11:433.
16. Puoane T, Fourie JM, Shapiro M, Rosling L, Tshaka NC, Oelofse A. 'Big is beautiful' - an exploration with urban black community health workers in a South African township. SAJCN 2005;18:6-15.
17. Mvo Z, Dick J, Steyn K. Perceptions of overweight African women about acceptable body size of women and children. Curationis 1999;June:27-31.
18. Thombs BD, Bennett W, Ziegelstein RC, Bernstein DP, Scher CD, Forde DR. Cultural sensitivity in screening adults for a history of childhood abuse: evidence from a community sample. J Gen Intern Med 2007;22:368-73.
19. Thombs BD, Lewis C, Bernstein DP, Medrano MA, Hatch JP. An evaluation of the measurement equivalence of the Childhood Trauma Questionnaire--Short Form across gender and race in a sample of drug-abusing adults. J Psychosom Res 2007;63:391-8.

CHAPTER 11

CHILDHOOD TRAUMA AND PTSD SYMPTOMS INCREASE THE RISK OF COGNITIVE IMPAIRMENT IN A SAMPLE OF FORMER INDENTURED CHILD LABORERS IN OLD AGE

ANDREA BURRI, ANDREAS MAERCKER, SANDY KRAMMER, AND KETI SIMMEN-JANEVSKA

11.1 INTRODUCTION

Early childhood adversity such as physical and sexual abuse, emotional neglect, parental loss, etc., are major risk factors for the development of a range of psychiatric disorders in adulthood, including posttraumatic stress disorder (PTSD) [1], [2]. PTSD occurs following exposure to a traumatic event and is defined by distinct symptom clusters of re-experiencing, avoidance and numbing, and arousal persisting for more than 1 month after trauma [3]. PTSD can have severe long-term consequences and in-

Childhood Trauma and PTSD Symptoms Increase the Risk of Cognitive Impairment in a Sample of Former Indentured Child Laborers in Old Age. © 2013 Burri A, Maercker A, and Kramer S, PLoS ONE 8(2): e57826. doi:10.1371/journal.pone.0057826. Licensed under Creative Commons Attribution 2.0 Generic License, http://creativecommons.org.

dividuals who develop PTSD have an increased risk of major depression, substance dependence, and other health conditions, as well as impaired role functioning and reduced life course opportunities [4], [5].

Recently, links between trauma, PTSD and increased risk of dementia have been suggested. According to several pieces of evidence from animal and human studies, stress experienced early in life induces structural, functional, and epigenetic changes in brain regions involved in cognition, predominantly in the frontal and temporal lobes and the hippocampus [6]. Animal studies demonstrated that early life stress-induced increase of glucorticoids significantly influenced the degree of cognitive impairment with age [7], which is in accordance with the glucocorticoid-cascade-hypothesis of aging [8]. The latter postulates that chronic stress can lead to an increase of cortisol-release which can cause hippocampal atrophy (central region for learning and memory processing). Similarly, several previous study findings have shown that mood disorders such as depression may be associated with a distinct pattern of cognitive impairment [9].

In humans, research has shown that around 70% of individuals suffering from dementia report at least one severe traumatic event before the onset of the disease, as reported by a study conducted at an Dementia Outpatient Clinic in Greece (n = 1,271) [10]. In the like way, in a seminal retrospective cohort study including n = 181,093 predominantly male US war veterans, those who had suffered a PTSD (n = 53,155) had a two-fold increased risk of developing dementia compared with their counterparts without PTSD (n = 127,938) [11]. In addition, PTSD did not appear to be associated with a particular dementia type but rather had an 'across-the-board effect' for all dementias, including vascular dementia and Alzheimer's disease. These findings were supported in another recent group comparison study conducted by Qureshi and colleagues, using n = 10,481 US war veterans recruited through the Veterans Integrated Service Network 16 [12]. Veterans aged 65 and older with a diagnosis of PTSD or who were recipients of a Purple Heart (PH) and a comparison group of the same age with no PTSD diagnosis or PH, were divided into four groups and prevalence of dementia was compared across these groups. Results indicated higher incidence and prevalence of dementia in veterans with

PTSD compared to veterans without PTSD [12]. Although these findings have important implications for preventive care, it remains to be investigated whether this association is due to a common risk factor underlying PTSD and dementia or to PTSD being a risk factor for dementia.

Overall, current literature suggests that PTSD is associated with cognitive impairment, and a greater incidence and prevalence of dementia. However, whether PTSD-related cognitive changes represent an early marker of dementia or whether they act as risk factors for later dementia needs to be further investigated. Whilst clear associations between adult trauma and cognitive impairment have been repeatedly found, only few studies have measured the long-term consequences of childhood trauma on cognitive function and PTSD in elder individuals. Although such an effect is very likely given that modifiable or stable biographical, psychological, genetic, individual and social factors are causal for the development of dementia, literature reporting on this topic is fairly inconsistent [13]. For example, in a recent study, Majer and colleagues investigated a group of healthy adults with significant exposure to early-life trauma and concluded that physical neglect and emotional abuse might be associated with long-term and working memory deficits in adulthood [14]. Since the authors did not include individuals suffering from PTSD or other trauma-related psychiatric disorders, their study does neither allow to draw conclusions on the association between these disorders and cognitive dysfunction nor does it provide information on the influence of the time-point of traumatization (i.e. adulthood, childhood) on the extent of cognitive symptoms. Moreover, their restricted sample size (n = 47) might have introduced a bias; therefore replication in bigger samples is needed. Two other studies investigating intelligence, memory and learning deficits in groups of trauma-exposed and non-exposed children and adolescents found no association between cognitive performance and traumatic events in early life [15], [16]. Saigh et al. compared the IQ scores of traumatized youth with PTSD to scores of trauma-exposed and non-exposed comparison groups without PTSD whilst controlling for other major childhood psychiatric disorders. The PTSD group consisting of n = 228 individuals scored significantly lower on the verbal, but not on the performance subtests compared to the n = 276 controls [15]. Furthermore, the scores of the trauma-exposed non-PTSD individuals and non-trauma exposed controls were not significantly different indicating that PTSD and not a history of trauma exposure (without PTSD) is associated with lower verbal IQ. Similarly, Yasik and colleagues found youth with PTSD (n = 29) to have significantly lower scores in verbal memory indices compared with non-traumatized control subjects (n = 40) but no significant differences for general memory or visual memory[16]. The studies expand on the literature documenting memory impairments among adults with PTSD. However, additional research is needed to explore the relation between trauma exposure, diagnostic status, and cognitive performance across a broader range of neuropsychological indices.

To further investigate the role of PTSD as a potential mediator or moderator variable in the association between trauma and cognitive impairment and to determine the influence of PTSD resilience, it is therefore crucial to not only compare cognitive function in individuals with and without prior traumatic experience, but also to look at individuals who developed a PTSD and those who did not. Given also the limited information and inconsistency of current literature, more research is needed to explore the links between cognitive performance and traumatic events early in life. It is likewise possible that the effects of childhood trauma on cognitive function differ in strength from traumas experienced in adulthood and therefore need to be analyzed separately.

The aim of this study was to investigate the association between childhood trauma exposure, PTSD symptoms and cognitive function in a sample of elder adults. To the best of our knowledge no other studies have investigated and compared levels of cognitive function of cohorts of individuals having been exposed to childhood trauma to cohorts of individuals with adulthood trauma. According to previous studies we hypothesized that exposure to childhood trauma, as well as PTSD symptoms would be significantly associated with poorer cognitive function, especially in memory-related domains. To test these hypotheses, childhood trauma exposure, PTSD status, and neurocognitive function was assessed in a unique sample of former Swiss indentured child laborers.

TABLE 1: Sample characteristics of the overall sample and by gender. T-tests were used for the comparison of continuous variables, two-sample tests of proportion for the comparison of categorical/binary variables.

	Overall (n = 96)			Men (n = 55, 57.3%)			Women (n = 41, 42.7%)			
	Mean	SD	Range	Mean	SD	Range	Mean	SD	Range	p
Age	77.6	6.3	60–95	77.7	5.3	69–90	77.5	7.5	60–95	ns
GDS	3.8	3.5	0–13	3.5	3.4	0–13	4.3	3.7	0–13	ns
MMS	26.9	2.9	4–30	26.9	3.3	14–30	26.8	2.6	20–30	ns
SISCO	46.2	6.5	22–55	46.8	6.8	22–55	45.5	5.9	34–54	ns
MHV	27.9	8.5	0–40	28.9	8.9	0–40	26.7	7.9	4–38	ns
	N	%		N	%		N	%		p
PTSD diagnosis	22	22.9		13	23.6		9	21.9		ns
Childhood trauma	53	56.4		29	53.7		24	60.0		ns
Physical abuse	17	21.3		14	25.9		6	15.0		*
Sexual abuse	11	14.9		3	5.6		11	27.5		*
Emotional abuse	11	11.7		4	7.4		7	17.5		ns
Self-experienced danger or death	2	7.5		6	11.1		1	2.5		ns
Alcohol addiction or abuse	2	2.1		2	3.6		–	–		ns
Substance addiction or abuse	1	1.0		–	–		1	2.4		ns

*Note: * = p<0.05; ns = non-significant. GDS = Geriatric Depression Scale; MMS = Mini Mental State Score; Sisco = Sidam score; MHV = Mill Hill Vocabulary Scale.*

11.2 MATERIALS AND METHODS

11.2.1 SAMPLE

The study sample consisted of a subsample (n = 96) of the Swiss 'Verdingkind'-cohort for which data was available. 'Verdingkinder' were indentured child laborers who during their childhood were removed from their usually poor family environment (e.g. parents) by the authorities and sent to work on farms. This was a common feature of Swiss life until the mid-1950's and a dark chapter of Swiss history. Historic studies have shown that many of these children were regularly beaten, and emotionally and sexually abused [17]. In the present study, the following inclusion criteria applied: (Swiss)-German speaking; a minimum age of 60 years; at least one experienced period of indentured child labor; voluntary participation. 57.3% (n = 55) of the participants were male. The mean age of the overall sample was 77.5 years, ranging from 60 to 95 years (Table 1, upper part). The project started in May 2010. Participants were recruited via advertisements in local and national newspapers and magazines, and via specific indentured child laborers' societies and associations. Also, individuals who had previously been mentioned by name in publications or who had talked publicly about their child labor experiences were contacted directly by the research team. All participants provided written consent stating their willingness to participate in this study.

11.2.2 ETHICS STATEMENT

The study was conducted following the ethical standards of the German and Swiss psychological associations. According to article §29.2–4 of the 'Patient law of the Canton Zurich, 5.4.2004', formal approval of the project was not necessary as no patients were recruited and strict standards of voluntariness, confidentiality and respondent protection were observed.

11.2.3 MATERIAL

Socio-demographic information was assessed with self-constructed questions.

11.2.4 CHILDHOOD ADVERSITY AND TRAUMATIC LIFE EXPERIENCES

As part of the clinical interview, the Composite International Diagnostic Interview (CIDI) trauma events list [18], [19] served as a guide to enquire the most severe traumatizing life experience participants had gone through. Additionally, the verbal descriptions of their most severe traumatic events were assessed and categorized into childhood (CT) or adulthood traumatic (AT) experience based on when the traumatizing event had occurred. Typically, periods of indentured laboring ended at the age of 18, therefore this is the cut-off chosen to distinguish between CT and AT. CT were further sub-classified into sexual abuse, emotional abuse/neglect, physical abuse, and self-experienced death threat, severe accident/illness, witnessing a severe accident, losing a close member of the family or reference person, and other/not specified (e.g. imprisonment). Apart from those subclasses AT further included: severe accident/illness, witnessing a severe accident, losing a close member of the family or reference person, and other/not specified (e.g. imprisonment).

In individuals reporting childhood adversity the most frequent type of trauma was physical violence (32.1%), followed by sexual abuse (20.8%) and emotional abuse/neglect (20.8). The most frequently reported traumas in adulthood were 'other' (25.6%), witnessing death/accident (20.9%) and death of a family member (16.3%). Only 6.9% reported physical or sexual violence and none of the individuals reported emotional abuse/neglect as their most severe traumatic event.

11.2.4.1 SYMPTOMS OF POST-TRAUMATIC STRESS DISORDER (PTSD)

The 7-item short screening scale for PTSD (SSS) is an empirically derived instrument used to discriminate individuals with a diagnosis of PTSD from healthy ones [20]. It was designed after the DSM-IV criteria for PTSD by an iterative series of sensitivity and specificity analyses and thus constitutes a short form of the Posttraumatic Diagnostic Scale (PDS) [21], [22]. Five of the seven symptoms relate to the avoidance and numbing symptom cluster and two to the hyper-arousal symptom cluster. Respondents rate each item as either 'yes' or 'no' and the overall score is computed by adding the number of 'yes' responses. The authors of the SSS suggest a cut-off score of 4 which best balances the scale's sensitivity (80%)—the ability to detect patients with PTSD—and specificity (97%)—the ability to detect patients who do not have PTSD. A German version of the scale is available [23]. The psychometric properties of the PDS from which the SSS was derived has been extensively investigated and been considered good to very good [21]. The specific performance characteristics of the SSS (including the German version) have recently been investigated in two studies [23], [24] and have been considered very good.

11.2.4.2 ASSESSMENT OF COGNITIVE FUNCTION

Cognitive function was assessed with the Structured Interview for Diagnosis of Dementia of Alzheimer Type, Multi-infarct Dementia and Dementia of other Etiology according to ICD-10 and DSM-III-R (SIDAM) [25]. The SIDAM comprises a test performance part, a section for clinical judgment and third party information to determine psychosocial impairment. The SIDAM test performance part consists of a range of cognitive tests that constitute a short neuropsychological battery with 55 questions, including all 30 items of the Mini-Mental State Examination (see below) [26]. Within the context of this study, only the performance part was conducted. It yields a maximum score of 55 (SIDAM score or SISCO). The SISCO can be subdivided into several cognitive domains including: orientation, immediate recall, delayed recall, long term memory, intellectual abilities, verbal abilities/calculation, visuo-spatial function, and aphasia/apraxia. The composite subscore 'memory' is derived by summing the performance in the subdomains 'immediate recall' (of numbers and words), 'delayed recall' (of verbal and figural material) and 'long term memory' (biographical memory).

The SIDAM has a high overall test-retest reliability which equally holds true on the diagnostic, criterion and item level. It separates reliably between subjects with DSM-III-R and ICD-10 dementia from those without such a disorder. Furthermore, good congruence was found between SIDAM diagnosis and corresponding ICD-9 expert diagnosis [25]. Age- and education-specifics norms for the assessment of dementia have been obtained in a German population-based sample of n = 1001 individuals aged >75 years [26]. Independent of education, a Sisco score of 36 for individuals >80 years, and a score of 38 for individuals aged 75 to 79 years were found to differentiate best (i.e. best specificity-sensitivity profile) between clinically demented and healthy individuals.

In the current study reliability coefficients for the various subscale of the SIDAM ranged from $\alpha = 0.51$ (for orientation) to $\alpha = 0.74$ (for short term memory).

The Mini-Mental State Exam (MMSE) is one of the most widely used screening measures of general cognitive ability [27]. The brief 30-point questionnaire is used to screen for levels of cognitive function, with items assessing six different domains including: cognition, including orientation, word recall, registration of new information, attention and calculation, language abilities, and visuo-spatial ability. Scores on the MMSE range from 0 to 30, with scores of 25 or higher being considered normal. The instrument has been used within different cultural and ethnic groups and translated into many languages. Good psychometric properties (reliability and validity) have repeatedly been demonstrated [27].

The 'Vocabulary Test' is the German version of the Mill Hill Vocabulary Scale (MHV) used for the measurement of acquired verbal knowledge [28], [29]. The MHV represents the verbal test part of the Raven's Progressive Matrices. Contrary to most other vocabulary tests which assess passive vocabulary or recognition performance, the MHV allows the assessment of active vocabulary. The test consists of a list of words divided into two parallel lists of 44 words (set A and B) and participants are asked to explain the meanings of the words. Alternatively, participants can chose a synonym from a selection of six words. The psychometric properties of the test have been extensively investigated and considered good to excellent, with internal consistencies are .93 and .91, respectively (for definition vs. synonym picking task) and good convergent and discriminant validity [29].

11.2.4.3 DEPRESSION

The Geriatric Depression Scale (GDS) is a commonly applied self-report instrument used to specifically identify depression in older people [30]. A short version of the original questionnaire (GDS-SF) containing 15 questions is available and was used within the context of this study. The short version has been found to be an adequate substitute for the original 30-

item scale. The questions are answered 'yes' or 'no', instead of a five-category response set. This simplicity enables the scale to be used with ill or moderately cognitively impaired individuals. Scores greater than 3 suggest the presence of depression. The test sensitivity ranges from 79% to 100%, specificity from 67% to 80%. Validation of the German version of the GDS found the instrument to be a reliable and valid screening instrument with an average item discrimination of 0.5, an average item difficulty of $P = 43$, low inter-item correlation $r = 0.2$ and a very high internal consistency (Cronbach's $\alpha = 0.9$) [31]. In the current study GDS showed adequate internal consistency reliability (Cronbach's $\alpha = 0.8$).

11.2.5 DESIGN

According to the information on PTSD symptoms (derived from the SSS) and whether participants experienced CT (including either sexual abuse, emotional abuse, physical abuse or near to death experiences that happened during the indentured child laboring period) or AT (additionally including near to death experiences, severe accident/illness, witnessing a severe accident, losing a close member of the family or reference person, and other/not specified) individuals were categorized as belonging to one of four groups: with CT and a PTSD (CT/PTSD+), with CT and no PTSD (CT/PTSD-), with AT and PTSD (AT/PTSD+), with AT and no PTSD (AT/PTSD-). Note that in all subsequent paragraphs PTSD+ does not refer to a clinical diagnosis of PTSD but solely describes traumatized individuals who screened positively for PTSD symptoms according to the SSS.

11.2.6 STATISTICAL ANALYSES

For descriptive statistics, two-sample tests of proportions to assess differences between gender on categorical and binary data were used. Student's t-tests were applied to assess differences between gender means on continuous variables. We used point-biserial correlation coefficient and logistic regression to examine the relationship between the binary variables representing PTSD symptoms and childhood trauma status and the various continuous variables measuring cognitive function. Because normality of the data could not be assumed, given the low sample size in some of the groups, univariate Kruskal-Wallis analyses (non-parametric test, equivalent to ANOVA) were calculated to compare the score differences between the groups for the continuous cognitive function variables. Bonferroni corrected, multiple sample contrasts were performed post-hoc to these analyses. To control for the influence of depression as a potential covariate on the cognitive function outcome variables, Kruskal-Wallis tests were performed on covariate-adjusted (i.e. GDS) residuals. Covariate-adjusted residuals were obtained from the overall regression line fit to the entire data set.

All tests were two-tailed. For all analyses, a P value less than0.05% or odds ratios (OR) with a 95% confidence interval (CI) not including '1' were considered statistically significant, unless stated otherwise. Data handling and analyses were undertaken using STATA (Version 10.0, 2008, StataCorp, College Station, TX, USA).

11.3 RESULTS

According to the SSS (cut-off score of 4), 22 individuals (22.9%) screened positively for PTSD symptoms. Thus, the 96 participants were assigned to the four groups as follows: n = 10 in the CT/PTSD+ group, n = 31 in the CT/PTSD- group, n = 12 in the AT/PTSD+ group, n = 43 in the AT/PTSD- group.

Participants further reported a high prevalence of depressive symptoms, with an average geriatric depression score of 3.8 (SD = 3.5; Table 1). Overall, participants showed mild to no cognitive impairment, with average MMS and SISCO scores of 26.9 (SD = 2.9) and 46.2 (SD = 6.45), respectively.

In terms of cognitive function variables and prevalence of PTSD symptoms, no significant gender differences could be detected (Table 1). Male and female participants, however, differed significantly in prevalence of sexual and physical abuse, with male more frequently reporting previous physical abuse (25.9% vs. 15.0%, P<0.01) and females more frequently sexual abuse (5.6% vs. 27.5%, P<0.01).

TABLE 2: Results of analysis of variance (Kruskal-Wallis test) for the means of the cognitive function variables across the four CT/PTSD groups.

	CT/PTSD+ (n = 10)		CT/PTSD– (n = 31)		AT/PTSD+ (n = 12)		AT/PTSD– (n = 43)		X^2	Contrasts
	Mean	SD	Mean	SD	Mean	SD	Mean	SD	5.5	–
Age	75.9	4.5	75.9	6.7	78.5	7.1	78.9	5.9	1.3	–
GDS	4.6	3.9	3.8	3.4	4.3	3.7	3.5	3.6	9.3*	1<4, 3<4
MMS	25.6	3.4	26.9	3.2	25.5	2.8	27.6	2.6	10.1*	1<4, 3<4
SISCO	42.3	6.4	46.7	6.7	43.0	6.5	47.8	5.7	1.6	–
Orientation	9.5	0.7	9.5	0.9	9.8	0.4	9.7	0.6	6.6	–
Memory total score	13.1	2.9	15.6	3.5	14.2	3.4	15.5	3.6	3.1	–
Memory immediate reproduction	4.1	0.3	4.4	0.6	3.8	1.1	4.3	0.6	4.4	–
Short term memory	4.6	2.1	5.7	2.4	4.8	2.1	5.6	2.3	3.8	–
Long term memory	4.4	1.8	5.5	1.4	5.6	0.9	5.5	1.3	1.3	–
Intellectual performance	4.5	0.9	4.9	0.6	4.3	1.5	4.7	0.7	**12.3****	3<4
Higher cortical function	15.2	2.2	16.6	2.9	14.7	2.4	17.4	2.6	**8.8***	3<4
Verbal numeracy	4.1	1.0	5.5	1.6	4.6	1.6	5.7	1.4	**6.3***	3<4
Construction skills	1.4	0.8	1.7	1.1	1.0	0.7	1.9	1.2	2.0	–
Aphasia aparaxia	9.5	6.6	9.3	0.9	9.1	1.3	9.6	0.8	7.5ᵃ	–
MHV	26.1		30.3	6.3	21.6	10.8	28.5	8.8		–

Note: $^a p<0.06$, *$p<0.01$, **$p<0.001$. GDS = Geriatric Depression Scale; MMS = Mini Mental State Score; Sisco = Sidam score; MHV = Mill Hill Vocabulary Scale.

The main analysis compared the four groups of childhood/adulthood trauma (CT/AT) and PTSD (+/−) for indicators of cognitive decline or dementia processes (Table 2). The mean age across all four groups was similar. Furthermore, the four groups did not differ significantly in terms of depressive symptoms. As expected there was a statistically significant difference between groups in levels of cognitive function as measured by the MMS and SISCO score (X^2 = 9.3, P<0.05 and X^2 = 10.1, P<0.05, respectively). Upon investigation of the specific cognitive sub-domains, significant group differences were detected for higher cortical function (X^2 = 12.3, P<0.001), verbal numeracy (X^2 = 8.8, P<0.05) and construction skills (X^2 = 6.3, P<0.05). The group differences in MHV scores fell short for significance (X^2 = 7.5, P<0.06). Overall, analyses showed that participants screening positively for PTSD symptoms were more likely to report poorer cognitive function compared to individuals without PTSD symptoms in both the main score and the three sub-domain scores.

To further investigate between which groups the differences in scores were significant we performed multiple sample contrasts. Post-hoc analyses indicated that individuals screening positively for PTSD symptoms reported poorer cognitive function, with significantly lower MMS and SISCO scores, compared to individuals without PTSD symptoms (Table 2). Especially individuals with PTSD symptoms and reporting CT showed poorer cognitive function. Similarly, these groups also differed significantly with respect to higher cortical function, verbal numeracy and construction skills.

Because previous literature has shown a moderating role of depressive symptoms on cognitive functioning, we included GDS scores as a confounder in the analyses of all available variables. Even after controlling for depression, the difference between the groups remained significant for the MMS and the Sisco score (X2 = 9.9, P<0.05 and X2 = 12.5, P<0.001, respectively), as well as for the sub-domains of higher cortical function and verbal numeracy (X2 = 12.9, P<0.001 and X2 = 8.2, P<0.05, respectively). Contrary to the initial results, the significant group difference for construction skills could not be detected when controlling for depression.

11.4 DISCUSSION

Early-life trauma is a major risk factor and elicitor for the development of PTSD, a condition which cardinal features are changes in cognitive function. So far, only a handful of studies have measured the long-term consequences of childhood trauma on cognitive function in healthy adults.

This is the first study ever conducted on former indentured Swiss child laborers and the first to investigate the relationship between childhood versus adulthood trauma levels of cognitive function in later life. In this present study we found associations between childhood trauma exposure, PTSD symptoms and cognitive performance. In particular, individuals who screened positively for PTSD symptoms showed lower levels of cognitive function in the SIDAM total score (SISCO), the MMS score and the specific cognitive domains of higher cortical function, construction skills and verbal numeracy compared to individuals without PTSD symptoms. As to be expected, cognitive function was consistently highest across all domains in individuals without reported childhood trauma and without PTSD symptoms. Furthermore, individuals with adulthood trauma and screening positively for PTSD symptoms were at a similarly high risk for poorer cognitive performance compared to individuals with childhood trauma and screening positively for PTSD symptoms. Finally, we found that all associations between PTSD symptoms and cognitive function—apart from construction skills—were moderated by depressive symptoms. In other words, accounting for depression led to stronger associations between PTSD symptoms and lower levels of cognitive function. No differences in any of the variables studied could be found between male and female individuals.

Our results add to a growing body of literature supporting a relationship between childhood trauma exposure, PTSD and the development of cognitive dysfunction in elder individuals. Qureshi et al. (2010) for example found a somewhat similar picture in an analogous group comparison design including individuals with ICD-9 diagnoses of dementia [12]. In their study, almost two-fold higher dementia prevalences were reported in the two PTSD groups compared to the non-PTSD groups. Additionally, their group most similar to our 'AT/PTSD+' group showed the highest prevalence of a dementia diagnosis. Similarly, the results of the most comprehensive Yaffe et al (2010) study indicated an association between PTSD and increased dementia risk [11]. The study used war veterans who usually combat at ages around 18–28 years, therefore relying on traumatization in early adulthood. Together with our findings this tentatively indicates that adulthood trauma-related PTSD may outweigh childhood-related PTSD in its relevance as a causal agent for cognitive decline. This assumption is further supported by a recent study on childhood Holocaust survivors conducted by the research group around Ravona-Springer who found no evidence for an increased risk for dementia at old age [32]. Although overall these preliminary findings cautiously point towards a more substantial influence of traumatic effects experienced in adulthood on cognitive decline, they need to be replicated and supported by other studies. In future it will be especially important to diligently assess the amount and severity of traumatic childhood and adulthood experiences. At this stage it is not possible to exclude the existence of cumulative or masking effects of different trauma types and times of occurrence which could be an explanation for the rather inconsistent research outcomes.

Our main analyses were supported and even strengthened when taking depressive symptoms into account (for additional analyses on depression in the current sample, see Kuhlman et al., 2012) [33]. These results are in line with findings from previous studies reporting an independent association between depressive symptoms and cognitive performance [34]. It has been argued that this relationship can be best explained by neurobiological models suggesting a link between depression, hypothalamo-pituitary-adrenal (HPA) axis dysfunction (i.e. depression-related cortisol hypersecretion) and cognitive dysfunction [34], [35].

A similar model has been proposed for symptom development and psychobiologic changes occurring in individuals with PTSD. Most of the post-traumatic symptoms have a biological correlate; this is particularly true for hyperarousal—one of the elementary characteristics of PTSD, defined as a heightened state of psychological and physiological tension. The body responds to increased acute physical or psychological stress by activating the HPA-axis which leads to the release of adreno-corticotrophin (ACTH) from the anterior pituitary and produces an increase of cortisol levels. Over the long term, such hyperarousal and the increased levels of corticosteroid secretion may disrupt somatic, cortical, cognitive and affective processing by having neurotoxic effects [8], [36]. Such hypercortisolemia has previously been associated with increased risk of dementia. It is very likely that PTSD-related or PTSD-symptom related (e.g. hyperarousal) alterations in the HPA-axis produce neuroanatomical changes including volume changes in the frontal lobe, lower neuronal density in the medial temporal lobe and hippocampal atrophy [37]–[39] and thereby evoke significant changes in cognitive functioning.

In another longitudinal validation study conducted by Bickel and colleagues (2007) the subdomains' predictive validities for dementia were explored. The authors found the SIDAM total score and the subscale 'memory' (especially 'short-term memory') and 'higher cortical function' to have the strongest predictive power for the development of later dementia [40]. This is somewhat in line with our findings, where significant group-differences could be detected for the SIDAM total score and the domains of higher cortical function, construction skills and verbal numeracy (as part of the higher cortical function subscale). This provides additional support for our findings of tentative effects of trauma and PTSD symptoms on cognitive function. To further explore whether such changes are static or develop progressively and how they correlate with disease (PTSD) duration, longitudinal designs are needed. In addition, there might be differences in the specific causes leading to cognitive decline in people with PTSD. Recent research, such as the study conducted by Dretsch et al. (2012) on 46 war veterans with PTSD, indicate that cognitive deficits appear to be partially attributed to anxiety and depression symptoms [41]. Although the mediating effects of depression were controlled for in our study, we cannot exclude a potential effect of other mediators (such as e.g. anxiety) on the detected group differences in neuro-cognitive functioning.

11.4.1 LIMITATIONS

Our results should be considered in light of several limitations. First, due to the uniqueness of the indentured child laborers sample, the overall, as well as the group-specific sample sizes were relatively small. This might have led to restricted power in statistical testing. The chi-square approximation of the Kruskal-Wallis test statistics, however, has been proven to be highly satisfactory also when sample sizes are small [42]. Given the singularity of our study sample, the possibility to recruit additional participants is unlikely. Nevertheless, replication of the study in other populations with childhood trauma and PTSD could allow more detailed group-comparison of cognitive function. Second, our sample is specific in terms of life histories or events' characteristics, thus the study might have limited generalizability to other populations and other subpopulations with histories of severe childhood trauma. However, long-lasting traumatic experiences during childhood are prevalent even in more common community samples [43]. Additionally, there might have been selectivity bias among the former child laborers who were willing to participate in a study asking about their traumatic experiences and the ones that were not. Similarly, trauma group studies have demonstrated that traumatized persons who have elevated PTSD-related avoidance symptoms tend to not participate in such studies. Third, we cannot exclude the possibility that our data are affected by biases (such as distortions due to forgetting, nondisclosure, mood states, reporting bias, etc.) given the fact that we relied on retrospective self-reports of childhood experiences. Previous evidence, however, has shown that the available standardized measurement instruments are sufficiently valid to warrant their use in retrospective recall studies [44]. As a fourth limitation, we did not consider effects of adulthood trauma and life stress that might have mediated the relationship between childhood trauma and cognitive decline. It is known that individuals with early trauma more frequently experience adulthood stress, and moreover, are sensitized to the effects of such stressors [45]. Fifth, several important variables that are known to affect cognition—such as duration, severity, and treatment of PTSD, medication use, years of education, and premorbid intelligence—could not be included in the analyses due to the unavailability of such data. Sixth, owing to the cross-sectional design the causal relationship between early adversity and cognitive dysfunction could not be determined. In the context of the second assessment wave, additional information on participants' cognitive status is currently being collected and will allow more specific statements regarding the relationship between earlier trauma and levels of cognitive function and potential long-term impairment. Finally, attention must be paid to the assessment of trauma type and severity, as well as PTSD status. The SSS is limited to measuring PTSD symptoms in persons who have experienced DSM-IV traumatic events, thus ascertainment of an index event in individuals exposed to multiple events is not covered by the scale. Also, the SSS is an efficient method to screen for PTSD in epidemiologic and clinical studies but does not substitute for a psychiatric diagnosis. Likewise, the SIDAM and MMSE solely allow assessment of cognitive function and decline. They do not permit a diagnosis of dementia which requires at least the exclusion of other psychiatric diseases and somatic disorders (such as hypovitaminosis, hypothyreodism, normal pressure hypdrocephalus), as well as multi time-point assessment for the identification of transient versus persistent cognitive impairments (i.e. dementia).

11.5 CONCLUSION

Findings from this study support the hypothesis that PTSD symptomatology affects cognitive function and may put individuals at risk for later dementia. These findings are consistent with previous reports of neuroanatomical changes in individuals suffering from PTSD or PTSD symptoms. This elevated risk for dementia seems to be particularly relevant, when trauma appeared in adulthood. Overall, our results suggest that poor cognitive function in late adulthood may be partly a consequence of PTSD symptoms but can also develop as a consequence to traumatization or be aggravated by them. Proposals for future research are given and longitudinal data providing more detailed information on the reported associations and to further investigate potential mediators and moderators is warranted.

REFERENCES

1. Anda RF, Felitti VJ, Bremner JD, Walker JD, Whitfield C, et al. (2006) The enduring effects of abuse and related adverse experiences in childhood. A convergence of evidence from neurobiology and epidemiology. Eur Arch Psychiatry Clin Neurosci
2. Maercker A (2004) Age of traumatisation as a predictor of post-traumatic stress disorder or major depression in young women. BJP 184: 482–487. doi: 10.1192/bjp.184.6.482
3. American Psychiatric Association (1994) Diagnostic and statistical manual of mental disorders, 4th edition. Washington, DC: American Psychiatric Association.
4. Subica AM, Claypoole KH, Wylie AM (2009) PTSD'S mediation of the relationships between trauma, depression, substance abuse, mental health, and physical health in individuals with severe mental illness: evaluating a comprehensive model. Schizophr. Res 136: 104–109. doi: 10.1016/j.schres.2011.10.018
5. Dedert EA, Green KT, Calhoun PS, Yoash-Gantz R, Taber KH, et al. (2009) Association of trauma exposure with psychiatric morbidity in military veterans who have served since September 11, 2001. J Psychiatr Res 43: 830–836. doi: 10.1016/j.jpsychires.2009.01.004

6. Lupien SJ, McEwen BS, Gunnar MR, Heim C (2009) Effects of stress throughout the lifespan on the brain, behaviour and cognition. Nat Rev Neurosci 10: 434–445. doi: 10.1038/nrn2639
7. Solas M, Aisa B, Mugueta MC, Del Río J, Tordera RM, et al. (2010) Interactions between age, stress and insulin on cognition: implications for Alzheimer's disease. Neuropsychopharmacology 35: 1664–1673. doi: 10.1038/npp.2010.13
8. Sapolsky RM, Krey LC, McEwen BS (1986) The neuroendocrinology of stress and aging: the glucocorticoid cascade hypothesis. Endocr Rev 7: 284–301. doi: 10.1210/edrv-7-3-284
9. Goodwin GM (1997) Neuropsychological and neuroimaging evidence for the involvement of the frontal lobes in depression. J of Psychopharmacol 11: 115–122. doi: 10.1177/026988119701100204
10. Tsolaki M, Papaliagkas, Kounti F, Messini C, Boziki M, et al. (2010) Severely stressful events and dementia: a study of an elderly Greek demented population. Psychiatr Res176: 51–54. doi: 10.1016/j.psychres.2009.06.001
11. Yaffe K, Vittinghoff E, Lindquist K, Barnes D, Covinsky KE, et al. (2010) Posttraumatic stress disorder and risk of dementia among US veterans. Arch Gen Psychiatry 67: 608–13, Jun, 2010. doi: 10.1001/archgenpsychiatry.2010.61
12. Qureshi SU, Long ME, Bradshaw MR, Pyne JM, Magruder KM, et al. (2011) Does PTSD impair cognition beyond the effect of trauma? J Neuropsych Clin N 23: 16–28. doi: 10.1176/appi.neuropsych.23.1.16
13. Forstmeier S, Maercker A (2009) Neurodegenerative Diseases Alzheimer' s Disease Potentially Modifiable Risk Factors in the Development of Alzheimer' s Disease. US Neurology 5: 18–21.
14. Majer M, Nater UM, Lin JMS, Capuron L, Reeves WC (2010) Association of childhood trauma with cognitive function in healthy adults: a pilot study. BMC Neurology 10: 61. doi: 10.1186/1471-2377-10-61
15. Saigh PA, Yasik AE, Oberfield RA, Halamandaris PV, Bremner JD (2006) The intellectual performance of traumatized children and adolescents with or without posttraumatic stress disorder. J Abnorm Psychol 115: 332–340. doi: 10.1037/0021-843x.115.2.332
16. Yasik AE, Saigh PA, Oberfield RA, Halamandaris PV (2007) Posttraumatic stress disorder: memory and learning performance in children and adolescents. Biol Psychiatr 61: 382–388. doi: 10.1016/j.biopsych.2006.06.005
17. Leuenberger LSM (2008) Versorgt und vergessen. Rotpunktverlag p 314.
18. Wittchen HU (1994) Reliability and validity studies of the WHO--Composite International Diagnostic Interview (CIDI): a critical review. J Psychiatr Res 28: 57–84. doi: 10.1016/0022-3956(94)90036-1
19. World Health Organization: Composite International Diagnostic Interview (CIDI), version 2.1. (2007) Geneva, Switzerland: World Health Organization.
20. Breslau N, Peterson EL, Kessler RC, Schultz LR (1999) Short screening scale for DSM-IV posttraumatic stress disorder. Am J Psychiatry 156: 908–911.
21. Foa K, Edna B Cashman L, Jaycox L (1997) The validation of a self-report measure of posttraumatic stress disorder: The Posttraumatic Diagnostic Scale. Psychol Assess 9: 445–451. doi: 10.1037/1040-3590.9.4.445

22. Steil A, Ehlers R (2000) Posttraumatische Diagnoseskala (PDS). Universitaet Jena: Psychologisches Institut.

23. Siegrist P, Maercker A (2010) Deutsche Fassung der Short Screening Scalefor DSM-IV Posttraumatic Stress Disorder. Aktueller Stand der Validierung. Trauma & Gewalt 4: 208–213.

24. Bohnert N, Breslau K (2011) Assessing the performance of the short screening scale for posttraumatic stress disorder in a large nationally representative survey. Int J Meth Psychiatr Res 20: 1–8. doi: 10.1002/mpr.331

25. Zaudig M, Mittelhammer J, Hiller W, Pauls A, Thora C, et al. (1991) SIDAM--A structured interview for the diagnosis of dementia of the Alzheimer type, multi-infarct dementia and dementias of other aetiology according to ICD-10 and DSM-III-R. Psychol Med 21: 225–236. doi: 10.1017/s0033291700014811

26. Busse M, Aurich A, Zaudig C, Riedel-Heller M, Matschinger S, et al. (2002) Age- and education-specific reference values for the cognitive test of the SIDAM (Structured Interview for the Diagnosis of Dementia of the Alzheimer type, Multi-infarct Dementia and Dementias of Other Etiology According to ICD-10 and DSM-IV). Zeitschrift für Gerontologie und Geriatrie 35: 565–574.

27. Folstein MF, Folstein SE, McHugh PR (1975) Mini-mental state'. A practical method for grading the cognitive state of patients for the clinician. J Psychiatr Res 12: 189–98. doi: 10.1002/(sici)1099-1166(199805)13:5<285::aid-gps753>3.3.co;2-m

28. Raven J (2000) The Raven's progressive matrices: change and stability over culture and time. Cog Psychol 41: 1–48. doi: 10.1006/cogp.1999.0735

29. Raven JH, Raven J, Court JC (1998) Manual for Raven's Progressive Matrices and Vocabulary Scales.: Section 5.The Mill Hill Vocabulary Scale. San Antonio, TX Harcourt Assessment.

30. Yesavage JA, Brink TL, Rose TL, Lum O, Huang V, et al. (1983) Development and validation of a geriatric depression screening scale: a preliminary report. J Psychiatr Res 17: 37–49. doi: 10.1016/0022-3956(82)90033-4

31. Gauggel B, Birkner S (1999) Validität und Reliabilität einer deutschen Version der Geriatrischen Depressionsskala (GDS). Zeitschrift für Klinische Psychologie und Psychotherapie 28: 18–27. doi: 10.1026//0084-5345.28.1.18

32. Ravona-Springer R, Beeri MS, Goldbourt U (2011) Exposure to the Holocaust and World War II concentration camps during late adolescence and adulthood is not associated with increased risk for dementia at old age. JAD 23: 709–716.

33. Kuhlmann K, Burri A, Maercker A (2013) Severe Childhood Trauma and Geriatric Depression. In preparation doi: 10.1016/j.chiabu.2013.04.013

34. McAllister-Williams RH, Ferrier IN, Young AH (1998) Mood and neuropsychological function in depression: the role of corticosteroids and serotonin. Psychol Med 28: 573–584. doi: 10.1017/s0033291798006680

35. Rubinow DR, Post RM, Savard R, Gold PW (1984) Cortisol hypersecretion and cognitive impairment in depression. Arch Gen Psychiatry 41: 279–283. doi: 10.1001/archpsyc.1984.01790140069008

36. Perlis ML, Kehr EL, Smith MT, Andrews PJ, Orff H, et al. (2001) Temporal and stagewise distribution of high frequency EEG activity in patients with primary and secondary insomnia and in good sleeper controls. J Sleep Res 10: 93–104. doi: 10.1046/j.1365-2869.2001.00247.x

37. Bremner JD, Randall P, Scott TM, Bronen RA, Seibyl JP, et al. (1995) MRI-based measurement of hippocampal volume in patients with combat-related posttraumatic stress disorder. Am J Psychiatry 152: 973–81.

38. Bremner JD, Randall P, Scott TM, Capelli S, Delaney R, et al. (1995) Deficits in short-term memory in adult survivors of childhood abuse. Psychiatr Res 59: 97–107. doi: 10.1016/0165-1781(95)02800-5

39. Stern Y (2006) Cognitive reserve and Alzheimer disease. Alzheimer Dis Assoc Disord 20: 112–117. doi: 10.1097/01.wad.0000213815.20177.19

40. Bickel H, Mösch H, Förstl E (2007) Screening of Cognitive Functions and the Prediction of Incident Dementia by Means of the SIDAM. Psychiatrische Praxis 34: 139–144. doi: 10.1055/s-2006-951973

41. Dretsch MN, Thiel KJ, Athy JR, Irvin CR, Sirmon-Fjordbak B, et al. (2012) Mood symptoms contribute to working memory decrement in active-duty soldiers being treated for posttraumatic stress disorder. Brain Behav 2: 357–64. doi: 10.1002/brb3.53

42. Conover WJ (1999) Practical Nonparametric Statistics (Wiley Series in Probability and Statistics). Wiley p. 592. doi: 10.1002/9780470168707.scard

43. Maercker A, Forstmeier S, Wagner B, Glaesmer H, Brähler E (2008) Post-traumatic stress disorder in Germany. Results of a nationwide epidemiological study. Der Nervenarzt 79: 577–86. doi: 10.1007/s00115-008-2467-5

44. Hardt J, Rutter M (2004) Validity of adult retrospective reports of adverse childhood experiences: review of the evidence. J Child Psychol Psyc 45: 260–273. doi: 10.1111/j.1469-7610.2004.00218.x

45. Heim C, Nemeroff CM (2001) The role of childhood trauma in the neurobiology of mood and anxiety disorders: preclinical and clinical studies. Biol Psychiatr 49: 1023–1039. doi: 10.1016/s0006-3223(01)01157-x

CHAPTER 12

ADVERSE CHILDHOOD EXPERIENCES, PSYCHOSOCIAL WELL-BEING, AND COGNITIVE DEVELOPMENT AMONG ORPHANS AND ABANDONED CHILDREN IN FIVE LOW INCOME COUNTRIES

MAYA ESCUETA, KATHRYN WHETTEN, JAN OSTERMANN, KAREN O'DONNELL, AND THE POSITIVE OUTCOMES FOR ORPHANS (POFO) RESEARCH TEAM

12.1 BACKGROUND

The plight of orphans[a] and abandoned children (OAC) is an increasing global problem that is particularly pervasive in Southeast Asia and sub-Saharan Africa [1]. Improving the educational attainment of the 153 million orphans and other vulnerable children worldwide is a key goal for development policymakers and practitioners. International declarations such as the Millennium Development Goals and the Education for All Movement indicate that the educational attainment of vulnerable children has become a global priority. Most recently, the 2011 Political Declaration on HIV/

Adverse Childhood Experiences, Psychosocial Well-Being and Cognitive Development among Orphans and Abandoned Children in Five Low Income Countries. © Escueta M, Whetten K, Ostermann J, O'Donnell K, and The Positive Outcomes for Orphans (POFO) Research Team; licensee BioMed Central Ltd. BMC International Health and Human Rights 14,6 (2014), doi:10.1186/1472-698X-14-6. Licensed under Creative Commons Attribution 2.0 Generic License, http://creativecommons.org/licenses/by/2.0/.

AIDS targeted increases in school attendance of orphans as an important and measureable indicator of progress [2].

To understand which policies can improve educational attainment for OAC, decision makers must first understand the determinants of and barriers to these outcomes. However, there are mixed results regarding which factors, including orphanhood itself, are significantly associated with educational attainment. Previous research shows that the loss of a parent can lead to a series of developmental disadvantages resulting in poor education [3-7], such as lags in grade for age and school attendance relative to non-orphans [3,7,8]. In contrast, other studies find little negative impact of parental death on child education [9-11] and instead find that alternative factors such as wealth, age, or the child's relationship to the head of household are better predictors of education outcomes [12]. Importantly, many of these studies are restricted to single country analyses, rendering results arguably context specific.

Additionally, few studies examining the educational attainment of orphans move beyond outcomes such as school enrollment, grade for age, and attendance to disentangle what factors contribute to a child's learning [13,14]. Other outcomes may provide more meaningful information. A recent study showed that tests of cognitive development can be a useful measure in understanding OAC learning and educational experience across settings. In particular, cognitive development was found to be positively associated with increases in exposure to formal education [15].

One factor that may offer some insight into the development of OAC is mental health. Previous research, though not focused on orphans, highlights the role of adverse childhood experiences in life outcomes [16]. Cumulative effects from multiple risk factors have been shown to be more predictive of compromised early cognitive development among vulnerable children than any one risk factor alone [17]. In the research on orphans, the role of psychosocial status on multiple outcomes has been studied, though not specifically in relation to learning outcomes. Research on OAC in low and middle income countries found that orphaned children are more susceptible than non-orphans to exposure to potentially traumatic events due to lack of adequate adult protection [18-21]. A recent study found that OAC anxiety and emotional difficulties increased with additional exposure to potentially traumatic events [22]. Another recent study found associations between orphan risk of psychosocial difficulties and subsequent risk of HIV infection [23].

While there is a clear need for mental health interventions among OAC, few investigators have examined the role of mental health in predicting OACs' cognitive development [24-26]. To our knowledge, no study has attempted to do a cross-country analysis of community based OAC to address these questions. Through these analyses, we aim to understand better the linkages between emotional difficulties and a child's ability to participate in and gain from education in a context where children are particularly vulnerable to adverse events and subsequent emotional difficulties. In this manuscript, we employ within-country and cross-country analyses to examine associations between exposure to adverse childhood events, the emotional difficulties that OAC face, and their cognitive development.

12.2 METHODS

12.2.1 STUDY DESCRIPTION

Positive Outcome for Orphans (POFO) is an ongoing longitudinal study following a cohort of children, starting ages 6 to 12, who live in institutional or community-based settings in 5 low income countries: Cambodia, Ethiopia, Kenya, India, and Tanzania. This analysis used 3 years of data from the community-based sample to address the relationships stated above.

12.2.2 STUDY SAMPLE

The detailed sampling strategy and general characteristics of the sample have been reported elsewhere [26,27]. The following describes the elements of the sampling strategy applicable to this analysis.

The POFO study utilized a two stage random sampling methodology to identify a representative sample of 1,480 orphaned and abandoned children living in community-based settings in six sites across five low and middle income countries. Within each site, geographic or administrative boundaries were used to define sampling areas (clusters), 50 clusters were randomly selected at each site, and up to five eligible children ages 6-12 years were selected from each cluster. Eligible children were defined as follows: orphans were those children for whom one or both parents had died [1] and an abandoned child was one whose parents had left with no expectation of return. Eligible children were randomly selected from available lists or through a house-to-house census. One child per household was selected to participate in the study. For households with multiple age-eligible children, the child whose name started with the earliest letter in the alphabet was selected to participate. Additionally, each site enrolled 50 community-based children who were not orphaned or abandoned at baseline as a comparison group.

12.2.3 DATA COLLECTION PROTOCOL

As previously published [22,26], the following describes the procedures of data collection relevant to this analysis. Children and each of their self-identified primary caregivers were contacted and interviewed twice per year for up to 3 years. Baseline and annual follow up surveys collected data on numerous characteristics including the child's exposure to traumatic events, symptoms of emotional and behavioral difficulties, cognitive development, and educational attainment. Additionally, caregivers reported on household socioeconomic characteristics. Ethical approval was obtained from the Duke University Institutional Review Board (IRB) and from local and national IRB's in each participating country.

The primary measures utilized in this study include child self-reports of emotional difficulties, tests assessing cognitive abilities, and child and caregiver reports of exposure to potentially traumatic events, all reported at baseline, and at 12-month, 24-month and 36-month follow ups. The measures used for trauma, emotional difficulties and cognitive development were previously validated for use across cultures (see below) and field-tested using pilot interviews.

12.2.4 STUDY MEASURES

12.2.4.1 MEASURING COGNITIVE DEVELOPMENT: KAUFMAN ASSESSMENT BATTERY FOR CHILDREN AND THE CALIFORNIA VERBAL LEARNING TEST

The KABC-II is an individually administered test of intelligence and achievement that was developed with the intention of "building in sensitivity to preschoolers, minorities and exceptional populations" [28]. Three nonverbal subtests from the Second Edition of the Kaufman Assessment Battery for Children (KABC-II), Hand Movements, Triangles and Pattern Reasoning, were assessed at annual child interviews in the POFO study. The KABC was chosen because it is one of the most frequently used tests of learning ability internationally. The three non-verbal subtests were chosen to be used across the five countries as they are less dependent on language differences.

The California Verbal Learning Test (CVLT-C) is a test of verbal memory, used by POFO researchers as an indicator of memory, attention and motivation [15]. POFO interviewers modified the memory list, referred to here as the Market List (ML). Locally relevant lists were developed at each site that contained 15 items a child might see at their respective markets. The test required children to encode and store information in order to repeat back what was read to them. The Market List was chosen based on observed variability of children's engagement with the tests during pilot work in East Africa, suggesting that a tool that reflects motivation and attention would be an important addition to the learning tasks on the KABC-II [15].

Previous analyses by POFO researchers validated these tests as measures of learning and performance for children living in LMIC [15]. The findings of this previous analysis provided support that across the five countries, the subtests functioned as one would expect measures of learning to function, that is, raw scores increased with chronological age. These tests were also strongly associated with years in school for age. Hence, the KABC II scores used here can be seen as an effective tool for measuring learning, which also reflects experience in the learning environment [15].

This analysis used the highest of the three KABC test standard scores (called topscore) for each child at each round as the primary outcome measure for cognitive development. This measure represents the best the child was able to do across the three subtests when tested by the interviewer. Standard scores of the KABC II range between 0 and 19, and each subtest has a mean of 10 and a standard deviation of 3 [28]. In this analysis, scores were scaled to US age standards to enable comparison across children and these five settings. The average number of items recalled in the first three repetitions on the Market List was used as an ancillary measure of learning, attention, and motivation.

12.2.4.2 MEASURING PSYCHOSOCIAL WELL-BEING AND EMOTIONAL DIFFICULTIES: THE STRENGTHS AND DIFFICULTIES QUESTIONNAIRE

The Strengths and Difficulties Questionnaire (SDQ) is a behavioral screening tool, designed for children ages 4-16, that measures psychosocial well-being across five dimensions: (1) emotional symptoms, (2) conduct problems, (3) hyperactivity/inattention, (4) peer relationship problems, and (5) prosocial behavior. Each subscale has 5 items, scored on a 3-point Likert scale (0-2). The four difficulties subscales add up to a Total Difficulties Score, while the fifth subscale provides assessment of prosocial behavior. POFO researchers chose the Strengths and Difficulties Questionnaire "for its brevity, its psychometric properties, and its frequent use in other international studies" [22]. The questionnaire can be completed in two versions, either by parents, teachers or caregiver report, or, for children ages 11 and older, by self-report [29]. With scoring from 0-2 on each individual item, the Total Difficulties scale ranges from 0 - 40. This analysis used the Total Difficulties score as a continuous variable, rather than using a clinical cutoff, which is not available across these sites. The validity of the self-reported Total Difficulties scale has been assessed and confirmed in multiple contexts (Cronbach's alpha ranging from 0.73-0.89), indicating that the scale itself is internally valid [1]. In the POFO sample, Cronbach's alpha was 0.73. These analyses used the Total Difficulties Score self-reported by the child as the primary measure of emotional difficulties.

Limiting the SDQ self report to ages 11 and older is in line with the recommendation of the SDQb.

12.2.4.3 MEASURING ADVERSE CHILDHOOD EXPERIENCES: THE LIFE EVENTS CHECKLIST

This analysis used the Life Events Checklist, first created by the National Center for Posttraumatic Stress Disorder (PTSD) to aid in the diagnosis of post traumatic symptoms [30]. This checklist, which inquires about exposure to potentially traumatic events such as natural disasters, witnessing someone being hurt or killed, experiencing physical or sexual abuse, or being forced to leave home, is one of the most commonly used research instruments to evaluate exposure to trauma across countries and cultures [31]. Caregivers and children were independently asked at each interview whether the child had ever witnessed or experienced each of 21 types of events. A child was counted as having experienced an event if either the caregiver or the child reported it. As described previously, four categories of events were excluded from this analysis [22].c A cumulative traumatic exposure variable was generated for this analysis, which sums the total count of up to 17 different traumatic event categories reported through any given round.

12.2.4.4 ADDITIONAL COVARIATES: HOUSEHOLD WEALTH, CAREGIVER ILLITERACY, AND RELATIONSHIP TO THE CHILD

An asset checklist and other elements from the Demographic and Health Surveys (DHS)d of each site were used to derive a wealth index score for each participating household [32-36]. Wealth index scores are continuous, standardized for comparability with wealth index scores in each country's DHS, and indicate greater affluence as the score increases. Caregiver illiteracy was assessed based on a literacy test administered at the time of each survey. Caregivers unable to read four short sentences in the local language were classified as illiterate. The child's relationship to the caregiver (parent versus non-parent) and orphan status (single or double orphan v. abandoned) were included in the analysis.

12.2.5 ANALYSES

A linear regression model was estimated to describe the relationship between emotional difficulties (SDQ Total Difficulties score) and various explanatory variables, including orphan status, exposure to potentially traumatic events, and household wealth. Additional linear regression models with the KABC topscore and Market lists as dependent variables were used to estimate the association between emotional difficulties and cognitive development. These models controlled for age, gender, orphan status, wealth and caregiver illiteracy, and the number of prior administrations of the KABC test to account for child learning over time. Models analyzed up to four time points for each child cross-sectionally; each model specification was run separately by site and jointly for all sites.

Child-level fixed effects models were estimated to describe the relationship between the SDQ Total Difficulties score and cognitive outcomes while controlling for time invariant characteristics of children that may affect outcomes. Models were run jointly across all sites and controlled for age as the only other observed time varying characteristics expected to be associated with the child's cognitive development during the study period. Additional models, run for sensitivity analysis, evaluated whether the association between emotional difficulties and cognitive outcomes differed by caregiver type (parent versus non-parent), OAC status, or study site. Effect estimates for subgroups were calculated as linear combinations of SDQ main effects and interactions with the respective indicator variables for each subgroup. Two additional fixed effects model analyzed the association of cognitive outcomes with the four SDQ subscales (which comprise the SDQ Total Difficulties score) and with caregiver reports of the SDQ.

All models were estimated with robust standard errors to account for error correlations within sites and between multiple observations from each child. Child-level fixed effects models accounted for clustering at the level of the child. Weights were constructed to account for differences in the number of children and their age and gender distributions across study sites and were used in all models.

TABLE 1: Descriptive statistics at baseline

	Cambodia	Ethiopia	Hyderabad	Kenya	Nagaland	Tanzania	ALL SITES
Topscore at baseline							
Mean (SD)	7.4 (2.57)	7.6 (2.57)	6.96 (1.86)	7.43 (2.68)	6.71 (2.15)	6.61 (2.27)	7.12 (2.40)
N	300	300	300	300	279	302	1781
Market list at baseline							
Mean (SD)	7.68 (2.59)	7.71 (1.97)	6.47 (1.78)	7.46 (2.17)	6.5 (2.40)	7.48 (2.06)	7.23 (2.23)
N	297	300	299	297	266	301	1760
Total difficulties self-reported at baseline							
Mean (SD)	14.22 (5.49)	10.0 (4.49)	13.74 (4.89)	8.41 (4.15)	8.25 (3.37)	5.27 (3.74)	10.17 (5.68)
N	122	34	50	69	68	85	428
Total difficulties caregiver reported at baseline							
Mean (SD)	13.26 (4.89)	12.81 (6.05)	13.04 (5.30)	9.63 (4.11)	8.77 (3.89)	6.90 (4.80)	10.71 (5.47)
N	292	295	253	300	259	300	1699
Exposure to potentially traumatic events at baseline							
Mean (SD)	2.93 (1.68)	2.64 (1.68)	2.87 (1.95)	0.87 (1.32)	0.81 (0.94)	2.54 (1.08)	2.12 (1.74)
N	300	297	252	299	263	300	1711
Wealth index mean (SD)	0.98 (0.50)	0.97 (0.56)	1.01 (0.36)	1.00 (0.69)	0.99 (0.55)	1.00 (0.62)	0.99 (0.56)
N	258	265	299	281	267	286	1656
Frequency of OAC status at baseline N (%)							
Single orphan	178 (59.33)	161 (53.67)	151 (50.33)	207 (69)	205 (73.48)	178 (58.94)	1080 (60.64)
Double orphan	60 (20)	60 (20)	22 (7.33)	31 (10.33)	17 (6.09)	67 (22.19)	257 (14.43)
Abandoned	13 (4.33)	33 (11)	78 (26)	15 (5)	7 (2.51)	6 (1.99)	152 (8.53)

TABLE 1: *Cont.*

	Cambodia	Ethiopia	Hyderabad	Kenya	Nagaland	Tanzania	ALL SITES
Non orphans	49 (16.33)	46 (15.33)	49 (16.33)	47 (15.67)	50 (17.92)	51 (16.89)	292 (16.4)
Total N	300	300	300	300	279	302	1781
Caregiver type N (%)							
Parent	135 (45)	117 (39)	96 (32)	110 (36.67)	90 (32.26)	131 (43.38)	679 (38.12)
Non-parent	165 (55)	183 (61)	204 (68)	190 (63.33)	189 (67.74)	171 (56.62)	1102 (61.88)
Total N	300	300	300	300	279	302	1781
Illiterate caregiver N (%)	95 (46.57)	100 (43.48)	173 (64.07)	174 (63.5)	116 (44.27)	52 (22.71)	710 (48.33)
N	204	230	270	274	262	229	1469
Age Mean (SD)	9.41 (1.97)	9.05 (1.76)	9.13 (1.52)	9.25 (1.84)	9.07 (1.86)	9.43 (1.90)	9.22 (1.82)
N	300	300	300	300	279	302	1781
Gender N (%)							
Male	149 (49.67)	160 (53.33)	149 (49.67)	155 (51.57)	160 (57.35)	157 (51.99)	930 (52.22)
Female	151 (50.33)	140 (46.67)	151 (50.33)	145 (48.33)	119 (42.65)	145 (48.01)	851 (47.78)
Total N	300	300	300	300	279	302	1781

12.2.6 ATTRITION

To evaluate the extent to which attrition may have biased our estimates, bivariable logistic regression models of baseline characteristics analyzed whether children who left the study differed significantly from those who stayed.

12.3 RESULTS

12.3.1 Descriptive statistics
Table 1 shows descriptive statistics at baseline, including proportion and frequency of OAC status, frequency of caregiver type (parent versus non-parent) and the mean and standard deviation of performance on the KABC II, child self-reported emotional difficulties, mean count of exposures to types of potentially traumatic events, and other characteristics.

Single orphans constitute the largest group within the sample (60.6%). While the average topscore at baseline is similar across sites (ranging from 6.6 to 7.6), there is more variation by site on the average level of self-reported emotional difficulties (range 5.3 to 14.2), with Cambodia and Hyderabad reporting the highest average scores. The average self-reported Total Difficulties score was 10.2 for the entire sample at baseline. On average, children had experienced 1.7 types of potentially traumatic events, in addition to their orphaning or abandonment. Nagaland and Kenya had the lowest average levels of reported exposure to potentially traumatic events at baseline.

12.3.2 PREDICTING EMOTIONAL DIFFICULTIES

Table 2 describes the relationship between the self-reported Total Difficulties score among children 11 and older and a host of explanatory variables, including age, gender, orphan status, wealth, and exposure to potentially traumatic events.[e]

TABLE 2: OLS estimate of total difficulties score predicted by orphan status

Variables	Cambodia total difficulties	Ethiopia total difficulties	Hyderabad total difficulties	Kenya total difficulties	Nagaland total difficulties	Tanzania total difficulties	ALL SITES§ total difficulties
Exposure to potentially traumatic events	0.25	0.12	0.17	0.33**	-0.27	0.60**	0.36**
	(0.14)	(0.1)	(0.07)	(0.15)	(0.21)	(0.06)	(0.06)
Wealth index	-0.63	-0.47	-0.53	-0.14	-0.69**	-0.44	-0.49**
	(0.34)	(0.36)	(0.22)	(0.26)	(0.46)	(0.09)	(0.09)
Single orphan	1.2	1.40**	0.56	0.12	-1.09*	4.52**	0.87
	(0.53)	(0.37)	(0.39)	(0.47)	(0.55)	(0.8)	
Double orphan	-0.01	0.72	0.98	-0.99	-1.75*	4.88**	0.68
	(0.75)	(0.39)	(0.86)	(0.66)	(2.22)	(0.60)	
Abandoned	-0.18	0.65	0.19	0.14	-1.53*	3.18	0.35
	(1.15)	(0.39)	(0.72)	(0.55)	(0.47)	(0.48)	
Non-parent caregiver	-0.09	0.72	0.25	0.36	0.24	-1.26	0.04
	(0.50)	(0.32)	(0.40)	(0.34)	(0.67)	(0.20)	
Age in months	-0.04**	-0.03**	-0.04**	-0.02*	-0.01	0	-0.03*
	(0.01)	(0.01)	(0.01)	(0.01)	(0.02)	(0.01)	
Female	-1.16*	-0.02	-1.01**	-0.03	-1.09**	-0.08	-0.61*
	(0.36)	(0.27)	(0.30)	(0.27)	(0.49)	(0.23)	
Constant	19.11**	12.61**	16.78**	10.64**	11.81**	0.69	15.34**
	(1.84)	(2.10)	(1.34)	(1.21)	(2.32)	(2.10)	
Observations	438	410	656	573	550	584	3,211
R-squared	0.11	0.18	0.18	0.16	0.09	0.16	0.28

*Robust standard errors in parentheses **$p<0.01$, *$p<0.05$. §Model also included site level and round level fixed effects (not shown).*

Several factors were associated with children's emotional difficulties, including child age and gender, exposure to trauma, and household wealth; however, associations varied across sites. In Cambodia, Ethiopia, Hyderabad and Kenya, Total Difficulties were lower for older children. Female gender was associated with lower levels of difficulties in Cambodia, Hyderabad, and Nagaland; wealth was negatively associated with higher levels of emotional difficulties in Nagaland. In two of the six sites, Kenya and Tanzania, exposure to potentially traumatic events was significantly and positively associated with higher levels of emotional difficulties.

There were mixed results for orphan status. Being a single orphan was associated with higher emotional difficulties relative to non-orphans in 2 sites, and being a double orphan was associated with higher emotional difficulties in one site. However orphaned and abandoned children in Nagaland reported lower rates of emotional difficulties relative to comparison children. While the wealth index, exposure to potentially traumatic events, gender and age were statistically significant when looking jointly across "All Sites", no orphan status held significant associations with emotional difficulties in this specification.

12.3.3 PREDICTING COGNITIVE DEVELOPMENT

Tables 3 and 4 show ordinary least squares (OLS) and fixed effects regressions of emotional difficulties predicting cognitive development. Since exposure to potentially traumatic events was highly correlated with emotional difficulties (rho=0.33; also see Table 2), exposure to trauma was not included in these models.

There was a significant negative association between emotional difficulties and the child's topscore on the KABC II tests in five of six study sites (Table 3). There is no evidence that orphan status holds a significant relationship to the child's topscore. Wealth is positive and significant in Cambodia and Kenya. Caregiver illiteracy is associated with lower performance on the KABC II tests, with significant associations in Kenya and Tanzania. Female gender was associated with lower KABC II scores in Cambodia and Kenya.

TABLE 3: OLS estimate of topscore predicted by total difficulties

Variables	Cambodia	Ethiopia	Hyderabad	Kenya	Nagaland	Tanzania	ALL SITES§
	Topscore	Topscore	Topscore	Topscore	Topscore	Topscore	
Total difficulties	-0.09**	-0.09*	-0.01	-0.07**	-0.11**	-0.08**	-0.09**
	(0.03)	(0.04)	(0.02)	(0.03)	(0.02)	(0.01)	(0.01)
Age in months	-0.01	0.01	-0.01*	0	-0.03**	0	-0.01
	(0.01)	(0.01)	(0.01)	(0.01)	0.00	0.00	(0.01)
Female	-1.20**	-0.24	0.07	-0.68**	-0.14	0	-0.36
	(0.25)	(0.22)	(0.17)	(0.22)	(0.15)	(0.14)	(0.17)
Single orphan	-0.09	-0.48	-0.26	0	0.09	-0.24	-0.1
	(0.34)	(0.42)	(0.23)	(0.27)	(0.19)	(0.20)	(0.09)
Double orphan	-0.56	-0.41	-0.51	-0.45	0.43	0.08	-0.08
	(0.44)	(0.46)	(0.34)	(0.41)	(0.41)	(0.23)	(0.14)
Abandoned	0.36	-0.39	-0.17	0.28	0.18	0.85	-0.03
	(0.83)	(0.55)	(0.25)	(0.57)	(0.40)	(0.66)	(0.11)
Illiterate caregiver	-0.01	-0.13	0	-0.56*	0.02	-0.36*	-0.16
	(0.28)	(0.22)	(0.18)	(0.23)	(0.15)	(0.18)	(0.09)
Wealth index	0.80**	-0.03	0.22	0.46*	0.1	0.13	0.31*
	(0.26)	(0.21)	(0.24)	(0.18)	(0.14)	(0.11)	(0.11)
Constant	10.00**	7.12**	8.69**	7.96**	10.05**	7.35**	9.07**
	(1.26)	(1.31)	(1.08)	(1.19)	(0.69)	(0.75)	(0.52)
Observations	371	390	675	569	543	553	3,101
R-squared	0.14	0.09	0.4	0.07	0.22	0.22	0.34

*Robust standard errors in parentheses **p<0.01, *p<0.05. §Model also included site level and round level fixed effects (not shown) Table 3. OLS Estimate of Topscore Predicted By Total Difficulties.*

TABLE 4: Fixed effects estimate of topscore predicted by total difficulties

		Main model	Model 2	Model 3	Model 4	Model 5	Model 6
					Sensitivity analysis		
		SDQ	SDQ	SDQ	Self report	Self report	Self report
		Self report	Subscales	CG report	by OAC status	by CG type	by site
SDQ self report	Total difficulties	-0.09**					
		(0.01)					
	Emotions		-0.08**				
			(0.03)				
	Conduct		-0.04				
			(0.04)				
	Hyperactivity		-0.12**				
			(0.03)				
	Peer relations		-0.13**				
			(0.03)				
SDQ caregiver report total difficulties				-0.07**			
				(0.01)			
Orphan status	Non-orphan				-0.04		
					(0.04)		
	Single orphan				-0.09**		
					(0.01)		
	Double orphan				-0.11**		
					(0.02)		
	Abandoned				-0.13**		
					(0.04)		
Caregiver	Parent					-0.10**	
						(0.01)	

TABLE 4: *Cont.*

		Sensitivity analysis					
		Main model	Model 2	Model 3	Model 4	Model 5	Model 6
		SDQ	SDQ	SDQ	Self report	Self report	Self report
		Self report	Subscales	CG report	by OAC status	by CG type	by site
	Non-parent					-0.09**	
						(0.01)	
Study site	Cambodia						-0.00
							(0.02)
	Ethiopia						-0.09**
							(0.04)
	Hyderabad						-0.18**
							(0.03)
	Kenya						-0.09**
							(0.03)
	Nagaland						-0.11**
							(0.03)
	Tanzania						-0.09**
							(0.02)
Observations		3,418	3,418	5,882	3,418	3,327	3,418
R-squared		0.14	0.14	0.13	0.14	0.14	0.15
Number of children		1,445	1,445	1,775	1,445	1,442	1,445

Robust standard errors in parenthesis **p<0.01, *p<0.05. Estimates from fixed effects linear regression models, controlling for child age, SDQ variable(s), and interactions of OAC status, caregiver type, or study site with SDQ Effects for subgroups calculated as linear combinations of SDQ main effects and interaction effect for the respective indicator variable.

Table 4 shows the results of a fixed effects model of the relationship between emotional difficulties and cognitive development, thus controlling for all time invariant characteristics within one child. Since most co-

variates in previous models are considered time invariant, age is the only
additional covariate included in the model.

TABLE 5: OLS estimate of market list predicted by total difficulties

Variables	Cambodia	Ethiopia	Hyderabad	Kenya	Nagaland	Tanzania	Tanzania ALL SITES§
	Market list	Market list	Market list	Market list	Market list	Market list	Market list
Total difficulties	0.01	-0.07**	-0.02	-0.03	0.04*	-0.20**	-0.09
	(-0.02)	(-0.02)	(-0.02)	(-0.02)	(-0.02)	(-0.01)	(-0.04)
Age in months	0.03**	0.03**	0.02**	0.02**	0.01*	0.01**	0.02**
	(-0.01)	(-0.01)	(0.00)	(-0.01)	(0.00)	(0.00)	(0.00)
Female	-0.01	0.17	0.16	0.17	0.15	0.15	0.05
	(0.20)	(0.15)	(0.11)	(0.15)	(0.11)	(0.13)	(0.03)
Single orphan	0.01	-0.23	0.09	-0.32	0.17	0.3	-0.07
	(0.30)	(0.25)	(0.14)	(0.18)	(0.15)	(0.23)	(0.09)
Double orphan	-0.31	-0.33	0.33	-0.78**	0.23	0.64*	-0.06
	(0.35)	(0.28)	(0.21)	(0.29)	(0.30)	(0.25)	(0.22)
Abandoned	0.22	-0.71*	-0.06	-0.78	0.44	0.43	-0.25
	(0.48)	(0.34)	(0.15)	(0.45)	(0.31)	(0.60)	(0.14)
Illiterate caregiver	0.19	-0.21	-0.23	-0.35*	-0.11	-0.39*	-0.19
	(0.21)	(0.15)	(0.12)	(0.16)	(0.12)	(0.18)	(0.09)
Wealth index	0.48*	0.04	0.07	0.1	0.11	0	0.1
	(0.22)	(0.14)	(0.14)	(0.11)	(0.11)	(0.12)	(0.05)
Constant	4.50**	5.95**	5.07**	6.09**	5.64**	6.88**	8.03**
	(0.98)	(0.89)	(0.72)	(0.80)	(0.52)	(0.61)	(0.97)
Observations	371	390	675	568	542	552	3098
R-squared	0.08	0.16	0.31	0.12	0.04	0.48	0.3

*Robust standard errors in parentheses **p<0.01, *p<0.05. §Model also included site level
and round level fixed effects (not shown).*

The relationship between emotional difficulties and cognitive development remains negative and significant in the fixed effects estimation (Table 4). In sensitivity analysis, the relationship also holds for three out of the four subscales of the self-reported SDQ (Emotions, Hyperactivity and Peer Relations) as well as the caregiver reported SDQ (Model 3). The negative and significant relationship also holds for most subgroups evaluated in the sensitivity analysis. The relationship between emotional difficulties and cognitive development remains negative and significant for each orphan type (with no significant effect for non-orphans), and across caregiver types (parent versus non-parent). The estimated effect was statistically significant in four out of the six study sites. Effects estimates for the association between SDQ and topscore did not differ between single and double orphans (p-value 0.711) or children with parent vs. non-parent caregivers (p-value 0.625; not shown).

The same models as in Tables 3 and 4 were estimated for the CVLT-T Market List to test whether associations held across multiple measures of learning. The correlation between the KABC II topscore and the CVLT-T Market List is 0.373, indicating that while there is some shared variance, the two indices still likely capture different aspects of the child's cognitive development. The relationship between emotional difficulties and scores on the Market List test was negative and significant in 3 of 6 sites for the OLS model. The relationship was also negative and significant across "All Sites" in the fixed effects model, with similar results for the sensitivity analysis as were found with the topscore measure. Results are presented in Tables 5 and 6.

12.3.4 ATTRITION AND MISSING DATA

Attrition differed significantly across study sites (p-value 0.00) and children living with parents (single or non-orphan) were less likely to drop out (p-value 0.046). Results in Tables 4 and 6 suggest that the observed associations do not differ between children living with parents and non-parents, thus it is unlikely that differential attrition between children residing with biological parents versus other children substantively biased our estimates. Further, the direction of the observed associations was similar in most study sites. There were no differences in rates of attrition across other relevant factors such as exposure to potentially traumatic events, cognitive development, socioeconomic status, gender, or the level of emotional difficulties.

Using the child self-report measure of the Total Difficulties scale resulted in a number of missing data points at baseline, since children did not self-report on the SDQ until they were 11 years old. To check whether missing data of this nature might change results, cross-sectional analysis was restricted to the 36-month follow up (when most children (84.3%) were old enough to self-report) controlling for baseline characteristics, with little change in results. Given that a) the caregivers of nearly half of all participating children were not their biological parents, b) caregivers may significantly under-report the behavioral effects of traumatic events experienced by children [37], and c) caregivers had been taking care of these children for variable amounts of time, the child self-reported difficulties were considered more accurate than caregiver reports.

12.4 DISCUSSION

This is the first cross-country study to examine the relationship between orphans' emotional difficulties and their learning. Moreover, conducting such an analysis on a unique sample of vulnerable children who are susceptible to multiple instances of adversity, including trauma, provides evidence of the nature of this relationship within a context of heightened adversity and potentially higher risk of mental health difficulties. This analysis showed that OAC exposure to potentially traumatic events is an important predictor of emotional difficulties, thus supporting previous literature that the number of adverse events matters for risk of mental health difficulties.

The most salient finding was a negative and significant relationship between a child's emotional difficulties and his/her cognitive development, within and across five of six study sites. Rates of exposure to adverse childhood events among the orphaned and abandoned children in this study were high, and exposure to adverse events, in addition to male gender, and lower household wealth, was associated with significantly higher rates of emotional difficulties. Interestingly, orphan status was only significantly associated with emotional difficulties in some sites and was not predictive of cognitive development, although the negative and significant relationship between emotional difficulties and cognitive development held within each orphan subgroup. These findings may suggest that when a child is more vulnerable to a number of adverse events, it is the context in which a child loses a parent, rather than the loss of a parent alone, that better explains mental health outcomes. Children who are vulnerable from orphaning and have experienced other adversity are at heightened risk of increased emotional difficulties, which is associated with lags in cognitive development. These findings offer insights into the relationship between vulnerable children's mental health and their ability to participate in and benefit from education.

In the context of multiple adversity, the loss of a parent, or orphan status, does not show statistical significance in the hypothesized relationship between mental health and learning. Nevertheless, the overall findings still underscore the importance of mental health intervention for children who are especially vulnerable. It is likely that the effect of parental loss is further affected by the additional adverse events to which the child is even more vulnerable. No trauma or potentially traumatic event happens in isolation.

Although causality cannot be inferred from this analysis, the results offer insight into the relationship between emotional difficulties and educational outcomes. The fixed effects model controls for unobserved time-invariant differences between children that may be correlated with emotional difficulties and may influence cognitive development. Consequently, the results in Table 4 give us an unbiased estimate of the relationship between a child's emotional difficulties and his/her cognitive development, controlling for these differences. The consistency of the association between these two factors across multiple contexts and measures and within different subgroups is striking. This underscores the importance of providing trauma support and focusing on the psychosocial development of vulnerable children as a means to alleviate strains inhibiting a child's learning.

Additionally, the associations found between wealth and emotional difficulties may indicate that interventions aimed at easing households' resource constraints could help alleviate emotional difficulties in some contexts. One may hypothesize that in less stable, resource poor settings, children who were exposed to trauma may be less likely to recover from emotional difficulties. Interventions on both the child and family levels may work in tandem to improve education outcomes for orphans. If policies and programs can improve economic and emotional stability for both children and families, orphans may have a greater chance of pushing past the challenges of losing a parent and the additional traumas to which orphanhood exposes them. While economic support does not treat mental health difficulties, it may provide families with the resources needed to keep children in school, which may aide their psychosocial development. Such support may improve a child's chances of overcoming the emotional challenges that are associated with lags in cognitive development. We acknowledge several limitations.

Children's cognitive development is described by only two measures, an aggregated score summarizing children's performance on three nonverbal KABC II subtests plus a measure verbal memory and attention based on the CVLT. While ability is likely not to change over time, the child's performance on the KABC II tests is not only an indication of the child's ability, but also a variety of other factors associated with motivation, self-confidence, response to authority and the child's developed non-verbal skillset [1]. We may interpret the association of test scores with the child's emotional difficulties to be related to changes in these additional factors. While this measure may not singularly isolate the child's cognitive development, knowledge of the critical role of emotional difficulties in the child's learning and subsequent academic attainment is an important insight for policies on global support for vulnerable children, including but not limited to those vulnerable due to parental death.

Further, the available data do not offer adequate statistical power to describe the temporal association between the variables of interest, and therefore cannot rule out possibilities of reverse causality. It is possible that the observed relationships are circular and that, even if higher emotional difficulties impede cognitive development, lags in cognitive development in turn may heighten emotional difficulties. With adversity, psychosocial manifestations, and cognitive delays spanning much of the life span of the children in this study, the three year follow-up period does not offer sufficient within-child variation to disentangle these effects. Regardless of the direction of causality, if we know that children who are exposed to more trauma also report more emotional difficulties and perform lower on tests of cognitive ability, interventions to provide emotional support for children living in adversity will help at least one or more of these difficulties. Even though we do not know whether emotional difficulties are driving lags in cognition or the other way around, we still need to address the emotional difficulties, specifically targeting potentially traumatic events.

Finally, the study findings may not be generalizable, as there are many other groups of OAC, including street children, institution-based orphans, and those that live in countries with widely different contexts than those in our sample. These associations may differ in those samples. The variability in the observed associations across the six study sites suggests that associations between trauma, emotional difficulties and cognitive development, and appropriate interventions, are likely context-specific. Nevertheless, this analysis offers new insight into the relationship between psychosocial factors, exposure to adverse childhood experiences, resource constraints and the cognitive development of orphans in wide variety of contexts and diverse settings in Southeast Asia and sub-Saharan Africa.

12.5 CONCLUSIONS

This study suggests that increased reports of exposure to potentially traumatic events among orphans and abandoned children are associated with higher emotional difficulties, and increases in emotional difficulties are associated with lags in cognitive development. Hence, exposure to trauma and emotional difficulties comprise important barriers to educational attainment for all such vulnerable children, including orphans. Higher socioeconomic status and better educated caregivers may offer buffers to these difficulties, since they are associated with fewer emotional difficulties and higher performance on tests of cognitive development. Interventions targeting both the psychosocial development of the child, vis a vis their exposure to adverse childhood events, and the socio-economic status of the caregiver may work in tandem to improve educational outcomes for vulnerable children in a more holistic sense. Further, family based interventions to stabilize socioeconomic conditions or increase caregiver education may help overcome psychosocial challenges that otherwise would present as barriers to the child's educational advancement. Most importantly, psychosocial status may be an important actor in a child's ability to profit from and stay in school, and one factor that influences this status is a child's exposure to traumatic and other adverse experiences. These findings may provide a guide to developmental strategies for those working to improve education outcomes for children in less wealthy areas.

12.5.1 ETHICAL APPROVAL

Ethical approval was provided by the Duke Medicine Institutional Review Board (IRB); the local review boards of SaveLives Ethiopia and Stand for Vulnerable Organization (Addis Ababa, Ethiopia), Sharan (Delhi, India), and Kilimanjaro Christian Medical Centre (Moshi, Tanzania); and national regulatory agencies in all participating countries including the National Ethics Committee for Health Research (Cambodia), the Ministry of Science and Technology (Ethiopia), the Indian Council of Medical Research (India), the Kenya Medical Research Institute (KEMRI), and the National Institute for Medical Research (Tanzania).

12.5.2 INFORMED CONSENT

Children under the age of 18 were asked for assent to participate in the study only after the guardian had first given permission for the child to participate, and for the interviewer to speak with the child. The project was explained to the child in an age-appropriate manner, and the child was given the opportunity to ask questions about the project before assent was requested. Children who were not competent (who had moderate to severe learning or mental health disorders) to give assent were not included in the study. Children who previously gave assent as minors were re-consented as adults when they reached age 18.

ENDNOTES

ᵃWhile the definition of "orphan" varies across cultures and settings, UNICEF provides a commonly accepted definition for orphan as "a child who has lost one or both parents" (UNICEF 2004).

ᵇFor more information, see sdqinfo.org.

ᶜ"Hearing about a family member who has died", "had a brother or sister die", "seeing a dead body in town", and "having a painful or scary medical treatment," were excluded from the trauma count variable. Almost all children had lost a family member, hence the first event did not add to the variation in the count. For the second event, it was not clear whether the child witnessed the event themselves. For the third event, in some sites, burials are open-casket so all kids had seen these events. For the latter event, event description was not specific enough. It seemed that for some children, this included blood draws or like events that were scary to the child but not comparable to the other categories.

ᵈData was compiled from a variety of country specific DHS data sets. See references for further information on data used.

ᵉConstants in linear regression models represent the estimated mean value for the (hypothetical) reference group for whom the values of all variables in the model are zero.

REFERENCES

1.   UNICEF: Children on the Brink 2004: A Joint Report of New Orphan Estimates and a Framework for Action. 2004. Population, Health and Nutritional Information Project. accessed at http://www.unicef.org/publications/cob_layout6-013.pdf
2.   UNAIDS: A Global AIDS Response Progress Reporting 2012: Construction of Core Indicators for Monitoring the 2011 Political Declaration on HIV/AIDS. 2011. Joint United Nations Programme on HIV/AIDS. accessed at http://www.unaids.org/en/

media/unaids/contentassets/documents/document/2013/GARPR_2013_guidelines_
en.pdf

3. Case A, Ardington C: The impact of parental death on schooling outcomes: longitu-
    dinal evidence from South Africa. Demography 2006, 43:401-420.
4. Makame V, Ani C, Grantham-McGregor S: Psychosocial Well-being of Orphans in
    Dar El Salaam, Tanzania. Acata Paediatr 2002, 91:459-465.
5. Cas AG, Frankenberg E, Suriastini W, Thomas D: The Impact of Parental Death on
    Child Well-Being. Working Paper: Duke University; 2011.
6. Chatterji M, Hutchinson P, Buek K, Murray N, Mulenga Y, Ventimiglia T: Evaluat-
    ing the Impact of Community-Based Interventions on Schooling Outcomes among
    Orphans and Vulnerable Children in Lusaka, Zambia. Vulnerable Children Youth
    Stud 2010, 5:130-141.
7. Evans D, Miguel E: Orphans and Schooling in Africa: a longitudinal analysis. De-
    mography 2007, 44:35-57.
8. Ainsworth M, Beegle K, Koda G: The impact of adult mortality and parental deaths
    on primary schooling in North-Western Tanzania. J Dev Stud 2005, 41:412-439.
9. Kamali A, Seeley JA, Nunn AJ, Kengeya-Kayondo JF, Ruberantwari A, Mulder
    DW: The orphan problem: experience of a Sub-Saharan Africa rural population in
    the AIDS epidemic. AIDS Care 1996, 8:509-515.
10. Lloyd CB, Blanc AK: Children's Schooling in Sub-Saharan Africa: The Role of Fa-
    thers, Mothers and Others. Popul and Dev Rev 1996, 22:265-298.
11. Ryder RW, Kamenga M: Aids Orphans in Kinshasa, Zaire: incidence and socioeco-
    nomic consequences. AIDS 1994, 8:673-679.
12. Kurzinger ML, Pagnier J, Kahn JG, Hampshire R, Wakabi T, Dye TD: Education
    status among orphans and non-orphans in communities affected by AIDS in Tanza-
    nia and Burkina Faso. AIDS Care 2008, 20:726-732.
13. Nelson CA, Zeanah CH, Fox NA, Marshall PJ, Smyke AT, Guthrie D: Cognitive re-
    covery in socially deprived young children: the Bucharist early intervention project.
    Science 2007, 318:1937-1940.
14. Van IJzendoorn MH, Juffer F, Poelhuis CWK: Adoption and cognitive development:
    a meta-analytic comparison of adopted and nonadopted children's IQ and school
    performance. Psychol Bull 2005, 131:301-316.
15. O'Donnell K, Murphy R, Ostermann J, Masnick M, Whetten RA, Madden E, Thiel-
    man N, Whetten K: A brief assessment of learning for orphaned and abandoned
    children in low and middle income countries. AIDS Behav 2012, 16:480-490.
16. Felitti VJ, Anda RF, Nordenberg D, Williamson DF, Spitz AM, Edwards V, Koss MP,
    Marks JS: Relationship of childhood abuse and household dysfunction to many of
    the leading causes of death in adults. Am J Prevent Med 1998, 14(4):245-258.
17. Sameroff AJ, Sefer R, Barocas R, Zax M, Greenspan S: Intellectual Quotient Scores
    of 4-year old children: social environmental risk factors. Pediatrics 1987, 79(3):343-
    350.
18. Ahmad A, Qahar J, Siddiq A, Majeed A, Rasheed J, Jabar F, Von Knorring AL: A 2
    year follow up of orphans competence, socio-emotional problems and post-traumat-
    ic stress symptoms in traditional foster care and orphanages in Iraqi Kurdistan. Child
    Care Health Dev 2005, 31(2):203-215.

19. Cluver L, Gardner F: The psychological well-being of children orphaned by AIDS in Cape Town, South Africa. Ann Gen Psychiatry 2006, 5:8.

20. Cluver L, Gardner F, Operario D: Psychological distress amongst AIDS-orphaned children in urban South Africa. J Child Psychol Psychiatry 2007, 48(8):755-763.

21. Cluver L, Finchman DS, Seedat S: Post-traumatic stress in AIDS-orphaned children exposed to high levels of trauma: the protective role of perceived social support. J Traumatic Stress 2009, 22(2):106-112.

22. Whetten K, Ostermann J, Whetten RA, O'Donnell K, Thielman N: More than the loss of a parent: potentially traumatic events among orphaned and abandoned children. J Traumatic Stress 2011, 24:174-182.

23. Puffer ES, Drabkin AS, Stachko AL, Broverman SA, Ogwang-Odhiambo RA, Sikkema KJ: Orphan status, HIV risk behavior, and mental health among adolescents in rural Kenya. J Pediatric Psychol 2012, 37:868-878.

24. Ebersohn L, Eloff I: The black, white and grey of rainbow children coping with HIV/AIDS. Perspect Educ 2002, 20:78-86.

25. Miller L, Chan W, Comfort K, Tirella L: Health of children adopted from Guatemala: comparison of orphanage and foster Care. Pediatrics 2005, 115:710-718.

26. Whetten K, Ostermann J, Whetten RA, Pence BW, O'Donnell K, Messer LC, Thielman N: A comparison of the well-being of orphans and abandoned children ages 6-12 in institutional and community based care settings in 5 less wealthy nations. PLoS ONE 2009, 4:e8169.

27. Positive Outcomes for Orphans (POFO) - A Five Country Study of the Wellbeing of Orphaned and Abandoned Children: Study Description. http://chpir.org/_homepage-content/research/pofo/study-design/

28. Narrett CM: Kaufman Assessment Battery for Children (K-ABC). Reading Teacher, Int Reading Assoc 1984, 37:626-631.

29. Goodman R: The strengths and difficulties questionnaire: a research note. J Child Psychol Psychiatry 1997, 38:581-586.

30. Gray M, Litz B, Hsu JL, Lombardo TW: Psychometric properties of the life events checklist. Assessment 2004, 11:330-341.

31. Elhai JD, Gray MJ, Kashdan TB, Franklin CL: Which Instruments are Most Commonly used to Assess Traumatic Event Exposure and Posttraumatic Effects?: a Survey of Traumatic Stress Professionals. J Traumatic Stress 2005, 18:541-545.

32. Central Statistical Agency [Ethiopia] and ICF International: Ethiopia Demographic and Health Survey 2011. Addis Ababa, Ethiopia and Calverton, Maryland, USA: Central Statistical Agency and ICF International; 2012.

33. International Institute for Population Sciences (IIPS) and Macro International: National Family Health Survey (NFHS-3) 2005-2006, India. 2007.

34. National Coordinating Agency for Population and Development (NCPD) [Kenya], Ministry of Medical Services (MOMS) [Kenya], Ministry of Public Health and Sanitation (MOPHS) [Kenya]: Kenya National Bureau of Statistics (KNBS) [Kenya], ICF Macro: Kenya Service Provision Assessment Survey 2010 . Nairobi, Kenya: National Coordinating Agency for Population and Development, Ministry of Medical Services, Ministry of Public Health and Sanitation, Kenya National Bureau of Statistics, and ICF Macro; 2011.

35. National Institute of Statistics, Directorate General for Health, and ICF Macro: Cambodia Demographic and Health Survey 2010. 2011.
36. National Bureau of Statistics (NBS) [Tanzania] and ICF Macro: Tanzania Demographic and Health Survey 2010. Dar es Salaam, Tanzania: NBS and ICF Macro; 2011.
37. Almqvist K, Brandell-Forsberg M: Refugee children in Sweden: post-traumatic stress disorder in Iranian pre-school children exposed to organized violence. Child Abuse Neglect 1997, 24(1):351-366.

Table 6 is not available in this version of the article. To view this additional information, please use the citation on the first page of this chapter.

PART IV

HOPE FOR THE FUTURE

CHAPTER 13

SCHOOL-BASED MENTAL HEALTH INTERVENTION FOR CHILDREN IN WAR-AFFECTED BURUNDI: A CLUSTER RANDOMIZED TRIAL

WIETSE A. TOL, IVAN H. KOMPROE, MARK J.D. JORDANS, ALINE NDAYISABA, PRUDENCE NTAMUTUMBA, HEATHER SIPSMA, EVA S. SMALLEGANGE, ROBERT D. MACY, AND JOOP T. V. M. DE JONG

13.1 BACKGROUND

The 2009 Machel report estimates that just over one billion children and adolescents live in countries and territories affected by armed conflict [1]. In 2011 alone, 37 armed conflicts were recorded globally, the majority in Africa (n = 15, 41%), Asia (n = 13, 35%), and the Middle East (n = 6, 16%) [2]. Epidemiological studies have shown that armed conflicts are associated with a wide range of child mental health outcomes. These may range from resilience, that is, maintained mental health in the face of adversity, to increased psychological distress and heightened prevalence of mental disorders including (symptoms of) post-traumatic stress disorder (PTSD), depression, and anxiety disorders [3].

To address the mental health burden in humanitarian settings, mental health and psychosocial support interventions are increasingly popular and consensus-based guidelines for such interventions have been developed [4,5]. These guidelines recommend implementing multi-layered packages of services, including preventive and treatment interventions, to take into account the diversity of mental health and psychosocial needs in humanitarian settings. The current study concerns a school-based mental health intervention implemented within a multi-layered package of services [6,7]. Within this package, the school-based intervention was aimed both at reducing psychological symptoms (treatment aim), as well as improving strengths and functioning in children with heightened symptomatology (preventive aim).

Despite consensus on best practices, little rigorous evidence is available on the effectiveness of child mental health interventions in humanitarian settings [8,9]. A recent meta-analysis of interventions with children affected by armed conflict in low- and middle-income countries, including six randomized controlled trials with no-intervention comparison groups, showed high heterogeneity of intervention effects across studies [10]. This high heterogeneity may be due to the diversity of interventions included in the meta-analysis (that is, specialized psychotherapeutic interventions and preventive interventions), but may also be associated with individual and contextual factors that influence intervention effects. To improve knowledge on what works for whom and under what circumstances, a crucial research direction is the identification of mediators and moderators of interventions. Mediators are variables that identify why and how interventions have effects, whereas moderators are variables that identify on whom and under what circumstances interventions have different effects [11]. Identification of mediators and moderators may assist in adapting interventions to make them more effective, or identifying the populations and contexts for which interventions are most beneficial.

This study was implemented with conflict-affected children in Burundi. Burundi is a landlocked country in the Great Lakes region of eastern Africa, with a population of 8.5 million. It is one of the poorest countries of the world, ranking 185 out of 187 countries on the Human Development

Index [12]. The country has experienced cyclical ethnic violence between Hutu and Tutsi ethnic groups since 1962. The most recent violence occurred in 1993, when the killing of the first elected Hutu president sparked a civil war that killed 300,000 people and displaced 1.2 million people. Although a peace agreement was signed by most warring parties in 2000, political instability and violence continued up to the time of the study [13].

We aimed to address three research questions. First, our treatment aim: What is the effectiveness of a school-based intervention to reduce psychological symptoms (primary outcomes: PTSD, depressive, and anxiety symptoms)? Second, our preventive aim: What is the efficacy of a school-based intervention to improve hope and improve functioning (secondary outcomes)? Finally, we wanted to address the question: What are the mediators and moderators of intervention outcomes? We hypothesized that the intervention would be associated with greater reductions in symptomatology and function impairment, as well as greater improvements of a sense of hope. Our hypotheses of mediators and moderators were based on the theoretical notion of 'ecological resilience,' that is we expected that intervention effects would be determined by protective and risk factors at various levels of children's social ecology (individual, family, peer, community) [14,15]. With regard to mediators, we were interested in coping and social support. We hypothesized that the intervention would be associated with larger improvements in coping and social support among children in the intervention condition, and that these improvements in turn would be associated with improvements on PTSD, depressive, and anxiety symptoms, and hope and function impairment. A systematic review on resilience and mental health in children affected by armed conflict found various studies supporting a relationship between coping and social support and lower levels of psychological symptoms, although these relations were often symptom-specific and varied by phase of conflict [16].

With regard to moderators, we hypothesized that intervention effects would vary by gender and age. Previous evaluation studies of psychosocial interventions in diverse settings have found differing effects by age and gender [17-21]. In addition, we were interested in the moderating roles of family-level variables, including household size, family connectedness, displacement status, and family composition. A longitudinal study with Afghan children found that quality of family life was an important predictor of psychological symptoms over time [22], as did a cross-sectional study in Lebanon [23]. An evaluation of a psychosocial intervention in conflict-affected areas in Indonesia found that household size influenced size of intervention effects [24]. Finally, we were interested in the potential moderating role of community-level variables, that is, social capital. In a longitudinal study with former child soldiers in Sierra Leone, a different but related variable (community acceptance) was associated with higher levels of prosocial behavior and lower levels of internalizing and externalizing symptoms over time [25]. Although the impact of armed conflict on supportive community relations has been a frequent theme in the literature on children and armed conflict [26], we are not aware of studies that have examined the role of social capital as a moderator of intervention efficacy. We hypothesized that children who perceived low levels of social capital would report stronger benefits from a psychosocial intervention, given its focus on improving supportive relations between peers.

13.2 METHODS

13.2.1 PARTICIPANTS AND SCREENING

Research was conducted in two northwestern provinces of Burundi (Bubanza and Cibitoke), between October 2006 and June 2007. This area suffered continued violence during the period of data collection despite peace agreements in 2000 and 2003, due to the presence of remaining rebel groups. Participants were selected in three steps. First, two of the 17 provinces in Burundi were selected (Bubanza and Cibitoke), because of their continued vulnerability to political violence, the relatively homogenous socio-cultural context in these provinces, and the existence of trained human resources due to previous implementation in the area. We randomly selected either Bubanza or Cibitoke province as the intervention province. We chose to stratify at the province level to avoid risks of contamination of intervention within provinces.

Second, we randomly selected schools within these provinces. We excluded all 'communes' (administrative unit below the province) where safety of research participants and staff could not be guaranteed, that is, forested areas populated by rebel forces (Rugazi, Musigati, Bukinyana) and communes close to restive areas in the Democratic Republic of the Congo (Mugina). We also excluded one commune in which mental health and psychosocial programs had previously been implemented. This resulted in a sampling frame of 60 schools out of the 159 schools in the two provinces (Figure 1). We chose to select 14 schools (seven per study condition) on the basis of a preceding power analysis. This power analysis was based on reported effect sizes for PTSD and depressive symptoms by Cohen et al. [27] and Layne et al. [28]. Although these studies focused on psychotherapeutic (group) interventions with trauma-affected children and our aim was to evaluate an intervention with dual aims, at the time of study design they represented the little available data on which power estimation could be based. Based on effect sizes of 1.10 for PTSD and 0.78 for depressive symptoms [27,28], a two-sided α equal to 0.02, and β equal to 0.05, we calculated that we needed a minimum of 18 and 35 children to detect changes in PTSD and depressive symptoms of similar size, respectively, per study condition. As recommended for cluster randomized trials [29], we accounted for intracluster correlation due to nested variance at the school level using the formula: $n(1+(m-1)\rho)$, with n = required non-corrected sample size, m = average cluster size and ρ = estimated intracluster correlation. In our sample: $35(1+(30-1)0.1)$. With a power of 95%, this resulted in an appropriate sample size of 137. Allowing for attrition, we estimated that one school would represent at least 25 to 30 eligible children, hence our choice of seven schools per study condition.

Third, we screened children within schools (class 4) for eligibility using standardized checklists. Children who were exposed to at least one potentially traumatic event, and who scored above the standard cut-off on symptom checklists for either PTSD (≥ 11), depression (≥ 15), or anxiety (≥ 5) were included in the intervention. Criterion validity of the PTSD and depression symptom measures was examined separately against a psychiatric diagnostic interview with the Schedule for Affective Disorders and Schizophrenia for School-Age Children [30]. Results showed that the PTSD symptom checklist had an area under the curve of 0.78 with an optimum cut-off for disorder of 26 (sensitivity: 0.71; specificity: 0.83). The depression checklist had an area under the curve of 0.85, with an optimal cut-off for disorder of 19 (sensitivity: 0.64; specificity: 0.88). However, because our interest was to evaluate the effects of the intervention on both preventive and treatment aims, the original cut-off scores were retained.

13.2.2 INTERVENTION

The classroom-based intervention (CBI) was part of a multi-layered care package implemented in schools that also included universal preventive activities (for example, structured social activities with those not screened into the CBI) and provision of mental health treatments (for example, psychosocial counseling and referral to mental health specialists) [7,31]. Within this care package, CBI was aimed at decreasing psychological symptoms and strengthening protective factors in children at risk, that is, those displaying heightened psychological symptoms. CBI entailed 15 sessions over five weeks implemented by locally identified non-specialized facilitators trained and supervised in implementing the intervention for one year prior to the study. Facilitators had at least a high school diploma and were selected for their affinity and capacity to work with children as demonstrated in role-plays and interviews. The manualized intervention consisted of cognitive behavioral techniques (psychoeducation, strengthening coping, and discussion of past traumatic events through drawing) and creative expressive elements (cooperative games, structured movement, music, drama, and dance) with groups of around 15 children. The intervention was structured to have specific themes across sessions with the following foci: information, safety, and control in week 1 (sessions 1 to 3); stabilization, awareness, and self-esteem in week 2 (sessions 4 to 6); the trauma narrative in week 3 (sessions 7 to 9); resource identification and coping skills in week 4 (sessions 10 to 12); and reconnection with the social context and future planning in week 5 (sessions 13 to 15). Each individual session was structured into four parts, starting and ending with structured movement, songs, and dance with the use of a 'parachute' (a large circular colored piece of fabric). The second part was based on a 'central activity' focused on the main theme of that week (for example, a drama exercise to identify social supports in the environment, or drawing of traumatic events), and the third part was a 'cooperative game' (that is, a game in which all children had to participate to promote group cohesion) [32].

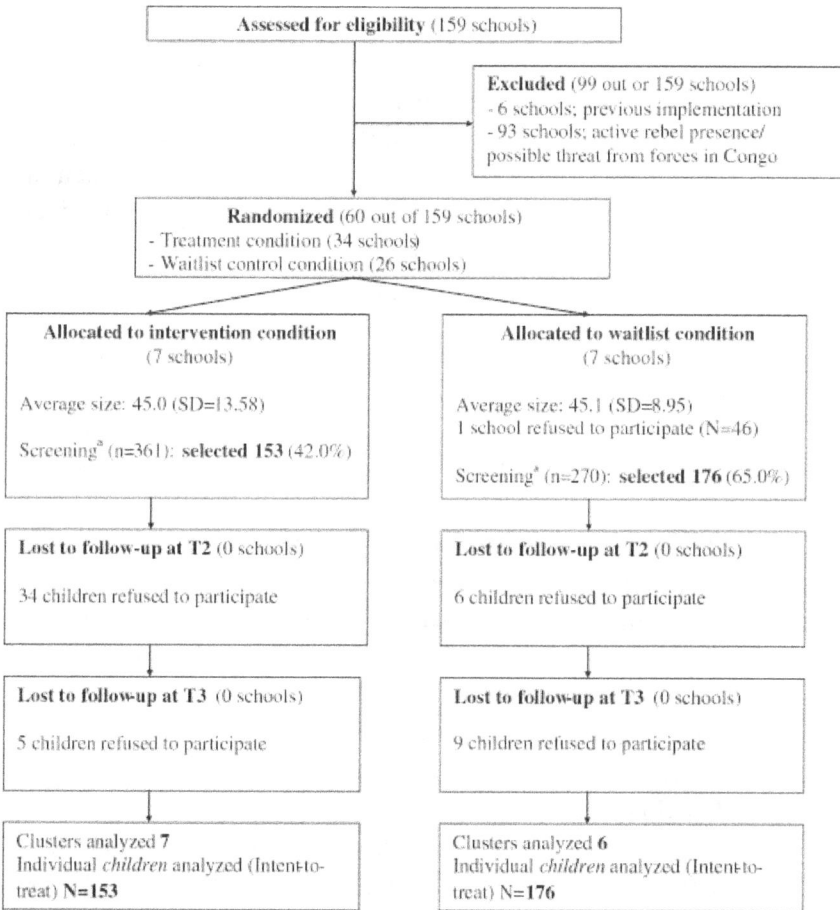

FIGURE 1: Participant flow diagram.

13.2.3 INSTRUMENTS

Instruments were selected based on previously conducted qualitative research in northwestern Burundi (data not shown, see [33]). This qualitative research entailed 14 focus group discussions, 40 semi-structured interviews with children and caregivers identified as affected by the civil war, and 32 key informant interviews (including traditional or religious healers, teachers, community health workers, clergy, and staff of organizations assisting war-affected children). Content analysis of verbatim recorded data evidenced an interrelated set of children's problems, including war-related problems at the individual, family (large-scale loss of parents, abuse by foster families, increased family conflicts over land), peer (distrust between Hutu and Tutsi peers), and community levels (loss of social solidarity, increased accusations of supernatural harm, ethnic hate and distrust) [15]. Often mentioned psychological problems included fears, sadness or despair, being reminded of bad events, loneliness, inactivity, anger and aggression, and grief-related problems. Based on this information, we selected standardized measures for PTSD, depressive, and anxiety symptoms (primary outcomes), and added context-specific items to the interviews.

Standardized measures were translated using a five-step method for preparation of instruments in transcultural research, which included bilingual translation, independent bi-lingual conceptual review, blind-back translation, focus groups, and piloting with target population [34]. Test-retest reliability (TRR) (Spearman-Brown correlation) was assessed over a two-week period with a convenience sample of 15 children.

We used the Child Posttraumatic Symptom Scale (17 items; four-point scale; range 0 to 51; internal reliability (IR, Cronbach Alpha)=0.84; TRR=0.59, P=0.032) to assess PTSD symptoms [35]. Depressive symptoms were assessed using the Depression Self-Rating Scale (18 items; three-point scale; range 0 to 36; IR=0.72; TRR=0.88, P <0.000) [36]. We measured anxiety using the five-item version of the Screen for Anxiety Related Emotional Disorders[37]. Although pre-trial piloting showed acceptable IR, Cronbach Alpha in the study was low (0.28), so we did not consider these items in further analyses.

To assess sense of hope, we used the Children's Hope Scale[38] (six items; six-point scale; range 6 to 36; IR=0.70; TRR=0.95, P <0.000). In this measure, hope is operationalized as a similar but different construct to self-esteem, and consists of agency (that is, the perception that children can initiate and sustain action towards a certain goal) and pathways (that is, perceived capability to produce routes to those goals). We also constructed a measure to assess function impairment using a previously applied mixed-methods approach that involved brief participant observation, collection of diaries, and focus groups [39]. The function impairment measure consisted of nine items and asked about impairment in such daily activities as hygiene, playing, household chores, studying, and religious activities (four-point scale; range 9 to 36; IR = 0.80; TRR = 0.73, P = 0.001).

13.2.4 MEDIATORS

We measured coping using the child-rated Kidcope[40]. The Kidcope contains 15 questions concerning use of 10 different coping strategies and satisfaction with used coping strategies. From this scale we derived a coping repertoire index, by summing the amount of coping strategies that were endorsed by children (dichotomous; range 0 to 15; TRR = 0.75, P = 0.003); and a coping satisfaction (three-point scale; range 15 to 45; IR = 0.68; TRR = 0.82, P < 0.000). Social support was assessed with the Social Support Inventory Scheme[41]. This measure asks children to list up to five people from whom they receive support and asks, for each of these people, whether they provided material (for example, giving food, clothes, helping with school fee), emotional (for example, cheering up, listening or attending to problems), guidance (for example, providing advice, teaching something), or play social support (singing, dancing, storytelling to feel better). For each support type, the child answers yes or no. From this measure we calculated a total social support measure by adding up the different types of support received (range 0 to 20; TRR not assessed).

13.2.5 MODERATORS

Gender, age, displacement status, household size, and family composition were all assessed through one-item questions as part of the demographics questionnaire. To measure exposure to traumatic events (11 items, dichotomous, range 0 to 11), we constructed a checklist locally through free listing. This consisted of asking 23 staff of implementing organization HealthNet TPO Burundi to list adverse events children may be exposed to as part of the armed conflict. We selected the traumatic events that were mentioned by five people or more for inclusion in the checklist. Finally, social capital was assessed with a locally constructed measure modeled after the Short Adapted Social Capital Assessment Tool[42]. Based on our qualitative data in which participants described how community ties were damaged by the conflict, we selected two items from the cognitive dimension of this instrument (trust in other children, children getting along), and added items asking about social solidarity, sense of community, sharing of child care, and perception of members' behavior towards each other (seven items; four-point scale; range 7 to 28; IR = 0.72).

13.2.6 PROCEDURES

All measures were interviewer-administered in private settings within schools, by interviewers trained over a four-week period. Instruments were applied one week before the intervention (T1), one week after the intervention (T2), and three months after the intervention (T3). After a complete description of the study to the participants, written informed consent was obtained from both children and parents. Ethical permission was granted by the Internal Review Board of the VU University Amsterdam. In addition, we obtained local permission from governors of provinces, all school principals, and village leaders in the areas where schools were located. One school in the waitlist condition discontinued participation after the baseline assessment (Figure 1).

13.2.7 DATA ANALYSIS

We assessed the comparability of study conditions (demographic characteristics, scores on moderators and mediators at baseline) by applying χ^2

with continuity correction or Fisher exact test for frequencies, and independent-sample t-tests for continuous measures.

Analyses of crude changes on the outcome measures, that is, mean changes not corrected for clustered variance at the school level, were conducted by computing pure change scores between baseline and follow-up scores (T1 to T3 for boys and girls separately on an intent-to-treat basis (last value carried forward). These pure change scores were compared using independent-sample t-tests.

To correct for clustering and examine the role of moderators and mediators, longitudinal changes on outcome measures were examined through latent growth curve modeling in a structural equation modeling framework [43]. Conditional growth models were used to estimate the intervention main effect and to model moderating effects while controlling for main effects accordingly. All models controlled for clustering at the school level. Latent growth curve modeling was conducted in two steps. First, we modeled growth curves, using 0, 6 and 20 weeks as time points, and estimated the effect of intervention on changes over time. Second, we added moderators and their main effects to explore potential variations in intervention effects. All growth models used maximum likelihood estimation to model all data available for dependent variables. Latent growth curve modeling was conducted using MPlus 4.21 [44].

13.3 RESULTS

13.3.1 CHARACTERISTICS AT BASELINE

We compared study conditions at baseline on demographic characteristics and scores on the outcomes measures, mediators and moderators (Tables 1 and 2). Children in the waitlist condition were exposed to fewer categories of traumatic events (0.5 type of event), and reported lower cognitive social capital at baseline. Children in the treatment condition had lower depressive scores at baseline and reported fewer coping strategies, smaller satisfaction with coping, and less social support than their counterparts in the waitlist condition.

TABLE 1: Clusters and baseline comparison of scores on moderators

		Intervention condition N (%)a	Waitlist condition N (%)a	Chi-square (df); P
Clusters	Number	7	6	
	Average Size	21.9	29.3	
	Total N (N=329)	153	176	
Moderators	Gender			0.457 (1); 0.509
	Boys	77 (50.3)	94 (53.4)	
	Girls	76 (49.7)	82 (46.6)	
	Age (years)			5.507 (2); 0.064
	<11	32 (20.9)	55 (31.3)	
	12 to 15	117 (76.5)	119 (67.6)	
	>16	3 (2.0)	1 (0.6)	
	Missing	1 (0.7)	1 (0.6)	
	Household size	Mean=6.9; SD=2.30	Mean=6.8; SD=2.17	t=0.435 (325); 0.664
	Displacement status			5.116 (4); 0.276
	Original village	76 (49.7)	77 (43.8)	
	Other village	37 (24.2)	51 (29.0)	
	Refugee camp	29 (19.0)	26 (14.8)	
	Bought new land	8 (5.2)	18 (10.2)	
	Other	3 (2.0)	2 (1.1)	
	Missing	0 (0.0)	2 (1.1)	
	Family composition			1.058 (3); 0.787
	Two parents in household	103 (67.3)	118 (67.4)	
	One parent in household	31 (20.3)	36 (20.6)	
	Other type of adult caregiver	15 (9.8)	19 (10.9)	
	No adult caregiver	4 (2.6)	2 (1.1)	
	Traumatic events	Mean=4.6, SD=2.05	Mean=4.1, SD=2.05	t=1.996 (327); 0.047*
	Social capital	Mean=18.4, SD=3.63	Mean=17.0, SD=2.92	t=3.924 (327); 0.000**

aPercentages may not add up to 100 due to rounding off. df, degrees of freedom; SD, standard deviation; *: statistically significant at a 0.01-0.05. **: statistically significant at α <0.01.

TABLE 2: Baseline comparisons of scores on outcome measures and mediators

		Intervention condition		Waitlist condition		T (df)	P	ICC
		(N=153)		(N=176)				
		Mean	SD	Mean	SD			
Outcomes	PTSD symptoms	15.62	9.42	16.30	7.35	−0.738 (327)	0.461	0.035
	Depressive symptoms	9.97	4.82	11.28	5.08	−2.396 (327)	0.017*	0.036
	Hope	15.97	5.77	15.03	5.81	1.471 (327)	0.142	0.038
	Function impairment	13.97	5.01	14.49	5.12	−0.934 (327)	0.351	0.035
Mediators	Coping repertoire	7.72	2.57	8.92	2.40	−4.354 (325)	0.000**	0.036
	Coping satisfaction	17.68	7.01	19.66	5.84	−2.793 (325)	0.006**	0.036
	Social support	10.51	5.10	12.63	4.46	−4.024 (327)	0.000**	0.031

df, degrees of freedom; ICC, intra cluster correlation; PTSD, posttraumatic stress disorder; SD, standard deviation; *: statistically significant at α 0.01-0.05, **: statistically significant at α <0.01.

We compared baseline mean values for children for whom complete follow-up was achieved (that is, T1, T2, and T3 participation) with children who dropped out at T2 (n=40, 12.2%) or T3 (n=14, 4.3%). No statistically significant differences were found with regard to exposure to traumatic events, depressive symptoms, hope, function impairment, or coping satisfaction. However, completers had lower baseline levels of PTSD (13.7 versus 16.4 in completers, T=2.27, P=0.024), higher levels of social capital (18.5 versus 17.5, T=-2.05, P=0.042), and lower levels of total social support (9.9 versus 12.0, T=2.64, P=0.010).

TABLE 3: Unadjusted comparison of differences in mean changes (baseline to three-month follow-up)

		Boys						Girls					
		Intervention (N=77)		Waitlist (N=94)		T; df=169	P	Intervention (N=76)		Waitlist (N=82)		T; df=156	P
		ΔT1 to T3 Mean	SD	ΔT1 to T3 Mean	SD			ΔT1 to T3 Mean	SD	ΔT1 to T3 Mean	SD		
Outcomes	PTSD symptoms	5.68	9.65	4.85	8.56	-0.597	0.551	5.85	10.97	5.18	11.46	-0.380	0.704
	Depressive symptoms	1.42	4.61	2.58	5.60	1.451	0.149	2.21	5.42	3.00	6.00	0.864	0.389
	Hope	-1.03	6.71	-0.47	6.59	0.546	0.586	-2.97	6.27	-1.93	6.17	1.058	0.292
	Function impairment	1.13	4.75	0.39	6.18	-0.865	0.388	1.76	5.06	1.95	4.93	0.237	0.813
Mediators	Coping repertoire	0.23	3.38	0.69	3.17	0.915	0.362	0.22	3.57	-0.05	3.81	-0.454	0.651
	Coping satisfaction	1.18	7.85	0.55	8.03	-0.514	0.608	1.48	7.41	0.89	8.38	-0.465	0.642
	Social support	-0.01	4.12	-1.32	4.85	-1.866	0.056	0.24	5.58	-0.62	5.67	-0.959	0.339

df, degrees of freedom; PTSD, posttraumatic stress disorder; SD, standard deviation.

13.3.2 COMPARISON OF CHANGES OVER TIME

Per illustration, Table 3 provides crude (unadjusted) t-test comparisons between the treatment and waitlist condition of changes on mental health outcomes and putative mediators over time by gender. No statistically significant differences were found for mean changes between study conditions on outcomes and mediators.

13.3.3 MAIN EFFECTS

For a true test of our hypothesis, we conducted latent growth curve modeling of changes over time that corrected for nested variance. As can be seen in Table 4, these analyses confirmed the lack of main effects of the intervention on outcome measures. Given that we did not find significant changes on the mediators over time, a first condition for establishing potential mediation effects, we did not pursue further analysis of mediation effects.

13.3.4 MODERATORS

Next, we compared trajectories of outcome measures between study conditions, while taking into account interaction effects with potential moderators of intervention. These analyses showed several instances where changes on outcome measures over time were different between study conditions in interaction with moderators. For ease of reading, these effects are summarized in Table 5. First, the effect of household size on depressive symptom and function impairment trajectories was statistically significantly different between study conditions. Children in the intervention condition living in larger households showed greater improvements for both depressive symptom and function impairment trajectories, whereas there were no effects of household size on either trajectory in the waitlist control condition (depressive symptoms: intervention condition estimate=-0.016, SE=0.004, Z=-3.640 (z-test and waitlist control condition estimate=0.002, SE=0.004, Z=0.509; function impairment:

intervention condition estimate=-0.009, SE=0.005, Z=-2.050 and wait-list control condition estimate=0.002, SE=0.005, Z=0.369). In addition, we found different trajectories between study conditions for PTSD and depressive symptoms when analyzing the interaction with family com-position. In the intervention condition, living with both parents was as-sociated with statistically significant decreases in PTSD and depressive symptoms (PTSD estimate=-0.158, SE=0.036, Z=-4.348; depressive symptoms estimate=-0.069, SE=0.020, Z=-3.371). There was no asso-ciation between living with both parents and PTSD in the waitlist condi-tion (estimate=0.039, SE=0.036, Z=1.080); however, living with both parents was associated with significant increases in depressive symptoms over time in the waitlist control condition (estimate=0.041, SE=0.020, Z=2.001).

TABLE 5: Overview of findings

Outcome	More favorable longitudinal trajectory	Moderator
PTSD	Intervention condition	Family composition (living with both parents)
Depression	Intervention condition	Family composition (living with both parents)
Intervention condition	More members in household	
Hope	Intervention condition	Younger age
Intervention condition	Lower trauma exposure	
Control condition	Displacementa	
Functioning	Intervention condition	More members in household
Control condition	Displacement	

aMore favorable outcomes in waitlisted children who lived on their own land or newly bought land. PTSD, posttraumatic stress disorder.

Second, for the outcome, hope, we found statistically significant dif-ferent trajectories between study conditions in interaction with three mod-erators: age, exposure, and displacement status. With regard to age, in the intervention condition younger age was associated with increased hope, whereas there was no association between age and hope in the waitlist condition (intervention condition estimate = -0.060, SE = 0.009, Z = -6.639; waitlist control condition estimate = -0.004, SE = 0.013, Z = -0.355). Hope also increased among children with fewer exposures in the intervention condition (estimate = -0.029, SE = 0.009, Z = -3.237), but there was no association between exposures and hope in the waitlist control condition (estimate = -0.001, SE = 0.009, Z = -0.142). Hope, however, also increased among children living in their original villages or who had bought new land in the waitlist control condition, but decreased over time among these children in the intervention condition (intervention condition estimate = -0.116, SE = 0.025, Z = -4.607; waitlist control condition estimate = 0.080, SE = 0.025, Z = 3.150).

Third, we also found differences in trajectories for function impairment by displacement status. In the intervention condition, function impairment increased for children living in their original villages or who had bought new land (estimate = 0.060, SE = 0.018, Z = 3.250) but decreased in the waitlist control condition (estimate = -0.056, SE = 0.018, Z = -3.062).

13.4 DISCUSSION

This study was aimed at identifying intervention outcomes, and mediators and moderators of a school-based mental health intervention for children in war-affected Burundi. The intervention was aimed both at the reduction of PTSD, depressive, and anxiety symptoms (treatment aim, primary outcomes), as well as the improvement of hope and functioning (preventive aim, secondary outcomes). We did not find any main effects on the primary and secondary outcome measures, that is, for either the treatment or preventive aims. Therefore, mediation analyses were not performed. However, we did find eight differences in longitudinal trajectories between study conditions in interaction with a number of moderators. These moderation effects are challenging to interpret clinically, as commonly applied effect size calculations do not take clustered variance into account and may obscure subgroup findings. However, moderation effects generally applied to larger groups of children in our sample (for example, children living with both parents, 67.2% of the sample; children with larger households,

54.3% had seven members or more; children with lower trauma exposure, 21.6% reported two or fewer events; children living in their original village or bought land, 54.8%).

Before discussing these findings in more detail, we highlight limitations of the study. First, we found statistically significant differences between the study conditions at baseline, which may have been the result of randomization by province before randomization of schools. It is unknown how these differences may have impacted findings on intervention effects, given that children in the intervention condition were doing better in some aspects (that is, lower depressive symptoms, higher social capital) but worse in other aspects (that is, higher trauma exposure, fewer coping strategies and coping satisfaction, lower social support) at baseline. Differences may also have been associated with the fact that relatively few schools were randomized, which the analyses controlled for. In addition, differences were found mainly for variables for which we did not find significant intervention effects, with the exception of trauma exposure and depressive symptoms (three of eight differences identified between study conditions). Second, drop-out may have affected study findings. As with the baseline differences between study conditions, it is difficult to say how these findings may have impacted study findings, because study completers had lower levels of PTSD and higher levels of social capital, but lower levels of social support. Third, we had to exclude our measure of anxiety due to low IR of the measure. Although our other measures had good IR and TRR, unmeasured factors that contributed to low IR of the anxiety measure may have impacted our other instruments in ways we did not measure. Fourth, our research assessors were working independently from the implementation team, but were not blinded to study condition because they had to visit schools to interview children. We emphasized in training of assessors that an objective evaluation was crucial. However, the lack of blinding assessors may have biased findings in favor of the intervention. Strengths of the study include the detailed translation and mixed methods procedures to prepare instruments, the inclusion of a broader range of measures to assess different aspects of mental health (symptoms, hope, functioning), the inclusion of a follow-up assessment three months after the intervention, and the examination of moderators.

Our current findings from Burundi add to a number of recent studies that have rigorously evaluated this school-based intervention with conflict-affected populations in Indonesia, Nepal, the occupied Palestinian territories, and Sri Lanka. Collectively, these studies provide emerging evidence-based answers to important questions on the practical benefit of this and similar interventions. First, given inconsistent results on primary outcome measures across settings, it now seems that this school-based intervention should not be recommended as a treatment for PTSD, depressive, and anxiety symptoms. Although the school-based intervention was associated with reductions in these symptoms in some settings (such as girls in Indonesia, boys and children with less ongoing trauma exposure in Sri Lanka, and children with both parents in Burundi), it was not associated with improvements in these symptoms in Nepal and the occupied Palestinian territories, and was associated with unfavorable effects on PTSD symptoms in Sri Lankan girls and older children in the occupied Palestinian territories. Rather, recent World Health Organization guidelines for non-specialized health settings in low- and middle-income countries recommend cognitive behavioral treatments with a trauma focus and eye movement desensitization reprocessing as treatments for PTSD in children and adolescents [45]. Although this school-based intervention incorporated cognitive behavioral elements (for example, working on coping skills, psycho-education, some discussion of trauma-related material through drawings), it did not comprise consistent trauma exposure, memory, or cognitive processing when compared to cognitive behavioral treatments with a trauma focus or to eye movement desensitization reprocessing. On the basis of findings in Indonesia and Sri Lanka, we previously argued that this intervention may nevertheless have a place in a spectrum of treatment options: despite smaller main effects, it can reach more children with fewer resources. Given the inconsistent results across settings, however, it may be better to start with World Health Organization recommendations for treatment of PTSD in children and adolescents. A remaining key research question here is how existing evidence-based interventions, often tested in more highly resourced research settings, can be effectively disseminated and implemented in real-world health-care settings [46-48].

When considering the benefit of the school-based intervention as a preventive intervention, that is, in strengthening resilience processes in conflict-affected children, the intervention seems to have more consistent results across settings. Intervention effects were found for hope, positive coping, social support, and function impairment in Indonesia; hope and prosocial behavior in Nepal; hope in Sri Lanka; hope and a range of other strengths in the occupied Palestinian territories; and hope and function impairment in this study. However, in this study in Burundi, displaced children in the intervention condition had worse trajectories on hope and function impairment. Further adaptation of this school-based intervention may focus on removing the trauma-focused elements (see [49]) and implementing it only as a preventive tool, as well as concentrating on more active involvement of families and communities. An important future direction would then be to examine whether changes in strengths in the shorter term translate to improvements in psychological symptoms and overall wellbeing and development in the longer term.

An important question concerns the differential intervention effects (both treatment and preventive) by gender, age, and a variety of contextual factors. We feel results across studies may best be explained from the theoretical perspective of ecological resilience. This theoretical framework aims to explain children's mental health by examining which resources (strengths) are available in children and their social contexts, at family, peer, and community levels. From this perspective, the complex differential effects of the intervention may be clarified by the extent to which the resources in children's environment may interact with intervention activities. The most positive intervention effects were observed in Central Sulawesi, Indonesia, which may be explained by the fact that children there were still living in generally supportive families and communities - although tension remained between the communities after the conflict [15,33]. In Indonesia, the children that benefited most from the intervention were the children who were socially more isolated [24]. It appears that in settings that are more volatile (for example, Burundi, Sri Lanka), the resilience of children that live in particularly stressful conditions may actually be undermined by the intervention (for example, girls and children exposed to higher levels of ongoing stressors in Sri Lanka, male adolescents in the occupied Palestinian territories, displaced children in Burundi). In these settings, a preliminary intervention recommendation would be to have a clearer separation between intervention aims and to implement interventions in more homogenous groups, so that only the positive preventive effects may be achieved with children in more stable situations, and more intensive treatments may reach those who are more vulnerable. Detailed pre-intervention assessments seem crucial to identify who the particularly socially vulnerable children may be.

From a scientific point of view, the identified differential effects from our studies call for a more detailed look at how context interacts with intervention effects in conflict-affected settings, particularly for evaluations of preventive interventions. This would require an adaptation of the randomized controlled trial (for example, with a cohort multiple randomized controlled trial design) to encompass the multi-disciplinary examination of family-, peer-, and community-level variables before and during implementation of interventions, and the study of how such variables interact over the longer term with psychological symptoms. Following advances that have been made in the field of treatment of PTSD symptoms, such scientific developments would aid in strengthening efforts to prevent long-lasting psychological symptoms and promote mental health in children affected by armed conflict.

Furthermore, a promising research direction for preventive efforts could be to intervene in earlier developmental periods, when parenting skills and parental mental health can be enhanced before negative patterns set in [50]. Given that development proceeds sequentially (that is, skills learned later in life build on skills learned earlier), researchers focusing on children growing up in adversity have emphasized the early childhood period as a particularly cost-effective period for intervention [51,52]. For example, in a randomized controlled trial with 87 displaced mother-child dyads (mean age of children, 5.5 years), Dybdahl found that a group intervention aimed at strengthening parental involvement, support, and education in mothers had promising benefits for their children [53].

13.5 CONCLUSIONS

Our evaluation of a school-based mental health intervention with children affected by armed conflict showed both benefits and unfavorable effects in interaction with moderators that included age, exposure to potentially traumatic events, family composition, size of household, and displacement status. For treatment purposes, other interventions may be more suitable. For preventive interventions, further multi-disciplinary studies are required to study how intervention at the family, peer, and community levels may best promote mental health and development, and prevent occurrence of psychological symptoms over time.

REFERENCES

1. Machel G: Children and Conflict in a Changing World: Machel Study 10-year Review. New York: UNICEF; 2009.
2. Themner L, Wallensteen P: Armed conflicts, 1946–2011. J Peace Res 2012, 49:565-575.
3. Attanayake V, McKay R, Joffres M, Singh S, Burkle FM Jr, Mills E: Prevalence of mental disorders among children exposed to war: a systematic review of 7,920 children. Med Confl Surviv 2009, 25:4-19.
4. The Sphere Project: Humanitarian Charter and Minimum Standards in Disaster Response - 2011 Edition. Geneva, Switzerland: The Sphere Project; 2011.
5. Inter-Agency Standing Committee (IASC): IASC Guidelines on Mental Health and Psychosocial Support in Emergency Settings. Geneva: IASC; 2007.
6. Jordans MJ, Komproe IH, Tol WA, Susanty D, Vallipuram A, Ntamatumba P, Lasuba AC, De Jong JT: Practice-driven evaluation of a multi-layered psychosocial care package for children in areas of armed conflict. Community Ment Health J 2011, 47:267-277.
7. Jordans MJ, Tol WA, Susanty D, Ntamatumba P, Luitel NP, Komproe IH, de Jong JT: Implementation of a mental health care package for children in areas of armed conflict: a case study from Burundi, Indonesia, Nepal, Sri Lanka, and Sudan. PLoS Med 2013, 10:e1001371.
8. Jordans MJD, Tol WA, Komproe IH, de Jong JTVM: Systematic review of evidence and treatment approaches: psychosocial and mental health care for children in war. Child Adolesc Ment Health 2009, 14:2-14.
9. Betancourt TS, Meyers-Ohki S, Charrow AP, Tol WA: Interventions for children affected by war: an ecological perspective on psychosocial support and mental health care. Harv Rev Psychiatry 2013, 21:70-91.
10. Tol WA, Barbui C, Galappatti A, Silove D, Betancourt TS, Souza R, Golaz A, van Ommeren M: Mental health and psychosocial support in humanitarian settings: linking practice and research. Lancet 2011, 378:1581-1591.
11. Kraemer HC, Wilson T, Fairburn CG, Agras WS: Mediators and moderators of treatment effects in clinical trials. Arch Gen Psychiatry 2002, 59:877-883.
12. United Nations Development Program (UNDP): Human Development Report 2011. New York, NY: UNDP; 2011.

13. Human Rights Watch: Pursuit of Power: Political Violence and Repression in Burundi. New York: Human Rights Watch; 2009.

14. Betancourt TS, Kahn KT: The mental health of children affected by armed conflict: protective processes and pathways to resilience. Int Rev Psychiatry 2008, 20:317-328.

15. Tol WA, Jordans MJD, Reis R, De Jong JTVM: Ecological resilience: working with child-related psychosocial resources in war-affected communities. In Treating Traumatized Children: Risk, Resilience, and Recovery. Edited by Brom D, Pat-Horenczyk R, Ford J. London: Routledge; 2009.

16. Tol WA, Song S, Jordans MJD: Annual research review: resilience in children and adolescents living in areas of armed conflict: a systematic review of findings in low- and middle-income countries. J Child Psychol Psychiatry 2013, 54:445-460.

17. Betancourt TS, Newnham EA, Brennan RT, Verdeli H, Borisova I, Neugebauer R, Bass J, Bolton P: Moderators of treatment effectiveness for war-affected youth with depression in northern Uganda. J Adolesc Health 2012, 51:544-550.

18. Jordans MJD, Komproe IH, Tol WA, Kohrt BA, Luitel N, Macy RD, de Jong JTVM: Evaluation of a classroom-based psychosocial intervention in conflict-affected Nepal: a cluster randomized controlled trial. J Child Psychol Psychiatry 2010, 51:818-826.

19. Tol WA, Komproe IH, Susanty D, Jordans MJD, Macy RD, De Jong JTVM: School-based mental health intervention for children affected by political violence in Indonesia: a cluster randomized trial. JAMA 2008, 300:655-662.

20. Tol WA, Komproe IH, Jordans MJ, Vallipuram A, Sipsma H, Sivayokan S, Macy RD, de Jong JTVM: Outcomes and moderators of a preventive school-based mental health intervention for children affected by war in Sri Lanka: a cluster randomized trial. World Psychiatr 2012, 11:114-122.

21. Bolton P, Bass J, Betancourt T, Speelman L, Onyango G, Clougherty KF, Neugebauer R, Murray L, Verdeli H: Interventions for depression symptoms among adolescent survivors of war and displacement in northern Uganda: a randomized controlled trial. J Am Med Assoc 2007, 298:519-527.

22. Panter-Brick C, Goodman A, Tol WA, Eggerman M: Mental health and childhood adversities: a longitudinal study in Kabul, Afghanistan. J Am Acad Child Adolesc Psychiatry 2011, 50:349-363.

23. Zahr RK: Effect of war on the behavior of Lebanese preschool children. Am J Orthopsychiatry 1996, 66:401-408.

24. Tol WA, Komproe IH, Jordans MJ, Gross AL, Susanty D, Macy RD, de Jong JT: Mediators and moderators of a psychosocial intervention for children affected by political violence. J Consult Clin Psychol 2010, 78:818-828.

25. Betancourt TS, Brennan RT, Rubin-Smith J, Fitzmaurice GM, Gilman SE: Sierra Leone's former child soldiers: a longitudinal study of risk, protective factors, and mental health. J Am Acad Child Adolesc Psychiatry 2010, 49:606-615.

26. Thurman TR, Snider L, Boris N, Kalisa E, Nkunda Mugarira E, Ntaganira J, Brown L: Psychosocial support and marginalization of youth-headed households in Rwanda. AIDS Care 2006, 18:220-229.

27. Cohen JA, Deblinger E, Mannarino AP, Steer RA: A multisite, randomized controlled trial for children with sexual abuse-related PTSD symptoms. J Am Acad Child Adolesc Psychiatry 2004, 43:393-402.

28. Layne CM, Pynoos RS, Saltzman WR, Arslanagić B, Black M, Savjak N, Popović T, Duraković E, Mušić M, Ćampara N, Djapo N, Houston R: Trauma/grief-focused group psychotherapy: school-based postwar intervention with traumatized Bosnian adolescents. Group Dyn, Theory, Res Pract 2001, 5:277-290.

29. Campbell MK, Elbourne DR, Altman DG: CONSORT statement: extension to cluster randomised trials. BMJ 2004, 328:702-708.

30. Ventevogel P, Komproe IH, Jordans MJD, Feo P, de Jong JTVM: Validation of the Kirundi versions of brief self-rating scales for common mental disorders among children in Burundi. BMC Psychiatry 2014, 14:36.

31. Jordans MJD, Tol WA, Komproe IH, Susanty D, Vallipuram A, Ntamutumba P, Lasuba AC, de Jong JTVM: Development of a multi-layered psychosocial care system for children in areas of political violence. Int J Ment Health Syst 2010, 16:4-15.

32. Macy RD, Johnson Macy D, Gross SI, Brighton P: Healing in familiar settings: support for children and youth in the classroom and community. New Dir Youth Dev 2003, 98:51-79.

33. Tol WA, Reis R, Susanty D, de Jong JT: Communal violence and child psychosocial well-being: qualitative findings from Poso, Indonesia. Transcult Psychiatry 2010, 47:112-135.

34. van Ommeren M, Sharma B, Thapa SB, Makaju R, Prasain D, Bhattarai R, de Jong JTVM: Preparing instruments for transcultural research: use of the translation monitoring form with Nepali-speaking Bhutanese refugees. Transcult Psychiatry 1999, 36:285-301.

35. Foa EB, Johnson KM, Feeny NC, Treadwell KR: The Child PTSD Symptom Scale: a preliminary examination of its psychometric properties. J Clin Child Psychol 2001, 30:376-384.

36. Birleson P: The validity of depressive disorder in childhood and the development of a self-rating scale - a research report.

37. J Child Psychol Psychiatry 1981, 22:73-88.

38. Birmaher B, Khetarpal S, Brent D, Cully M, Balach L, Kaufman J, Neer SM: The Screen for Child Anxiety Related Emotional Disorders (SCARED): scale construction and psychometric characteristics. J Am Acad Child Adolesc Psychiatry 1997, 36:545-553.

39. Snyder CR, Hoza B, Pelham WE, Rapoff M, Ware L, Danovsky M, Highberger L, Rubenstein H, Stahl KJ: The development and validation of the Children's Hope Scale. J Pediatr Psychiatry 1997, 22:399-421.

40. Tol WA, Komproe IH, Jordans MJ, Susanty D, de Jong JT: Developing a function impairment measure for children affected by political violence: a mixed methods approach in Indonesia. Int J Qual Health Care 2011, 23:375-383.

41. Spirito A, Stark LJ, Williams C: Development of a brief coping checklist for use with pediatric populations. J Pediatr Psychol 1988, 13:555-574.

42. Paardekooper B, de Jong JT, Hermanns JM: The psychological impact of war and the refugee situation on South Sudanese children in refugee camps in Northern Uganda: an exploratory study. J Child Psychol Psychiatry 1999, 40:529-536.

43. de Silva MJ, Harpham T, Tuan T, Bartolini R, Penny ME, Huttly SR: Psychometric and cognitive validation of a social capital measurement tool in Peru and Vietnam. Soc Sci Med 2006, 62:941-953.

44. Duncan TE, Duncan SC: An introduction to latent growth curve modeling. Behav Ther 2004, 35:333-363.
45. Muthen LK, Muthen BO: MPLUS User's Guide: Fifth Edition. Los Angeles, CA: Muthen & Muthen; 2008.
46. Tol WA, Barbui C, van Ommeren M: Management of acute stress, PTSD and bereavement: WHO recommendations. JAMA 2013, 310:477-478.
47. Murray LK, Familiar I, Skavenski S, Jere E, Cohen J, Imasiku M, Mayeya J, Bass JK, Bolton P: An evaluation of trauma focused cognitive behavioral therapy for children in Zambia. Child Abuse Negl 2013, 37:1175-1185.
48. Jordans MJ, Tol WA: Mental health in humanitarian settings: shifting focus to care systems. Int Health 2013, 5:9-10.
49. Ertl V, Pfeiffer A, Schauer E, Elbert T, Neuner F: Community-implemented trauma therapy for former child soldiers in Northern Uganda: a randomized controlled trial. JAMA 2011, 306:503-512.
50. Ager A, Akesson B, Stark L, Flouri E, Okot B, McCollister F, Boothby N: The impact of the school-based psychosocial structured activities (PSSA) program on conflict-affected children in northern Uganda. J Child Psychol Psychiatry 2011, 52:1124-1133.
51. Tol WA, Rees SJ, Silove D: Broadening the scope of epidemiology in conflict-affected settings: opportunities for mental health prevention and promotion. Epidemiol Psychiatr Sci 2013, 22:197-203.
52. Shonkoff JP, Richter L, van der Gaag J, Bhutta ZA: An integrated scientific framework for child survival and early childhood development. Pediatrics 2012, 129:e460-e472.
53. Heckman JJ: Skill formation and the economics of investing in disadvantaged children. Science 2006, 312:1900-1902.
54. Dybdahl R: Children and mothers in war: an outcome study of a psychosocial intervention program. Child Dev 2001, 72:1214-1230.

Table 4 is not available in this version of the article. To view this additional information, please use the citation on the first page of this chapter.

CHAPTER 14

TRAUMA-FOCUSED COGNITIVE BEHAVIORAL THERAPY FOR CHILDREN AFFECTED BY SEXUAL ABUSE OR TRAUMA

CHILD WELFARE INFORMATION GATEWAY

14.1 FEATURES OF TF-CBT

Trauma-Focused Cognitive Behavioral Therapy (TF-CBT) addresses the negative effects of sexual abuse, exposure to domestic violence and other traumatic events by integrating several therapeutic approaches and treating both child and parent in a comprehensive manner.

14.1.1 TF-CBT ADDRESSES THE EFFECTS OF SEXUAL ABUSE AND TRAUMA

In the immediate as well as long-term aftermath of exposure to trauma, children are at risk of developing significant emotional and behavioral difficulties (see, for example, Berliner & Elliott, 2002; Briere & Elliott,

Child Welfare Information Gateway. (2012). Trauma-Focused Cognitive Behavioral Therapy for Children Affected by Sexual Abuse or Trauma. Washington, DC: U.S. Department of Health and Human Services, Children's Bureau.

2003; Chadwick Center, 2004). For example, victims of sexual abuse often experience:

- Maladaptive or unhelpful beliefs and attributions related to the abusive events, including:
  - A sense of guilt for their role in the abuse
  - Anger at parents for not knowing about the abuse
  - Feelings of powerlessness
  - A sense that they are in some way "damaged goods"
  - A fear that people will treat them differently because of the abuse
- Acting out behaviors, such as engaging in age-inappropriate sexual behaviors
- Mental health disorders, including major depression
- Posttraumatic stress disorder (PTSD) symptoms, which are characterized by:
  - Intrusive and reoccurring thoughts of the traumatic experience
  - Avoidance of reminders of the trauma (often places, people, sounds, smells, and other sensory triggers)
  - Emotional numbing
  - Irritability
  - Trouble sleeping or concentrating
  - Physical and emotional hyperarousal (often characterized by emotional swings or rapidly accelerating anger or crying that is out of proportion to the apparent stimulus)

These symptoms can impact the child's daily life and affect behavior, school performance, attention, self-perception, and emotional regulation. To date, numerous studies have documented the effectiveness of TF-CBT in helping children overcome these and other symptoms following child sexual, domestic violence, and similar traumatic experiences (see Empirical Studies at end of paper). This treatment helps children to process their traumatic memories, overcome problematic thoughts and behaviors, and develop effective coping and interpersonal skills (see Effectiveness of TF-CBT, below).

14.1.2 TF-CBT TREATS NONOFFENDING PARENTS IN ADDITION TO THE CHILD

Recognizing the importance of parental support in the child's recovery process, TF-CBT includes a treatment component for parents (or caregivers) who were not abusive. Treatment sessions are divided into individual meetings for the children and parents, with about equal amounts of time for both. The parent component teaches stress management, parenting and behavior management skills, and communication skills. As a result, parents are better able to address their own emotional distress associated with the child's trauma, while also supporting their children more effectively.

14.1.3 TF-CBT INTEGRATES SEVERAL ESTABLISHED TREATMENT APPROACHES

TF-CBT combines elements drawn from:

- Cognitive therapy, which aims to change behavior by addressing a person's thoughts or perceptions, particularly those thinking patterns that create distorted or unhelpful views
- Behavioral therapy, which focuses on modifying habitual responses (e.g., anger, fear) to identified situations or stimuli
- Family therapy, which examines patterns of interactions among family members to identify and alleviate problems

TF-CBT uses well-established cognitivebehavioral therapy and stress management procedures originally developed for the treatment of fear, anxiety, and depression in adults (Wolpe, 1969; Beck, 1976). These procedures have been used with adult rape victims with symptoms of PTSD (Foa, Rothbaum, Riggs, & Murdock, 1991) and have been applied to children with problems with excessive fear and anxiety (Beidel & Turner, 1998). The TF-CBT protocol has adapted and refined these procedures to target the specific difficulties exhibited by children who are experiencing PTSD symptoms in response to sexual abuse, domestic violence, or other childhood traumas. In addition, well-established parenting approaches (e.g., also are incorporated into treatment to guide parents in addressing their children's behavioral difficulties.

14.1.4 TF-CBT SHOWS RESULTS IN VARIOUS ENVIRONMENTS AND CULTURAL BACKGROUNDS

TF-CBT has been implemented in urban, suburban, and rural environments and in clinics, schools, homes, residential treatment facilities, and inpatient settings. TF-CBT has demonstrated effectiveness with children and families of different cultural backgrounds (including Caucasian, African-American, and Hispanic children from all socioeconomic backgrounds) (e.g., Weiner, Schneider, & Lyons, 2009). Therapy has been adapted for Latino, Native American, and hearing-impaired populations. It is a highly collaborative therapy approach in which the therapist, parents, and child all work together to identify common goals and attain them.

14.1.5 TF-CBT IS APPROPRIATE FOR MULTIPLE TRAUMAS

Recent research findings suggest that TF-CBT is more effective than non-directive or client-centered treatment approaches for children who have a history of multiple traumas (e.g., sexual abuse, exposure to domestic violence, physical abuse, as well as other traumas) and those with high levels of depression prior to treatment (Deblinger, Mannarino, Cohen, & Steer, 2006). The model also has been tested with children who are experiencing traumatic grief after the death of a loved one (Cohen, Mannarino, & Knudsen, 2004; Cohen, Mannarino, & Staron, 2006).

14.2 KEY COMPONENTS

TF-CBT is a short-term treatment typically provided in 12 to 18 sessions of 50 to 90 minutes, depending on treatment needs. The intervention is usually provided in outpatient mental health facilities, but it has been used in hospital, group home, school, community, residential, and in-home settings.

The treatment involves individual sessions with the child and parent (or caregiver) separately and joint sessions with the child and parent together. Each individual session is designed to build the therapeutic relationship while providing education, skills, and a safe environment in which to address and process traumatic memories. Joint parent-child sessions are designed to help parents and children practice and use the skills they learned and for the child to share his/her trauma narrative while also fostering more effective parent-child communication about the abuse and related issues.

14.2.1 GOALS

Generally, the goals of TF-CBT are to:

- Reduce children's negative emotional and behavioral responses to the trauma
- Correct maladaptive or unhelpful beliefs and attributions related to the traumatic experience (e.g., a belief that the child is responsible for the abuse)
- Provide support and skills to help nonoffending parents cope effectively with their own emotional distress
- Provide nonoffending parents with skills to respond optimally to and support their children

14.2.2 PROTOCOL COMPONENTS

Components of the TF-CBT protocol can be summarized by the word "PRACTICE":

- P: Psychoeducation and parenting skills—Discussion and education about child abuse in general and the typical emotional and behavioral reactions to sexual abuse; training for parents in child behavior management strategies and effective communication
- R: Relaxation techniques—Teaching relaxation methods, such as focused breathing, progressive muscle relaxation, and visual imagery
- A: Affective expression and regulation—Helping the child and parent manage their emotional reactions to reminders of the abuse, improve their ability to identify and express emotions, and participate in selfsoothing activities
- C: Cognitive coping and processing—Helping the child and parent understand the connection between thoughts, feelings, and behaviors; exploring and correcting of inaccurate attributions related to everyday events
- T: Trauma narrative and processing—Gradual exposure exercises, including verbal, written, or symbolic recounting of abusive events, and processing of inaccurate and/or unhelpful thoughts about the abuse
- I: In vivo exposure—Gradual exposure to trauma reminders in the child's environment (for example, basement, darkness, school), so the child learns to control his or her own emotional reactions
- C: Conjoint parent/child sessions—Family work to enhance communication and create opportunities for therapeutic discussion regarding the abuse and for the child to share his/her trauma narrative
- E: Enhancing personal safety and future growth—Education and training on personal safety skills, interpersonal relationships, and healthy sexuality

and encouragement in the use of new skills in managing future stressors and trauma reminders

14.3 TARGET POPULATION

TF-CBT is appropriate for use with sexually abused children or children exposed to trauma ages 3 to 18 and parents or caregivers who did not participate in the abuse.

14.3.1 APPROPRIATE POPULATIONS FOR USE OF TF-CBT

Appropriate candidates for this program include:

- Children and adolescents with a history of sexual abuse and/or exposure to trauma who:
  - Experience PTSD
  - Show elevated levels of depression, anxiety, shame, or other dysfunctional abuse-related feelings, thoughts, or developing beliefs
  - Demonstrate behavioral problems, including age-inappropriate sexual behaviors
- Children and adolescents who have been exposed to other childhood traumas (e.g., exposure to community violence, traumatic loss of a loved one) and show symptoms of depression, anxiety, or PTSD
- Nonoffending parents (or caregivers)

Meaningful assessment is important in selecting which children may benefit from TF-CBT and to inform the focus of the intervention. The assessment should specifically address PTSD, depressive and anxiety symptoms, and sexually inappropriate behaviors and other behavior problems, as these have been found to be most responsive to TF-CBT in multiple studies.

14.3.2 LIMITATIONS FOR USE OF TF-CBT

TF-CBT may not be appropriate or may need to be modified for:

- Children and adolescents whose primary problems include serious conduct problems or other significant behavioral problems that existed prior to the trauma and who may respond better to an approach that focuses on overcoming these problems first.
- Children who are acutely suicidal or who actively abuse substances. The gradual exposure component of TF-CBT may temporarily worsen symptoms. However, other components of TF-CBT have been used successfully to address these problems. It may be that, for these children, the pace or order of TF-CBT interventions needs to be modified (as has been done in the Seeking Safety model; Najavits, 2002), rather than that TF-CBT is contraindicated for these populations.
- Adolescents who have a history of running away, serious cutting behaviors, or engaging in other parasuicidal behavior. For these teens, a stabilizing therapy approach such as dialectical behavior therapy (Miller, Rathus, & Linehan, 2007) may be useful prior to integrating TF-CBT into treatment.

14.4 EFFECTIVENESS OF TF-CBT

The effectiveness of TF-CBT is supported by outcome studies and recognized on inventories of model and promising treatment programs.

14.4.1 DEMONSTRATED EFFECTIVENESS IN OUTCOME STUDIES

To date, at least 11 empirical investigations have been conducted evaluating the impact of TF-CBT on children who have been victims of sexual abuse or other traumas (see Empirical Studies at end of paper). In addition, there have been studies specifically showing the effectiveness of TF-CBT with children exposed to domestic violence (Cohen, Mannarino, & Iyengar, 2011; Weiner, Schneider, & Lyons, 2009). The findings consistently demonstrate TF-CBT to be useful in reducing symptoms of PTSD as well as symptoms of depression and behavioral difficulties in children who have experienced sexual abuse and other traumas. In randomized clinical trials comparing TF-CBT to other tested models and services as usual (such as supportive therapy, nondirective play therapy, child-centered therapy), TF-CBT resulted in significantly greater gains in fewer clinical sessions. Follow-up studies (up to 2 years following the conclusion of therapy) have shown that these gains are sustained over time.

Children showing improvement typically:

- Experience significantly fewer intrusive thoughts and avoidance behaviors
- Are able to cope with reminders and associated emotions
- Show reductions in depression, anxiety, disassociation, behavior problems, sexualized behavior, and trauma-related shame
- Demonstrate improved interpersonal trust and social competence
- Develop improved personal safety skills
- Become better prepared to cope with future trauma reminders (Cohen, Deblinger, Mannarino, & Steer, 2004)

Research also demonstrates a positive treatment response for parents (Cohen, Berliner, & Mannarino, 2000; Deblinger, Lippmann, & Steer, 1996). In TF-CBT studies, parents often report reductions in depression, emotional distress associated with the child's trauma, and PTSD symptoms. They also report an enhanced ability to support their children (Deblinger, Stauffer, & Steer, 2001; Cohen, Deblinger, et al., 2004; Mannarino, Cohen, Deblinger, Runyon, & Steer, in press).

14.4.2 RECOGNITION AS AN EVIDENCE-BASED PRACTICE

Based on systematic reviews of available research and evaluation studies, several groups of experts and Federal agencies have highlighted TF-CBT as a model program or promising treatment practice. This program is featured in the following sources:

- *Closing the Quality Chasm in Child Abuse Treatment: Identifying and Disseminating Best Practices* (Chadwick Center, 2004) at http://www.chadwickcenter.org/kauffman/kauffman.htm
- The National Child Traumatic Stress Network's (2005) *Empirically Supported Treatments and Promising Practices*, supported by the Substance Abuse and Mental Health Services Administration (SAMHSA), at http://www.nctsn.org/resources/topics/treatments-that-work/promising-practices
- *Child Physical and Sexual Abuse: Guidelines for Treatment* (Saunders et al., 2004) at http://academicdepartments.musc.edu/ncvc/resources_prof/OVC_guidelines04-26-04.pdf
- The California Evidence-Based Clearinghouse for Child Welfare (2011) at http://www.cebc4cw.org
- *SAMHSA Model Programs: National Registry of Evidence-Based Programs and Practices* at http://nrepp.samhsa.gov

- *Journal of Clinical Child and Adolescent Psychology* (Silverman et al., 2008).

14.5 WHAT TO LOOK FOR IN A THERAPIST

Caseworkers should become knowledgeable about commonly used treatments before recommending a treatment provider to families. Parents or caregivers should receive as much information as possible about the treatment options available to them. If TF-CBT appears to be an appropriate treatment model for a family, the caseworker should look for a provider who has received adequate training, supervision, and consultation in the TF-CBT model. If feasible, both the caseworker and the family should have an opportunity to interview potential TF-CBT therapists prior to beginning treatment.

14.5.1 QUESTIONS TO ASK TREATMENT PROVIDERS

In addition to appropriate training and thorough knowledge of the TF-CBT model, it is important to select a treatment provider who is sensitive to the particular needs of the child, caregiver, and family. Caseworkers recommending a TF-CBT therapist should ask the treatment provider to explain the course of treatment, the role of each family member in treatment, and how the family's specific cultural considerations will be addressed. The child, caregiver, and family should feel comfortable with and have confidence in the therapist with whom they will work.

Some specific questions to ask regarding TF-CBT include:

- What is the nature of the therapist's TF-CBT training (when trained, by whom, length of training, access to follow-up consultation, etc.)? Is this person clinically supervised by (or did he or she participate in a peer supervision group for private practice therapists with) others who are TF-CBT trained?
- Is there a standard assessment process used to gather baseline information on the functioning of the child and family and to monitor their progress in treatment over time?

- What techniques will the therapist use to help the child manage his or her emotions and related behaviors?
- How and when will the therapist ask the child to describe the trauma?
- Will the therapist use a combination of individual and joint child-parent sessions?
- Is the practitioner sensitive to the cultural background of the child and family?
- Is there any potential for harm associated with treatment?

14.5.2 TF-CBT TRAINING

TF-CBT training sessions are appropriate for therapists and clinical supervisors with a master's degree or higher in a mental health discipline, experience working with children and families, and knowledge of child sexual abuse dynamics and child protection. Therapists may benefit from sequential exposure to different types of training:

- Completing the 10-hour web-based training on TF-CBT on the Medical University of South Carolina website (http://tfcbt.musc.edu)
- Reading the program developer's treatment book(s) and related materials
- Participating in intensive skills-based training (2 days)
- Receiving ongoing expert consultation from trainers for 6 to 12 months
- Participating in advanced TF-CBT training for 1 to 2 days

See Training and Consultation Resources, below, for contact information.

14.6 CONSIDERATIONS FOR CHILD WELFARE AGENCY ADMINISTRATORS

Agency administrators considering promoting the use of TF-CBT with children who have suffered trauma and their families will want to research several variables:

- Agency-level adjustments to support successful TF-CBT with families, such as modifications in policy, practice, and data collection
- Identification of therapists or mental health agencies with experience offering TF-CBT and who can work with children from child welfare populations (see above)
- Projected costs

When introducing TF-CBT as a referral option that child welfare workers may consider for children and families in their caseload, administrators will want to ensure that workers have a clear understanding of how TF-CBT works, the values that drive it, and its efficacy. Training for child welfare staff on the basics of TF-CBT, how to screen for trauma, and how to make appropriate referrals can expedite parent and child's access to effective treatment options (see the National Child Traumatic Stress Network's Child Welfare Trauma Training toolkit at http://www.nctsn.org/products/child-welfare-trauma-training-toolkit-2008).

Research has shown that TF-CBT works best under the following organizational conditions:

- Organizational leadership that supports the use of evidence-based interventions, which, in turn, promote acceptance by workers and supervisors
- Provision of ongoing supervision to help child welfare workers make informed referrals to trauma-informed services and supervision for trained clinicians providing treatment

14.7 CONCLUSION

TF-CBT is an evidence-based treatment approach for children who have experienced sexual abuse, exposure to domestic violence, or similar traumas. Despite the impressive level of empirical support for TF-CBT and an established publication track record, many professionals remain unaware of its advantages, and many children and parents who could benefit do not receive such treatment. Further, in many communities around the nation, there may not yet be any TF-CBT trained therapists. The current demand for such evidence-based treatments, however, will encourage other professionals to acquire the needed training and to implement the TF-CBT model. Increased availability of TF-CBT, along with increased awareness among those making treatment referrals, can offer significant results in helping children to process their trauma and overcome emotional and behavioral problems following sexual abuse and other childhood traumas.

REFERENCES

1. Beck, A. T. (1976). Cognitive therapy and the emotional disorders. Oxford, England: International Universities Press.
2. Beidel, D. C., & Turner, S. M. (1998). Shy children, phobic adults: Nature and treatment of social phobia. Washington, DC: American Psychological Association.
3. Berliner, L., & Elliott, D. M. (2002). Sexual abuse of children. In J. E. B. Myers, L. Berliner, J. Briere,
4. C. T. Hendrix, C. Jenny, & T. A. Reid (Eds.), The APSAC handbook on child maltreatment (pp.55- 78). Thousand Oaks, CA: Sage Publications.
5. Briere, J., & Elliott, D. M. (2003). Prevalence and psychological sequelae of self-reported childhood physical and sexual abuse in a general population sample of men and women. Child Abuse & Neglect, 27, 1205-1222.
6. Chadwick Center. (2004). Closing the quality chasm in child abuse treatment: Identifying and disseminating best practices. San Diego, CA: Author.
7. Cohen, J. A., Berliner, L., & Mannarino, A. P. (2000). Treatment of traumatized children: A review and synthesis. Journal of Trauma, Violence and Abuse, 1(1), 29-46.
8. Cohen, J. A., Deblinger, E., Mannarino, A. P., & Steer, R. (2004). A multisite, randomized controlled trial for children with sexual abuse-related PTSD symptoms. Journal of the American Academy of Child & Adolescent Psychiatry, 43, 393-402.
9. Cohen, J. A., Mannarino, A. P., & Iyengar, S. (2011). Community treatment of posttraumatic stress disorder for children exposed to intimate partner violence. Archives of Pediatrics & Adolescent Medicine, 165(1), 16-21.
10. Cohen, J. A., Mannarino, A. P., & Knudsen, K. (2004) Treating childhood traumatic grief: A pilot study. Journal of the American Academy of Child & Adolescent Psychiatry, 43, 1225-1233.
11. Cohen, J. A., Mannarino, A. P., & Staron ,V. (2006). A pilot study of modified cognitive behavioral therapy for childhood traumatic grief (CBT-CTG). Journal of the American Academy of Child & Adolescent Psychiatry, 45(12), 1465-1473.
12. Deblinger, E., Lippmann, J., & Steer, R. (1996). Sexually abused children suffering posttraumatic stress symptoms: Initial treatment outcome findings. Child Maltreatment, 1(4), 310-321.
13. Deblinger, E., Mannarino, A. P., Cohen, J. A., & Steer, R. A. (2006). A multisite, randomized controlled trial for children with sexual abuse-related PTSD symptoms: Examining predictors of treatment response. Journal of the American Academy of Child and Adolescent Psychiatry, 45, 1474-1484.
14. Foa, E., Rothbaum, B. O., Riggs, D. S., & Murdock, T. B. (1991). Treatment of posttraumatic stress disorder in rape victims: A comparison between cognitive-behavioral procedures and counseling. Journal of Consulting & Clinical Psychology, 59(5), 715-723.
15. Forehand, R., & Kotchick, B. A. (2002). Behavioral parent training: Current challenges and potential solutions. Journal of Child & Family Studies, 11(4), 377-384.
16. Mannarino, A. P., Cohen, J. A., Deblinger, E., Runyon, M., & Steer, R. (in press). Trauma-focused cognitive-behavioral therapy for children: Sustained impact 6 and 12 months later. Child Maltreatment.

17. Miller, A. L., Rathus, J. H., & Linehan, M. M. (2007). Dialectical behavior with suicidal adolescents. New York: The Guildford Press.
18. Najavits, L. M. (2002). Treatment of posttraumatic stress disorder and substance abuse: Clinical guidelines for implementing Seeking Safety therapy. Alcoholism Treatment Quarterly, 22(1), 43-62.
19. Patterson, G. R. (2005). The next generation of PMTO models. Behavior Therapist, 28(2), 27-33.
20. Saunders, B. E., Berliner, L., & Hanson, R. F. (Eds.) (2003). Child physical and sexual abuse: Guidelines for treatment (Final Report: January 15, 2003). Charleston, SC: National Crime Victims Research and Treatment Center.
21. Silverman, W. K., Ortiz, C. D., Viswesvaran, C., Burns, B. J., Kolko, D. J., Putnam, F. W., & Amaya-Jackson, L. (2008). Evidence-based psychosocial treatments for children and adolescents exposed to traumatic events. Journal of Clinical Child & Adolescent Psychology, 37(1), 156-183.
22. Weiner, D. A., Schneider, A., & Lyons, J. S. (2009). Evidence-based treatments for trauma among culturally diverse foster care youth: Treatment retention and outcomes. Children and Youth Services Review, 31(11), 1199-1205.
23. Wolpe, J. (1969). Basic principles and practices of behavior therapy of neuroses. American Journal of Psychiatry, 125(9), 1242-1247.

EMPIRICAL STUDIES

1. Cohen, J. A., Deblinger, E., Mannarino, A. P., & Steer, R. (2004). A multisite, randomized controlled trial for children with sexual abuse-related PTSD symptoms. Journal of the American Academy of Child & Adolescent Psychiatry, 43, 393-402.
2. Cohen, J. A., & Mannarino, A. P. (1996). A treatment outcome study for sexually abused preschool children: Initial findings. Journal of the American Academy of Child and Adolescent Psychiatry, 35(1), 42-50.
3. Cohen, J. A., & Mannarino, A. P. (1997). A treatment study of sexually abused preschool children: Outcome during one year follow-up. Journal of the American Academy of Child and Adolescent Psychiatry 36(9), 1228-1235.
4. Cohen, J. A., Mannarino, A. P., & Knudsen K. (2005). Treating sexually abused children: One year follow-up of a randomized controlled trial. Child Abuse & Neglect, 29, 135-146.
5. Deblinger, E., Lippmann, J., & Steer, R. (1996). Sexually abused children suffering posttraumatic stress symptoms: Initial treatment outcome findings. Child Maltreatment, 1(4), 310-321.
6. Deblinger, E., Mannarino, A. P., Cohen, J. A., Runyon, M. K., & Steer, R. A. (2011). Trauma-Focused Cognitive Behavioral Therapy for children: Impact of the trauma narrative and treatment length. Depression and Anxiety, 28, 67–75.
7. Deblinger, E., Mannarino, A. P., Cohen, J. A., & Steer, R. A. (2006). A multisite, randomized controlled trial for children with sexual abuse-related PTSD symptoms: Examining predictors of treatment response. Journal of the American Academy of Child and Adolescent Psychiatry, 45, 1474-1484.

8. Deblinger, E., Stauffer, L., & Steer, R. (2001). Comparative efficacies of supportive and cognitive behavioral group therapies for children who were sexually abused and their nonoffending mothers. Child Maltreatment 6(4), 332-343.
9. Deblinger, E., Steer, R. A., & Lippmann, J. (1999). Two year follow-up study of cognitive behavioral therapy for sexually abused children suffering post-traumatic stress symptoms. Child Abuse and Neglect, 23(12), 1371-1378.
10. King, N., Tonge, B. J., Mullen, P., Myerson, N., Heyne, D., Rollings, S., et al. (2000). Treating sexually abused children with post-traumatic stress symptoms: A randomized clinical trial. Journal of the American Academy of Child and Adolescent Psychiatry, 59(11), 1347-1355.
11. Stauffer, L., & Deblinger, E. (1996). Cognitive behavioral groups for nonoffending mothers and their young sexually abused children: A preliminary treatment outcome study. Child Maltreatment, 1(1), 65-76.

ONLINE RESOURCES

1. Center for Traumatic Stress in Children & Adolescents http://www.pitts-burghchildtrauma.net
2. Medical University of South Carolina. Guidelines for Treatment of Physical and Sexual Abuse of Children http://academicdepartments.musc.edu/ncvc/resources_prof/OVC_guidelines04-26-04.pdf
3. Chadwick Center for Children and Families. Closing the Quality Chasm in Child Abuse Treatment: Identifying and Disseminating Best Practices http://www.chad-wickcenter.org/Kauffman/kauffman.htm
4. National Child Traumatic Stress Network. Empirically Supported Treatments and Promising Practices http://www.nctsn.org/resources/topics/treatments-that-work/promising-practices
5. University of Medicine & Dentistry of New Jersey, School of Osteopathic Medicine. CARES Institute. http://www.caresinstitute.org
6. SAMHSA Model Programs. National Registry of Evidence-Based Programs and Practices. http://nrepp.samhsa.gov
7. The California Evidence-Based Clearinghouse for Child Welfare. http://www.cebc-4cw.org/program/trauma-focused-cognitive-behavioral-therapy
8. Interventions Addressing Child Exposure to Trauma: Part 1 – Child Maltreatment and Family Violence Agency for Healthcare Research and Quality, U.S. Department of Health and Human Services http://effectivehealthcare.ahrq.gov/search-for-guides-reviews-and-reports/?mode=&pageaction=displayproduct&productid=846
9. Blueprints for Violence Prevention. University of Colorado Boulder's Center for the Study and Prevention of Violence. http://www.colorado.edu/cspv/blueprints

TRAINING AND CONSULTATION RESOURCES

WEB-BASED TRAINING

1. Medical University of South Carolina (MUSC). Distance learning course on TF-CBT http://tfcbt.musc.edu Web-based training in TF-CBT is available as an adjunct or precursor to attending training workshops. The website training may be accessed free of charge. Therapists typically benefit from a 2-day intensive initial training course, as well as advanced training seminars after some experience implementing the model. Access to written resources such as books and treatment manuals (listed below), ongoing consultation or clinical mentoring, and regular clinical supervision are important complements to any web-based training.
2. Medical University of South Carolina (MUSC). Distance Learning course on Child Traumatic Grief http://ctg.musc.edu Web-based training is available on the application of TF-CBT principles and interventions to child traumatic grief along with presentation of grief-related interventions.
3. National Child Traumatic Stress Network. Child Welfare Trauma Training Toolkit http://www.nctsn.org/products/child-welfare-trauma-training-toolkit-2008 This course is designed to teach basic knowledge, skills, and values about working with children in the child welfare system who have experienced traumatic stress. It also teaches how to use this knowledge to support children's safety, permanency, and well-being through case analysis and corresponding interventions tailored for them and their biological and resource families.

WEB-BASED CONSULTATION

1. Medical University of South Carolina (MUSC). Distance Learning Consultation on TF-CBT http://etl2.library.musc.edu/tf-cbt-consult/index.php This web-based consultation tool provides information about frequently asked questions by providers implementing TF-CBT.

IMPLEMENTATION GUIDE

1. Child Sexual Abuse Task Force and Research & Practice Core, National Child Traumatic Stress Network. (2008). How to implement trauma-focused cognitive behavioral therapy. http://www.nctsnet.org/nctsn_assets/pdfs/TF-CBT_Implementation_Manual.pdf

ONSITE TRAINING CONTACTS

1. Judith Cohen, M.D. Center for Traumatic Stress in Children & Adolescents. Allegheny General Hospital. Pittsburgh, PA. Phone: 412.330.4321. Email: JCohen1@wpahs.org
2. Anthony P. Mannarino, Ph.D. Center for Traumatic Stress in Children & Adolescents. Allegheny General Hospital. Pittsburgh, PA. Phone: 412.330.4312. Email: amannari@wpahs.org
3. Esther Deblinger, Ph.D. CARES Institute. University of Medicine & Dentistry of NJ - School of Osteopathic Medicine. Stratford, NJ. Phone: 856.566.7036. Email: deblines@umdnj.edu

PRACTITIONER'S GUIDES

1. Cohen, J. A., Mannarino A. P. & Deblinger, E. (2006). Treating trauma and traumatic grief in children & adolescents. New York: Guilford Press.
2. Deblinger, E. & Heflin, A. H. (1996). Treating sexually abused children and their nonoffending parents: A cognitive behavioral approach. Newbury Park, CA: Sage Publications.
3. Cohen, J. A., Mannarino, A. P., & Deblinger, E. (2012). Trauma-focused CBT for children and adolescents: Treatment applications. New York: Guilford Press.

The following children's books by Stauffer & Deblinger also may be useful in teaching personal safety and other coping skills:

4. Stauffer, L. B., & Deblinger, E. (2003). Let's talk about taking care of you: An educational book about body safety. Hatfield, PA: Hope for Families, Inc.
5. Stauffer, L., & Deblinger, E. (2005). Let's talk about coping and safety skills: A workbook about taking care of you. Hatfield, PA: Hope for Families, Inc.

AUTHOR NOTES

CHAPTER 2

Competing Interests
The authors declare that they have no competing interests.

Author Contributions
BI performed the statistical analyses and interpretation of findings, and drafted the manuscript. EB participated in the conception and design of the study, and data collection. FN made substantial contributions to the statistical analyses and interpretation of findings, helped to draft and revised the manuscript. WH participated in the conception and design of the study, and data collection. HG participated in the conception and design of the study, collected data, made substantial contributions to the statistical analyses and interpretation of findings, and revised the manuscript. All authors read and approved the final manuscript.

Acknowledgments
We acknowledge support of the publication fee by Deutsche Forschungsgemeinschaft and the Open Access Publication Funds of Bielefeld University.

CHAPTER 3

Competing Interests
This research was funded by Health Canada and the Mental Health Commission of Canada. The views expressed herein solely represent the authors. The authors declare no competing interests.

Author Contributions
MLP drafted the manuscript and oversaw data collection; AM conducted the statistical analyses; JMS contributed to study design and critical edit-

ing of the manuscript. All authors reviewed the final draft. All authors read and approved the final manuscript.

Acknowledgments
The authors thank the At Home/Chez Soi Project collaborative at both national and local levels; National project team: J. Barker, PhD (2008–2011) and C. Keller, National Project Leads; P. Goering, RN, PhD, Research Lead; approximately 40 investigators from across Canada and the US; 5 site coordinators; numerous service and housing providers; and persons with lived experience.

CHAPTER 4

Competing Interests
The authors declare that they have no competing interests.

Author Contributions
ASS, carried out the design of the study, collected the data, completed all statistical analyses, interpreting the data, and drafted the manuscript. ASH, has been actively involved in drafting the manuscript and revising it critically for important intellectual content; and has given final approval of the version to be published.

CHAPTER 5

Competing Interests
The authors declare they have no competing financial interests.

Author Contributions
JH contributed to design, execution, analysis and writing of the study. GG and WM were responsible for the study design and approval of the submitted and final version. ZW and BIN contributed to revising the paper and approval of the final version. All authors read and approved the final manuscript.

Acknowlegements

The study was supported by the Science and Technology Commission of Shanghai Municipality (12DZ1202600), Gong-Yi Program of China Meteorological Administration (GYHY201206027), Program for Technological Ventures of the Shanghai Meteorological Bureau (YJ201101), Shanghai Public Health 3-year Action Programme. We thank class teachers in grade one and two, out of four schools for their distributing and collecting the questionnaires. Special acknowledgment is due to Jianping Pan for providing the measures of neglect subtypes. We also thank all other researchers such as Zhang and Duan who had conducted the studies on child neglect in Chinese.

CHAPTER 6

Competing Interests

Authors declare they have no conflict of interests.

Author Contributions

MR carried out the realization and supervision of the study in Rwanda, performed statistical analysis and drafted the manuscript. FN and TE participated in planning design of the examination and supplemented the manuscript. All authors had full access to the data in the study. The first author takes responsibility for the integrity of the data and the accuracy of the data analysis. All authors read and approved the final manuscript.

Acknowledgments

We are grateful to all mothers and children, who participated in this study, and to the B.A. psychologists Primitive Mukantwari, Télesphore Nambajimana, Marthe Niyomsaba, Agnes Nyirabizimana, Anatole Nzabakurana, and Pierre Bisengimana, who conducted the interviews and supported the study with valuable discussions and personal engagement. The study was supported by DFG (Deutsche Forschungsgemeinschaft) and the European Refugee Fund. The authors would like to thank Prof. Jean-Pierre Duzingizemungu, Department of Psychology and Education at the National University of Rwanda, for helpful advices. Furthermore, the authors would like to thank Anna Mädl, Susanne Schaal, Heide Rieder and Katy Robjant for editing and valuable criticisms.

CHAPTER 7

Competing Interests
The authors declare that they have no competing interests.

Author Contributions
DD reviewed the literature and wrote the initial draft. MB, DO, ES, and JW critically reviewed and amended it. All authors read and approved the final manuscript.

Acknowledgments
Ruwan Ratnayake, The International Rescue Committee, advised on the content and commented on a draft version. There was no specific funding for this research. D Devakumar (092121) and D Osrin (091561) are supported by Wellcome Trust Research fellowships.

CHAPTER 8

Competing Interests
The authors have declared that no competing interests exist.

Author Contributions
Conceived and designed the experiments: ZZ PQ ZY. Performed the experiments: ZZ ZY PQ. Analyzed the data: SY ZY. Contributed reagents/ materials/analysis tools: PQ ZZ ZY. Wrote the paper: MC ZY SY ZZ PQ.

Acknowledgments
The authors acknowledge strong support and valuable inputs from Drs. Xu Yang, Caizhi Wu, Cuiying Fan, and Ersheng Zhou, all from Central China Normal University, in the conduction of the present study.

CHAPTER 9

Competing Interests
The authors have declared that no competing interests exist.

Author Contributions
Conceived and designed the experiments: KSK SS Yiping Chen JF. Performed the experiments: JC Y. Cai EC Y. Liu JG Youhui Li MT KZ Xumei Wang CG LY KL J. Shi GW LL JZ BD G J J. Shen ZZ WL J. Sun JH Tiebang Liu Xueyi Wang GM HM Yi Li CH Yi Li GH GL BH HD QM HZ SG HS YZ XF FY DY Tieqiao Liu Yunchun Chen XH WW GC MC YS JP JD RP WZ ZS ZL DG Xiaoping Wang XL QZ. Analyzed the data: Yihan Li KSK JF JC. Wrote the paper: JC. Made critical revision of the manuscript: JF.

CHAPTER 10

Acknowledgments:
The authors would like to thank the research volunteers for their participation in the study, Erin Le Roux and Khutjo Ledwaba for assistance with data collection and input, Nandipha Sinyanya for her field work, and Linda Bewerunge for the DXA scans. The study was funded by the South African Medical Research Council and the University of Cape Town.

CHAPTER 11

Acknowledgments
We thank all our participants for their invaluable contribution to this study. We also thank the students for their help in assessing the data and conducting the interviews.

Author Contributions
Conceived and designed the experiments: AB AM SK KS. Performed the experiments: SK KS. Analyzed the data: AB AM. Contributed reagents/materials/analysis tools: AM. Wrote the paper: AB AM.

Competing Interests

The authors have declared that no competing interests exist.

CHAPTER 12

Competing Interests

The authors declare that they have no competing interests.

Author Contributions

ME conceived of the analysis, analyzed the dataset, conducted the literature review and wrote the manuscript. KW assisted with conceptualization of the analysis models and interpretation of the results, and provided manuscript feedback. JO assisted with conceptualization and implementation of the analysis, data analysis, interpretation of the results, and provided manuscript feedback. KOD selected the measures of emotional difficulties and learning and assisted with study implementation and interpretation of the results. All authors read and approved the final manuscript.

Acknowledgments

This work was supported by the National Institute of Child Health and Human Development (NICHD), grant No. 5R01HD046345-04. The funders had no role in study design, data collection and analysis, decision to publish or preparation of the manuscript.

We thank all the children and caregivers who participated in this study. We appreciate the support that has been provided by the partner organizations: KIWAKKUKI and TAWREF in Moshi, Tanzania; ACE Africa in Bungoma, Kenya; Stand for Vulnerable Organization (SVO) and Save Lives Ethiopia in Addis Ababa, Ethiopia; Homeland Meahto Phum Ko'Mah in Battambang, Cambodia; and Sahara Centre for Rehabilitation and Residential Care in Delhi, Hyderabad and Nagaland, India.

The POFO Research Team consists of Chris Bernard Otieno Agalaa,b,c, Frehiwot Alebachewe, Sisay Woldeyohannes Ameyae, Robin Briggsa, Sopheak Chang, Haimanot Diroe,f, Rama Devi Durgamh, Belaynesh Engidaworke, Amy Hobbiea, Dafrosa Itembab,c, Venkata Gopala Krishna Kazah, Becky Kinotid, Rajeswara Rao Konjarlah, Mao Langg, Dean Lewish, Ira Madanh, Cyrilla Manyad, Max Masnicka, Sabina Mtwewei, Restituta

Mvungib,c, Laura Kathleen Murphy-McMillana, Robert Mujerad, Kokeb Badma Negatue,f, Imliyanger Pongenh, Pelevinuo Raih, John Shaoi, Neville Selhoreh, Amani Sizyab,c, Vanroth Vanng, and Augustine Wasongad. aDuke University, Durham, NC, USA; bKIWAKKUKI, Moshi, Tanzania; cTAWREF, Moshi, Tanzania;dACE Africa, Bungoma, Kenya; eSave-Lives Ethiopia, Addis Ababa, Ethiopia; fSave the Vulnerables Organization, Addis Ababa, Ethiopia; gHomeland Meahto Phum Ko'Mah, Battambang, Cambodia;hSahara Centre for Rehabilitation and Residential Care, Delhi, Hyderabad, and Nagaland, India;iKiliman jaro Christian Medical Centre, Moshi, Tanzania. In addition to the listed authors, the POFO Research Team members are listed in the Acknowledgments.

CHAPTER 13

Competing Interests
The authors declare that they have no competing interests.

Author Contributions
WT, IK, MJ, RM, JdJ designed the study. WT, AN, ES supervised data collection. MJ and PN supervised implementation of the intervention. WT, HS analyzed the data, with critical inputs from IK, MJ, JdJ. WT wrote a first draft of the manuscript. WT, IK, MJ, AN, PN, HS, ES, RM, JdJ revised the manuscript for important intellectual content. All authors read and approved the final manuscript.

CHAPTER 14

Acknowledgments:
The original (2007) and current versions of this issue brief were developed by Child Welfare Information Gateway, in partnership with the Chadwick Center for Children and Families at Rady Children's Hospital San Diego. Contributing Chadwick authors include Cambria Rose Walsh, Anthony P. Mannarino, and Charles Wilson. The conclusions discussed here are solely the responsibility of the authors and do not represent the official views or policies of the funding agency. The Children's Bureau does not endorse any specific treatment or therapy

INDEX

For Product Safety Concerns and Information please contact our EU
representative GPSR@taylorandfrancis.com
Taylor & Francis Verlag GmbH, Kaufingerstraße 24, 80331 München, Germany